The Unofficial Guide to Medical and Surgical Emergencies

The Unofficial Guide to Medical and Surgical Emergencies

Series Editor

Zeshan Qureshi, BM, BSc (Hons), MSc, MRCPCH, FAcadMEd, MRCPS(Glasg)
Paediatric Registrar
London Deanery
United Kingdom

Editors

Varshini Manoharan, MBChB, FRCOphth
Calderdale & Huddersfield NHS Foundation Trust
Yorkshire and the Humber
United Kingdom

Vijaytha Muralidharan, MBChB, MRCP, PGCert in Medical Education
Sandwell and West Birmingham NHS Trust
Birmingham
United Kingdom

Agalya Ramanathan, MBBS, MA Cantab (Hons), MRCGP
Imperial College London;
Stonecot Surgery, London
United Kingdom

Associate Editors

Jameela Sheikh, BMedSc (Hons)
University of Birmingham
United Kingdom

Anna Kathryn Taylor, BSC(Hons), MBChB, MRCPsych, PGDip, PGCert, FHEA
Leeds and York Partnership NHS Foundation Trust;
University of Leeds
United Kingdom

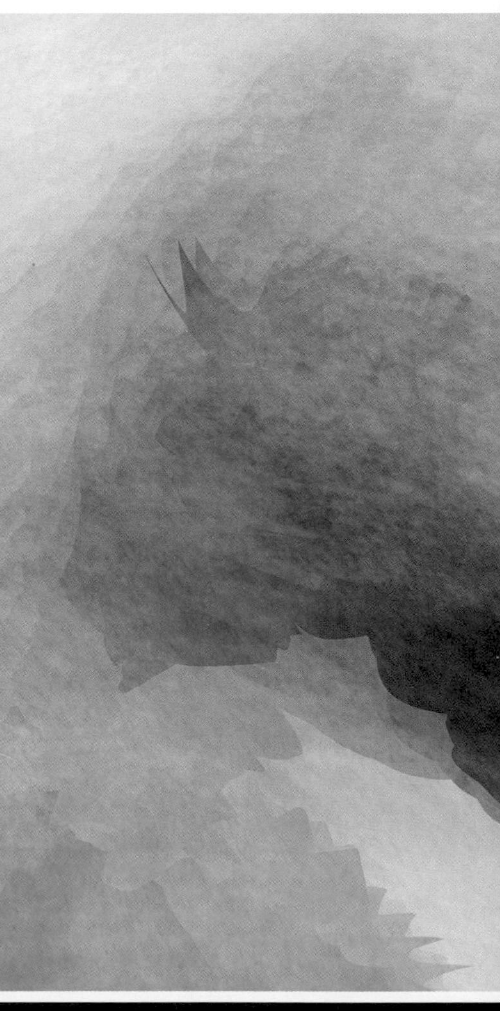

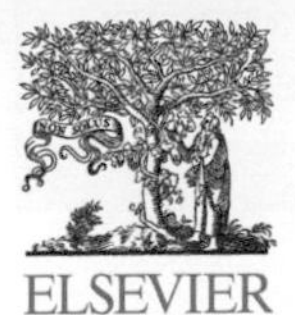

ELSEVIER

Notices

Practitioners and researchers must always rely on their own experience and knowledge in evaluating and using any information, methods, compounds or experiments described herein. Because of rapid advances in the medical sciences, in particular, independent verification of diagnoses and drug dosages should be made. To the fullest extent of the law, no responsibility is assumed by Elsevier, authors, editors or contributors for any injury and/or damage to persons or property as a matter of products liability, negligence or otherwise, or from any use or operation of any methods, products, instructions, or ideas contained in the material herein.

ISBN: 978-0-323-93674-3

Content Strategist: Jeremy Bowes
Content Project Manager: Shubham Dixit
Design: Miles Hitchen
Marketing Manager: Deborah Watkins

Printed in India by Replika Press Pvt. Ltd.

Last digit is the print number: 9 8 7 6 5 4 3 2 1

In loving memory of Dr Vaishnavi Kumar, a true believer in the beauty of medical practice, the strength of teamwork, the power of patience and a non-judgmental approach to colleagues and patients alike. May she rest in peace and her kindness seep through these pages to inspire the next generation of health professionals.

Series Editor Foreword

The Unofficial Guide to Medicine is not just about helping students study, it is also about allowing those that learn to take back control of their own education. Since its inception, it has been driven by the voices of students, and through this, democratised the process of medical education, blurring the line between learners and teachers.

Medical education is an evolving process, and the latest iteration of our titles has been rewritten to bring them up to date with modern curriculums, after extensive deliberation and consultation. We have kept the series up to date, incorporating new guidelines and perspectives from a wide range of students, junior doctors, and senior clinicians. There is greater consistency across the titles, more illustrations, and through these and other changes, I hope the books will now be even better study aids.

These books though are a process of continual improvement. By reading this book, I hope that you not only get through your exams but also consider contributing to a future edition. You may be a student now, but you are also the future of medical education.

I wish you all the best with your future career and any upcoming exams.

Zeshan Qureshi
November 2022

Foreword

Have you ever come across a book and instantly wish you'd discovered it years ago? This book is indeed one of those rare and important finds – to be valued by both clinicians in training and seasoned doctors alike.

Though I now work as a Specialist Consultant Geriatrician within the NHS, somewhere during my training a younger me came to the sound conclusion that knowledge does not always equate to usefulness. In fact, knowledge without understanding and application can be about as useful as a handbrake on a canoe. That is where this book differs from the rest.

The Unofficial Guide to Medical and Surgical Emergencies takes a sea of medical knowledge and complexity and makes it simple, practical and easy to follow. It has been written by doctors, for doctors and in doing so, adopts a real-world, pragmatic and concise approach to the common medical and surgical emergencies that doctors are likely to face. The sheer breadth of content synchronises perfectly well with the expansive and rotational nature of medical training and demonstrates that complicatedness is a choice – one this book chooses to avoid.

The unique qualities outlined above reflect heavily on the expertise of the editors involved, some of whom I have been very privileged to work alongside, and whose clinical nous and experience lend credit to the wonderful content of the book. There is an art to demonstrating both an eye for detail, as well as communicating the important broader messages – something the editors have managed to achieve with aplomb.

Whilst *The Unofficial Guide to Medical and Surgical Emergencies* is an excellent accessory to those in the early stages of their medical careers, the clarity and depth of information within are of a such high standard that this book will also serve as an excellent reminder to more seasoned doctors and advanced clinical practitioners keen to consolidate the key fundamentals of medical and surgical care.

Grace Shorthouse
Consultant Geriatrician, NHS
United Kingdom

Introduction

It has been wonderful to work on this book with such a fantastic team of doctors.

Acute medical and surgical emergencies are hugely varied, with presentations from every bodily system and from different age groups. All students and doctors will care for patients who are acutely unwell, even if they do not specialise in acute medicine or surgery. The difficulty is correctly identifying the acutely unwell patient, knowing how to commence the management plan in a structured manner and when to escalate to seniors or involve other specialities with appropriateness. It is therefore crucial for all students and doctors to have a strong foundation in acute medicine and surgery, and in the situations that they may encounter in clinical practice.

Whilst there is no substitute for clinical experience, we hope this book will give you theoretical knowledge and practical tips to help you make the transition to working in clinical settings. Managing acute emergencies can be busy and stressful. Experiencing the pace and challenges of triage, prioritisation, diagnosis and management, while maintaining good communication with both your team and your patients, are vital in helping you to become a better doctor. This book aims to give you a fun and accessible breakdown of the salient points of knowledge and practice in acute medicine and surgery. We hope that it is of great use to you in your practice.

Varshini Manoharan, Vijaytha Muralidharan and Agalya Ramanathan
November 2022

About the Editors

Varshini Manoharan is currently working as an ophthalmology registrar in the Yorkshire and Humber deanery. She has always had a passion for medical education. She has previously organised regional ophthalmology interview courses and has been a faculty lead for a national virtual ophthalmology taster course for junior doctors. This book has given her the opportunity to further influence and aid junior colleagues during their early training years. She hopes doctors reading this book find it a useful companion for their day-to-day work.

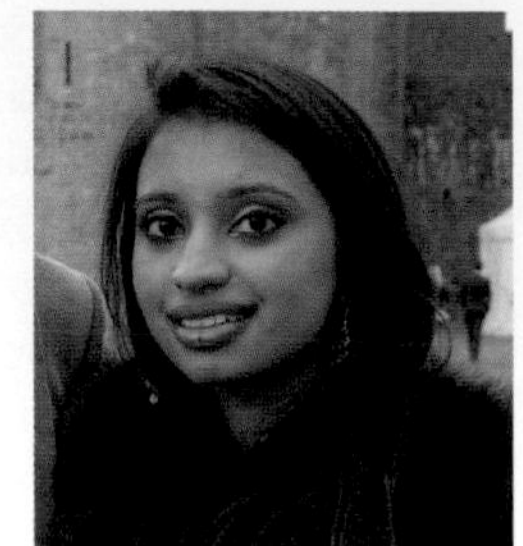

Vijaytha Muralidharan was a Core Medical Trainee whilst writing this book, and is now on her trajectory to specialising in Dermatology, currently undertaking a research fellowship in the United States. She has a passion for medical education, having worked as a Clinical Teaching Fellow at the University of Birmingham and has organised several teaching programmes from pharmacology to the simulation of acute scenarios. She believes that having a firm and practical grounding to emergencies on the ward can make early training years far less daunting, and hopes that this book will provide peace and comfort to readers during their transition into clinical practice.

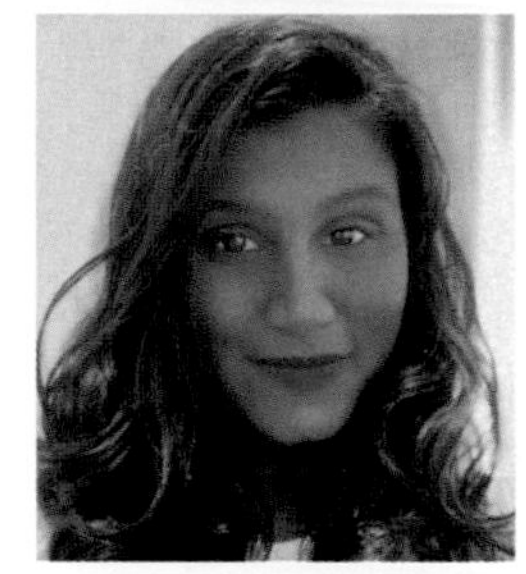

Agalya Ramanathan is a practising general practitioner (GP) in South London and Clinical Teaching Fellow at Imperial College London, having completed her GP training and Academic Clinical Fellowship at UCL/Royal Free. Outside of work her interests include travelling and cooking. She began working on this book as a foundation doctor when she and her co-editors were working at East Lancashire Hospitals NHS Trust. She has a keen interest in medical education and hopes that students reading this book will find it useful to draw links between their education and clinical practice.

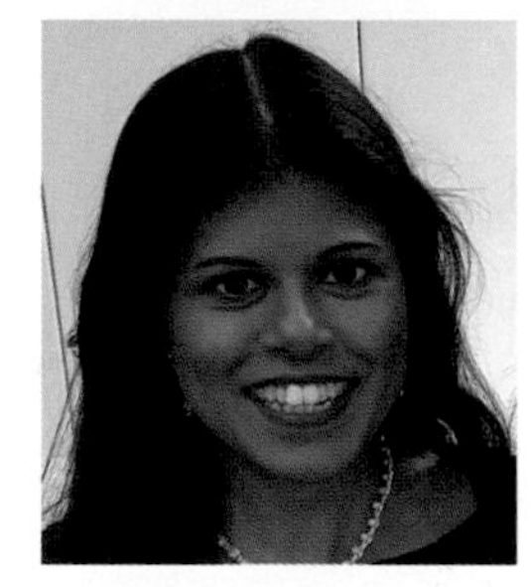

Jameela Sheikh is a final year medical student at the University of Birmingham, having completed her intercalation degree in Clinical Sciences: Reproduction and Women's Health in 2021. She is passionate about Obstetrics and Gynaecology, Surgery and Medical Education. She began working on this book as a clinical medical student and has thoroughly enjoyed contributing to this comprehensive and clinically relevant textbook. She hopes this book will continue to be useful for fellow medical students and junior doctors in the future.

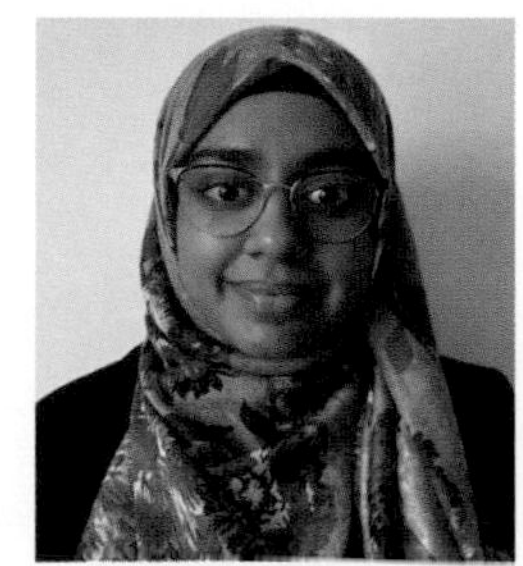

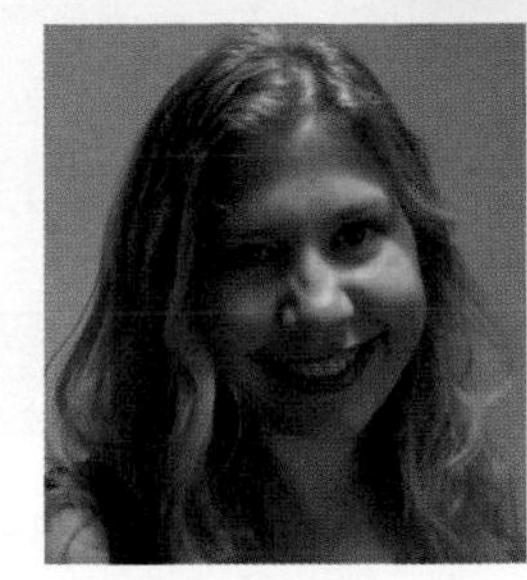

Anna Kathryn Taylor is an Academic Clinical Fellow in Psychiatry at Leeds. She also has a PGCert in Health Research, a PGDip in Clinical Education, and is a Fellow of the Higher Education Academy. Her primary research interest is in psycho-oncology, but she also has experience and expertise in research around workforce wellbeing and other areas of liaison psychiatry. Her work has been cited over 600 times across more than 30 publications, and she has been awarded both local and national prizes. Prior to commencing core psychiatry training she worked as a Clinical Teaching Fellow and has continued her teaching and mentoring work across both clinical and academic settings.

Contributors

Richard Barlow, MBBS, BSc, MRCP
University Hospital of Coventry and Warwickshire
United Kingdom

Kevin Beatson, MBChB, MRCS, PGDip
Maidstone and Tunbridge Wells
United Kingdom

Isaac Chan, MD
Westmead Hospital
Sydney, Australia

Dean Connolly, MA (Cantab), MBBS, MSc
East London NHS Foundation Trust
United Kingdom

Rebecca Edwards, MBChB, MRCP
Sandwell and West Birmingham NHS Trust
United Kingdom

Carys Fleming, MBChB, MRCP
Surrey and Sussex Healthcare NHS Trust
United Kingdom

Anjali Gangadharan, MBChB, MRCGP
NHS Greater Glasgow and Clyde
United Kingdom

Aryeh Greenberg, BSc, MBBS, MRCP(UK), PG Cert (Medical Education)
University College London Hospitals NHS Foundation Trust
United Kingdom

Jennifer Anne Hancox, MBChB (Hons), MRCP (UK)
University Hospitals Birmingham NHS Foundation Trust
United Kingdom

Richard James, MBChB (Leeds), MA (Oxford), MPH (York)
Leeds Teaching Hospitals Trust
United Kingdom

Alan Joseph, MBChB
Sandwell and West Birmingham NHS Trust
United Kingdom

Sanjana Kattera, MBChB, MRCPCH, MPH
Pediatrician at NHS
Liverpool, United Kingdom;
Research Assistant at Taimaka
Gombe, Nigeria

Arun Kirupakaran, MB BChir, MA (Cantab), PGDip (MedEd), FRCOphth
Barts Health NHS Trust
United Kingdom

Vaishnavi Menon, MBChB, Bsc (Hons)
University Hospitals Coventry & Warwickshire
United Kingdom

Amy Nelson, MBChB, BMedSci (Hons) Pharmacology
Senior Research Associate, University College London
United Kingdom

Tammy Oxley, BSc (Hons), MBChB, MRCP, PG Cert, MRCP (UK)
Leeds Teaching Hospital NHS Foundation Trust
United Kingdom

Elizabeth Peterknecht, MBChB (Hons)
University Hospitals Birmingham NHS Foundation Trust
United Kingdom

Naresh Rajasekar, MBChB (Hons), FRCA, FFPMRCA
Calderdale & Huddersfield NHS Foundation Trust
United Kingdom

Vikram Rajasekar, MBChB (Hons)
Calderdale & Huddersfield NHS Foundation Trust
United Kingdom

Alistair J. Roddick, MBBS, BSc
Oxford Health NHS Foundation Trust
United Kingdom

Demi Thompson, MBChB, PG Cert
Mid-Yorkshire Hospitals NHS Trust
United Kingdom

Megan Ugwu-Jones, BSc, PhD, MBChB
East Suffolk and North Essex NHS Foundation Trust
United Kingdom

Reviewers

Feaz Babwah
Endocrinology
University Hospitals Birmingham NHS Foundation Trust
United Kingdom

Natarajan Balaji
ENT
University Hospital Monklands
United Kingdom

Sanjay Banypersad
Cardiology
East Lancashire Hospitals NHS Trust
United Kingdom

Jonathan Cowie
Orthopaedics
NHS Fife
United Kingdom

Edward Fogden
Gastroenterology
Sandwell and West Birmingham NHS Trust
United Kingdom

Jonathan Hulme
Intensive Care
Medicine Sandwell and West Birmingham NHS Trust
United Kingdom

Bhupinder Kaur
Dermatology
East Lancashire Hospitals NHS Trust
United Kingdom

Anna Lock
Palliative Care
Sandwell and West Birmingham NHS Trust
United Kingdom

Meyyammai Mohan
Ophthalmology
East Lancashire Hospitals NHS Trust
United Kingdom

Michael Macmahon
Critical Care
NHS Fife
United Kingdom

Deepak Nama
Respiratory / Acute Medicine
East Lancashire Hospitals NHS Trust
United Kingdom

Huma Naqvi
Elderly Care Medicine
Sandwell and West Birmingham NHS Trust
United Kingdom

Kumar Periasamy
Orthopaedics
University Hospital Hairmyers
United Kingdom

Ravi Ravindran
General and HPB Surgery
NHS Lothian
United Kingdom

Sadasivam Selvakumar
Vascular
East and North Hertfordshire NHS Trust
United Kingdom

Jennifer Smith
General Surgery
East Lancashire Hospitals NHS Trust
United Kingdom

Subramanian Kanaga Sundaram
Urology
Mid Yorkshire Hospitals NHS Trust
United Kingdom

Ranji Thomas
Psychiatry
East Lancashire Hospitals NHS Trust
United Kingdom

Contents

Starting the Job

1

Content Outline

STATION 1.1: PRIORITISATION

The Bleep Scenario

You are a FY1 doctor doing a night shift in general surgery. Your list of jobs is given in Table 1.1. Think about how you would prioritise these tasks.

As a junior doctor, you will receive numerous tasks at the start of your shift and throughout the day. You may initially find it challenging to complete all your tasks and may even feel guilty about handing over to the next team. With experience, you will realise that some tasks are more urgent than others and that your priority is ultimately patient safety. Learning the skills of effective prioritisation will also help to prevent burnout and increase job satisfaction.

TYPES OF TASKS AND HOW TO PRIORITISE

Tasks assigned to junior doctors include:

- Reviews of sick patients
- Assessing stable patients
- Initiating management plans
- Discussions with other specialties
- Requesting, interpreting and actioning investigations
- Completing prescription charts and discharge letters
- Teaching other members of staff or medical students
- Non-clinical activities such as audit and quality improvement projects
- Talking to patients and their relatives
- Procedures such as insertion of cannulas

One approach is to distinguish between a routine and an emergency task. If you are asked to review a patient who has chest pain and to rewrite a drug chart for another patient, the unwell patient is your priority. This is an obvious example, but there are more difficult situations. Whilst discharge summaries can seem tedious, they are a crucial part of the patient journey and, when done well, prove immensely useful for continuity of care and future admissions. A delayed discharge significantly impacts the flow of acute admissions through the system and can even affect elective activity.

OTHER ASPECTS OF PRIORITISATION

Whilst you have to complete jobs for your own team, you should also be aware of the roles of other hospital teams and the impact on the wider hospital. For example, if you know you need to request a computed tomography (CT) scan for a patient to help your seniors plan treatment, you should ask for this as early as possible as there will be more slots available during the day time and there is more likely to be a radiologist on site. As you can see, prioritisation is dependent on the information you receive (Table 1.2). If you were told the cannula was for a patient who was bleeding profusely, then this would be more urgent.

Never forget that you are working in a team. If you feel you cannot manage or need help, do not hesitate to ask. Unless you ask, people may not know you need help.

Table 1.1 List of tasks

1	Review a patient on the surgical admissions unit with right-sided abdominal pain
2	Cannulate a patient who needs fluids because she has bowel obstruction and the previous cannula has stopped working
3	Rewrite a drug chat for a stable patient
4	Review a patient in accident and emergency who is hypotensive, tachycardic and has a distended abdomen
5	Review blood results for patients on the upper gastrointestinal ward as they were not back before handover

Table 1.2 Potential order of tasks with explanation

4	This comes first. This patient is in shock and will need emergency interventions. You will also need to escalate to senior team members
1	The patient will need to be assessed to decide if he needs emergency treatment or is stable enough to wait overnight
5	Review the bloods for the upper gastrointestinal patient – there is nothing to suggest that these might be urgent
2	After that, you should put the cannula in to avoid delaying fluid replacement and preventing electrolyte abnormalities
3	The last thing you would do is rewrite the drug chart for the stable patient

STATION 1.2: HANDOVER AND ESCALATION

The Bleep Scenario

You have come to the end of your shift as a FY1 doctor. There are 12 patients on the ward, 3 of whom need a review, 2 of whose blood tests need to be chased, and there is one who is waiting to be seen in ED. Please hand them over in an SBAR fashion.

WHY ARE THEY IMPORTANT?

As a junior doctor, your role involves assessing and making plans for acutely unwell patients as well as more stable patients. Thus, it is important to learn the art of effective handover. You also need to know when to escalate to a senior, for support or interventions that you are not trained to perform yourself. This is a brief guide to help you hand over properly. The more you do this, the easier and more natural it will become.

WHAT IS HANDOVER?

The process of handover includes a number of scenarios, including formal handover meetings in a dedicated room at the start and end of a shift (or sometimes in between), board rounds that involve discussing patients before (or after) a ward round, discussing patients over the phone or discussing patients face to face with a senior colleague. The person you are handing over to may not be based on site or may not know anything about the patient in question so it is important that you convey all pertinent information in a structured and concise manner.

HOW DO YOU HAND OVER A PATIENT?

There are a number of systems that are recommended for effective handovers. One that is commonly used in the NHS is SBAR: situation, background, assessment and response.

EXAMPLES AND EXPLANATION

Fig. 1.1 provides examples of handovers for you to judge.

SITUATION

Whilst the first example suggests that there is an unwell breathless patient, it does not provide specific information. This is important because you could have a patient who is short of breath but not desaturating.

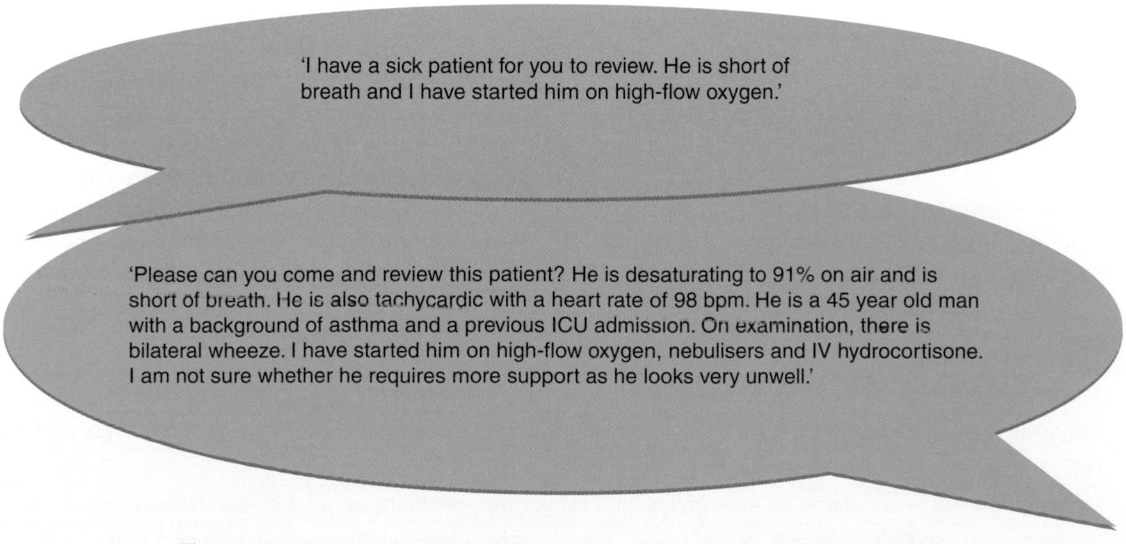

Fig. 1.1 Two speech bubbles giving examples of handover. ICU, intensive care unit.

BACKGROUND

The first example does not give any background. The patient's age and comorbidities are crucial to determining the diagnosis and guiding appropriate management. For example, the target saturation for this patient with asthma is >94% whereas in a patient with chronic obstructive pulmonary disease it may be 88–92%.

ASSESSMENT

The second case tells you about examination findings. This section could also include observations and other key information such as the results of blood tests, electrocardiogram (ECG) or imaging findings.

RESPONSE

This last section should tell the person you are handing over to what you have done so far and what you need them to do. The first example in Fig. 1.1 does not specify what you expect. This is important because the person you are handing over to may not be the best person for the specific scenario, but may be able to guide you to the right person. This part also allows you to ask for guidance on what to do before help arrives.

There are other methods of handover you can use instead of SBAR, such as I-PASS or SIGNOUT. They are all similar but feel free to experiment and pick the one that works well for you or that is recommended by your trust.

ESCALATION

Sometimes, there may not be enough time for escalation or handovers, for example if you have a rapidly deteriorating patient. In this situation, the best approach is to call the medical emergency team or cardiac arrest team. There will be specific teams for adult, paediatric and obstetric emergencies so make sure you are aware of how to call them. The standard 'cardiac arrest call' telephone number in Europe is 2222.

When escalating a patient, make sure you have the information stated above. Although not always the case, if you do not accurately convey the urgency of the scenario, this may influence whether you receive the support you need promptly. If you are not aware of the diagnosis or the severity of the situation, you should be honest as it shows the person you are speaking to that you do need help.

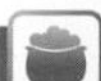
Clinical Tip

Some trusts or teams also use methods such as patient lists, which may be paperless or printed out. Other useful sources of information include ward round summaries which enable on call teams to have a better idea of the background of patients they are reviewing without needing to read through all of their notes. If these methods do not exist in your hospital, it may be an idea to introduce them and perform a quality improvement project.

MULTIDISCIPLINARY TEAM (MDT) MEMBERS

As a junior doctor, it is crucial to have an understanding of the roles and functionality of different aspects of the team. Listed below are some examples:

- Ward nursing staff
- Specialist nurses
- Healthcare assistants
- Physiotherapists
- Dieticians
- Occupational therapists
- Speech and language therapists
- Intensive care outreach team
- Chaplain service
- Psychologists
- Palliative care team
- Pharmacists
- Physician associates

Note that some referrals to allied health professionals are made by doctors and others by the nursing staff. Each department functions differently, so it is important to clarify this upon your arrival.

STATION 1.3: AN INTRODUCTION TO CLINICAL DECISION MAKING

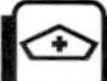
The Bleep Scenario

You are bleeped to review a 72 year old man with inoperable lung cancer, who is complaining of back pain. He has a background of chronic obstructive pulmonary disease, intravenous drug use and smokes cigarettes. He has recently started anticipatory palliative medication and is on slow background fluids only. He is not for cardiopulmonary resuscitation but there is no documented decision about escalation of care in his notes. His respiratory rate is 22 breaths per minute, heart rate 116 bpm, temperature 37.4°C and blood pressure is 98/68 mmHg. I think he is septic.

The art of clinical decision making is one that will be honed, changed and refined throughout your learning trajectory as a doctor.

We hope that being aware of the different factors that influence decision making will empower you by:

- Increasing your awareness of how a diagnosis is reached
- Showing you examples of how complex and holistic management plans are formulated
- Introducing you to concepts and theories that show how sometimes, despite best efforts, errors of judgement can occur

Figs 1.2 and 1.3 illustrate aspects of this process.

STATION 1.4: CLERKING

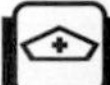
The Bleep Scenario

You are bleeped by a nurse on the acute medical unit. A new patient has arrived onto the ward following transfer from the accident and emergency (A&E) department. He informs you that a 64 year old man has been admitted with shortness of breath. You are asked to come and clerk the patient.

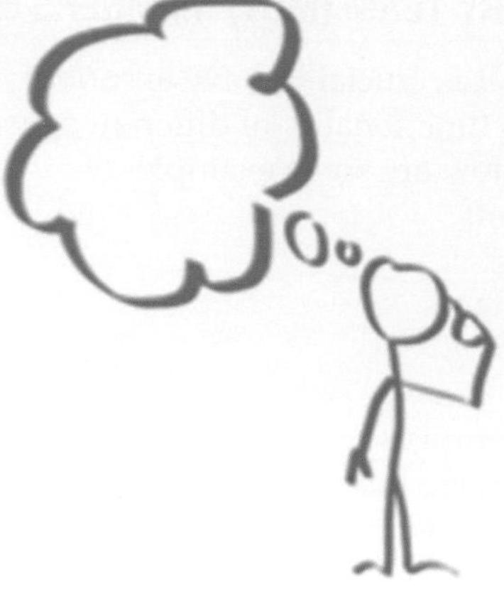

Initial thoughts

i. *Type 1 thinking*: Immediately start planning management of sepsis; rapid, reflexive, pattern recognition almost like autopilot mode

ii. *Type 2 thinking*: Demands more cognitive effort, is slower and focuses on deductive reasoning weighing up all the possibilities. This is the ideal diagnostic approach, however can be difficult to achieve consistently throughout a shift

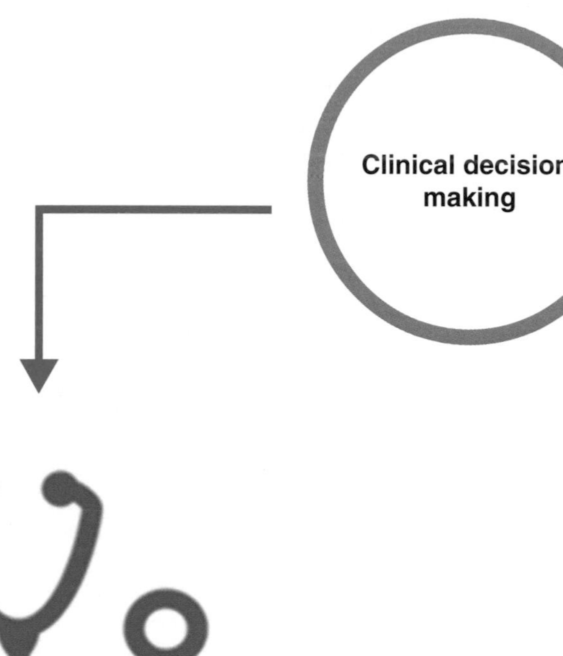

Investigations, management and escalation

This scenario has a wide differential and therefore a broad investigative plan which will dictate management. Additionally, in a patient like this, it is paramount to decide ceilings of care in case of deterioration.

It's also important to be aware of your own limitations, capabilities and knowledge, and ask for help when needed. It becomes much more problematic when we are not familiar with what we do not know

Scientific methodical approach (type 2 thinking)

Differential, assessment and resuscitation

1. *Generate hypothesis* from initial information
2. *Data gathering* from history and examination
3. *Refine hypothesis* by utilising patient's notes and investigations
4. *Implement intervention* if relevant, i.e. execute management plan

Worst case

Another approach is to rule out the worst-case scenario. This may be safe but often won't yield a cause or fully exercise our capacity to diagnose and can delay the correct management

Fig. 1.2 Thinking patterns.

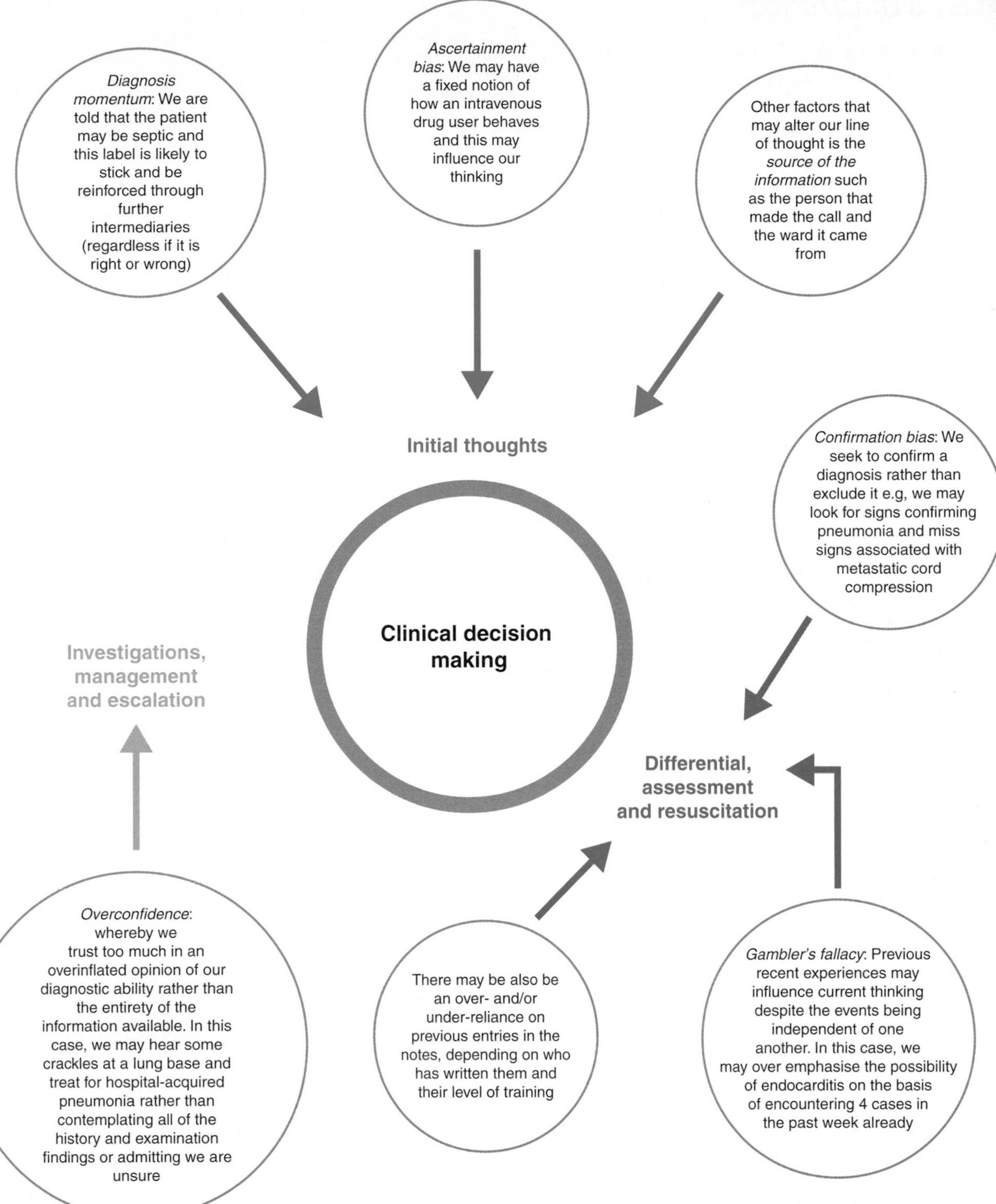

Fig. 1.3 Biases that occur in decision making.

WHAT IS EXPECTED OF YOU?

As a junior doctor you will often be involved in clerking new patients who have come in through various pathways, including A&E departments, direct general practitioner (GP) referrals, hospital transfers, elective surgical admissions or via clinic.

It is useful to develop a system so that you do not forget crucial information. Some hospitals have proformas in their admissions unit(s) for this purpose. It is vital that your documentation is clear and well presented. This is so that other team members can follow your diagnostic process and management plan (or the plan of the person for whom you are documenting).

SUGGESTED HEADINGS

The method shared below is one way of doing this, which the authors of the book have found to be effective. You may find a different way which is more comfortable for you.

1. Patient information, date and time of admission, doctor name and grade, location (department) and name of on call consultant
2. Presenting complaint
3. History of presenting complaint
4. Past medical and surgical history, including information about recent admissions
5. Drug history, including allergies
6. Social history, including type of accommodation, carers, assistance needed for activities of daily living, baseline mobility aids needed, smoking/drinking, drug use and who the patient lives with
7. Family history (if relevant; for example, a young patient presenting with weight loss and per rectum bleeding may have a family history of inflammatory bowel disease)
8. Observations
9. Examination findings (depending on the setting, this may include full-body plus neurological examination)
10. Relevant investigations (blood tests, including blood gas, imaging, microbiology results, previous results of significance, e.g. previous echocardiograms, biopsy results, etc.)
11. Plan

You may also find further sections for senior review and subsequent plan in the clerking proforma, if there is one.

WARD ROUND

The above format can also be used for ward rounds, and again some hospitals use ward round proformas particularly for consultant ward rounds. However, there are some differences. The version below is adapted and can be used on ward rounds.

1. Name and grade of doctor; date and time of ward round; patient name, age, hospital number
2. Active issues (for example, urinary sepsis, acute kidney injury [AKI], metabolic acidosis)
3. Old or resolved issues
4. Past medical history
5. Observations
6. Relevant investigations
7. Examination findings
8. Plan

Remember to sign your name and give your bleep number at the end. Some trusts will give you a stamp that you can also use and in some places it is expected that you will sign with your General Medical Council number.

Feel free to experiment with the above. You will soon find an approach that works for you and your team. The information you include will depend on the specific context of the patient you are seeing.

SUMMARY

Clerking is a common task and can feel quite daunting. It is important to be methodical so that vital information is not omitted. Any documentation will be reviewed if there is a complaint or investigation, so do make sure your documentation is as clear as possible.

It can be daunting when you begin seeing patients independently, but your confidence will grow as you see more patients. Try to see your patients on the post-take ward round wherever possible (where the new patients are reviewed by senior team members), as this is an excellent way to learn and to follow up on the plans you have made.

STATION 1.5: DISCUSSING 'DO NOT ATTEMPT CPR' ORDERS

The Bleep Scenario

A 78 year old female was admitted to your ward with pneumonia. She has a background of COPD, heart failure and renal failure. She is on home oxygen, and lives alone with carers that visit three times a day. She has been started on intravenous antibiotics, and your consultant has asked you to talk to her about a 'Do not attempt CPR' order.

Ideally, every patient should have an escalation plan from the start of their admission. These decisions are typically made at registrar level or above, but all members of the team should consider these discussions to be part of their management.

Try to make it part of your clerking process to consider escalation; gathering the past medical history and social history will give you an idea of someone's frailty levels, morbidity and functional status. If a 'do not attempt cardiopulmonary resuscitation' (DNACPR) order would be appropriate, having agreed it with a senior, you should start by discussing it with the patient themselves before including their family (if appropriate to do so and the patient consents). If the patient lacks capacity to have these discussions you may need to discuss with someone who has lasting power of attorney (LPA) for health or have a best interests meeting, or even involve the Court of Protection. If unsure, ask your senior colleagues.

RAISING THE TOPIC

This is a sensitive issue so it is good to introduce the topic with care. However, ambiguity is unhelpful and you should not be afraid to be specific. The structure of the conversation for patients and their relatives can be similar and you can adapt it to each specific situation. Below are some examples of phrasing.

I want to discuss a topic with you that is sensitive but is also very important. I wonder if anyone has spoken to you before about the subject of resuscitation?

Check understanding of terms early:

Do you know what I mean when I say 'resuscitation' or use the phrase 'CPR'?

CPR describes a number of actions which we as medics can take in an attempt to restart someone's heart if it has stopped for a reversible reason. It often includes drugs, chest compressions and inserting a breathing tube into the windpipe to allow machines to breathe for you. In some circumstances it may also include administering an electric current through the body to shock the heart.

Seek to normalise the topic and reassure people that they are not being singled out.

We try to have these discussions with most people who come into the hospital so you can have a say in your care going forward.

Get to the point. It is easy to come across as underprepared if you take too long to address the true agenda. Be reassuring, however, if this is not an immediate concern.

We are not anticipating any imminent deterioration in your health. However, given what you've already told me about your list of medical problems, if at any stage during this admission or in the future you were to become so sick that your heart stopped beating, it would not be appropriate to undertake CPR. As a team, we believe that if your body had reached this stage, it would not be reversible and so CPR would be futile.

Be kind and reassure them that management will otherwise be unchanged. This is a difficult conversation and it may bring about a degree of upset. It can be helpful to paint an alternative picture so they can begin to register the difference between CPR and other routes.

This decision will not otherwise change your management. As a team, we agree that in the event that your heart stops beating and you stop breathing, we would rather you have your family around you, holding your hand, than a team of people trying to poke and prod you to no avail.

It is strongly recommended that you don't ask the patient or relative 'do you agree?' as this gives them an impression of shouldering the burden. Instead, check 'do you understand the rationale for this decision?' Following this, open up the floor to questions.

DOCUMENTATION

Document the discussion in a summary form on your patient record. Depending on local trust protocol, you may also have to fill out a paper DNACPR form and have this signed by a senior clinician.

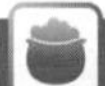 **Clinical Tip**

Review pre-existing wishes e.g. advanced directive/Coordinate My Care (CMC) record, Recommended Summary Plan for Emergency Care and Treatment (ReSPECT) form or community DNACPR forms.

STATION 1.6: UPDATING RELATIVES

 **The Bleep Scenario**

An 83 year old female was admitted to your ward with sudden-onset dysphasia and right hemiparesis. She has a background of dementia, hypertension, type 2 diabetes and angina. She lives at home with family and pre-admission was mobile with a frame, requiring assistance with her activities of daily living. The ward clerk tells you that her son called to ask for an update.

This is a job you will encounter daily. Whether it is an update in person or via telephone, there are several things you can do to maximise the effectiveness of your updates and ensure you are adequately prepared. It can also be useful to collect some stock phrases.

INITIAL THOUGHTS

Preparation is everything. Make sure you know the details of the admission: why the patient presented, what tests have been done, the results and ongoing management plan. Taking 10 minutes to read through the notes will make you feel more prepared before you begin. Simple measures can make the conversation more likely to be successful and should include taking consent from the patient to update their relative, identification of a suitable location and taking measures to avoid interruption.

CONVERSATION

INTRODUCTION

If the Conversation is via Telephone

Confirm the identity of the person at the other end of the phone as well as introducing yourself. Make sure it is clear early in the conversation that you are calling for a non-emergent update so that the relative is not unduly stressed.

Hi, my name is Dr ______, I'm calling from ______. I understand that you are the son of ______. I'm calling to give you an update on your mum, if you are free for a few minutes. Can I start by asking you to confirm your mother's date of birth?

In Person

Similarly, introduce yourself and the nature of the conversation.

I've asked you to come in today so we can discuss your mum's diagnosis and ongoing care.

CONTENT

The keystone of conversations with relatives is to establish their knowledge and understanding early. This gives you the opportunity to identify misunderstandings or gaps in their comprehension and correct these before you offer further information.

To start with, how much do you understand about what has been happening so far?

When you have established their baseline knowledge, it helps to go back to the reason the patient came to hospital. This is an opportunity to get a collateral history of what happened and to understand their perspective. What did they see? Did they have their own ideas about what the symptoms represented?

When your mum came in, we noticed that her speech was jumbled and she wasn't moving as well on the right side compared to the left. Does that tie in with what you saw at home?

Mention your diagnostic suspicions and the tests your team did as a result. This can act as a warning shot by bringing up your suspected diagnosis early in the conversation.

When someone has weakness on one side, or a new change to their speech, the first thing we have to think about is a stroke. The initial step is to do a CT scan of the brain.

It's OK to pause the narrative to check their understanding of any new terms you introduce.

You may have heard the word 'stroke' used before; what is your understanding of it?

Correct any misconceptions and fill gaps in knowledge before you continue on to explain what the tests have shown or ruled out. Talk about the plan in the short and longer term. It may be useful to anticipate the results of the tests but this will depend on your degree of diagnostic certainty.

The CT head has ruled out any bleeding in the brain, but we need to keep your mum in hospital for a more detailed scan of the brain, called a magnetic resonance imaging or MRI scan. We expect this will confirm that your mum has had a stroke. While we do more tests, she will also be seen by our therapy teams so they can assess the degree of deficit and start rehabilitation.

CLOSING

Check their understanding. Ask open and closed questions to ensure that they have processed the key points. It can be helpful to ask them to repeat things back to ensure retention of important details.

This has been a lot of information. What have you taken from the things we have talked about? Are you clear on what we expect to happen over the next few days?

You should then give them the opportunity to ask anything they are unsure about. Encouraging this will tease out any concerns or expectations that have not yet been uncovered.

Thank you so much for your time today, I hope this conversation has helped to make things clearer for you. Do you have any questions for me?

Finally, suggest when they should next expect an update so they have realistic expectations.

Document a summary of the discussion in the patient record, including the names of the relatives you spoke to, the information you relayed and any feedback or questions they had.

STATION 1.7: APPLICATION OF KEY ETHICAL PRINCIPLES

DEFINITION

Medical ethics describes the moral code by which doctors should practise; the key principles are autonomy, justice, beneficence and non-maleficence.

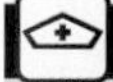

The Bleep Scenario

A 45 year old male presented with an open tibia and fibula fracture following a fall. He was due to have surgery today but this has been delayed. He is agitated and demanding to be discharged. You are on call and the nurse asks you to speak with him.

INITIAL THOUGHTS

The safety of the patient and staff should be your prime concern, as an agitated patient can pose risks to himself and others. Information gathering is crucial: you need to understand his reasons for wanting to leave and whether he is capable of making that decision. Meanwhile, the patient needs to understand the risks associated with discharging himself against medical advice.

ASSESSMENT

This is three-pronged:

- Safety: if there is a concern that the patient's behaviour represents a risk of harm to himself or others, call for help. It may be appropriate to inform senior ward staff and/or security staff urgently for support.
- ABCDE assessment: ensure that the patient is haemodynamically stable by checking vital signs and observing the patient. Could a physical health deterioration be contributing to their agitation? Be vigilant and ask to examine the patient if you have concerns, but ensure your own safety. Similarly, if there is any question about the patient's mental health, an urgent mental health team review may be indicated.
- Capacity: it is imperative that you assess this patient's capacity to make decisions about his medical care, specifically to discharge himself against medical advice. The Mental Capacity Act 2005 dictates that, in order to have capacity, patients must be able to do all of the following:
  - Understand relevant information conveyed to them
  - Retain the information
  - Weigh the risks and benefits of the different options
  - Communicate their decision

A conversation in which you discuss a patient's concerns, answer the patient's questions and explain the risks and benefits of each option will often demonstrate capacity or lack thereof. You may need to ask specific questions to supplement this.

In many cases, patients will agree with the medically recommended course of action when their questions and concerns have been addressed. However, a patient may make a decision which you do not agree with; this alone does not represent a lack of capacity.

In patients who lack capacity, a decision must be made by the medical team in their best interests.

Hospital inpatients who lack capacity to make a decision on their healthcare and for whom limitations on their liberty are in their best interests can be treated under the Mental Capacity Act. If a patient lacks capacity, you should seek the views of their next of kin, or make decisions with the person with lasting power of attorney for healthcare decisions and/or respect previously expressed views made in advanced directives.

However if their liberty must be deprived and they are not eligible to be treated under the Mental Health Act, Deprivation of Liberty Safeguards (commonly referred to as DoLS) paperwork must be completed as per the local trust protocol. This ensures that the least restrictive, most appropriate measures are used to keep patients safe.

Clinical Tip

If you are making a 'best interests' decision for a patient, it is a good idea to involve other members of the MDT who can provide different perspectives and areas of expertise.

Clinical Tip

If someone has a mental health problem that is affecting their decision making, and therefore putting them at risk, you should organise urgent psychiatry review. They may need to be assessed under the Mental Health Act rather than the Mental Capacity Act.

FOUR PILLARS OF MEDICAL ETHICS

These four guiding principles are applicable to each and every decision you make and together they can act as a foundation for your medical practice.

BENEFICENCE

Your intention should always be to bring about benefit to your patients. This could represent managing an acute condition or giving lifestyle advice to prevent health problems.

For example, ideally, this patient would decide to stay in hospital and undergo operative management, as this would be beneficial for his short- and long-term health. If the patient had fallen due to intoxication, you might offer lifestyle advice in addition to routine post-operative rehabilitation.

NON-MALEFICENCE

This essentially means 'do no harm'. Whilst it obviously precludes deliberate injury to a person in your care, it can be more complex and must be used in context. A degree of risk is unavoidable in almost every aspect of medical management, but this must be weighed against potential benefit.

In this case, non-maleficence could apply to the use of sedatives. This should be avoided unless someone poses a threat to themselves or others. Sedatives must never be given with the intention of harming a patient or if there are contraindications which would make their use unsafe.

AUTONOMY

This is the promotion of a patient's role in their own healthcare. It involves providing all necessary information required by a patient to make decisions about their care. Capacity is closely linked to this pillar; someone must be found to have capacity to be able to make such decisions.

For example, if a patient with capacity decides to discharge themself against medical advice, it is not your role to stop them, but to inform them regarding the risks and benefits of this decision and to support the patient in making a decision. In this scenario, the patient must be informed of the risks and benefits of surgery in order to consent.

JUSTICE

This predominantly applies to fairness and equality of patients. Patients should be treated with equality irrespective of their gender, ethnicity, background, age, disability and other protected characteristics. Distribution of resources must also be fair.

In this case, a more unwell or emergent patient has been prioritised for surgery over a stable patient. Limited resources mean that it is not possible to operate on both patients at once and so the available theatre and staff have been allocated according to need.

MANAGEMENT

Address the patient and suggest discussion in an area that is private but from which you can easily exit if required for your safety. Respect the patient's personal space. Establish what the patient understands and what he would like from you.

You should use a calm voice as well as displaying non-aggressive body language. Discuss options and try to reach a mutually agreed conclusion. If the patient has capacity and wishes to discharge himself against medical advice, ask him to sign an AMA (against medical advice) form (if used in your trust) and document the discussion in the notes.

If the patient lacks capacity to make a decision about discharge or ongoing management, you should discuss it with a senior (ideally the consultant) and the MDT. In some cases you will need to initiate the DoLS process to limit their freedom in order to treat them, if it is in their best interests. Ensure you are familiar with your trust processes for this.

STATION 1.8: DISCHARGE SUMMARIES

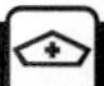

The Bleep Scenario

You are on weekend ward cover and receive a bleep from one of the medical wards. An 81 year old female who was admitted with chest pain several days ago is going home today. Unfortunately, the discharge letter was not prepared by the day team during the week and you are asked to complete it.

INITIAL THOUGHTS

Prioritisation is a vital part of ward cover shifts. It can be frustrating to have to fill out a discharge letter for someone you do not know. However, with a structured approach you can produce a concise summary of the main events of admission, overall diagnosis and plan on discharge. Everyone writes discharge summaries slightly differently and you will develop your own style over time.

Clinical Tip

When you start a new rotation, check with senior members of your team if there are specific requirements for your specialty. This could be for a certain investigation result, a prognostication score or the physiotherapy review outcome.

ASSESSMENT

The first task is to confirm that the patient is fit to be discharged. In most trusts, staff members at registrar level or above decide on discharge. However, after it has been documented by a senior that the patient is 'medically fit for discharge', there may be delays in arranging equipment or a package of care. Check that criteria for safe discharge have been met (whether this is equipment or clinical observations) and no new concerns have been recorded. When you are satisfied that the patient is safe to be discharged, begin the paperwork. In some circumstances, particularly for patients who have had lengthy inpatient admissions, it is worth preparing discharge summaries early on.

TTOS

TTO stands for 'To Take Out', and this is used to document and prescribe the medications with which patients are sent home. Each trust has different TTO protocols; whether these are online or on paper, familiarising yourself with these protocols may save you a lot of time. Some trusts require both pre-admission and new medications to be recorded, whereas others allow you to record just newly prescribed drugs as long as the admission is less than 48 hours or so. Trusts will also vary in the default duration of medication supplied.

AN APPROACH TO COMPLETING TTOS

- Start by reviewing the inpatient drug chart to see which medications the patient is on.
- Compare this with the list of admission medications: if there are discrepancies, you should refer to the notes to establish whether medications have been deliberately paused, discontinued or omitted in error.
- Depending on local procedure, proceed to document (at least) the new medications that the patient requires.

Clinical Tip

If you are struggling to piece together an accurate list, your colleagues are useful resources, as are the patients themselves. For example, patients may have been told why a medication has been stopped. Meanwhile, pharmacists can advise on medication course durations or drug interactions, as well as any discrepancies with medication the patient was on before admission.

WRITING A DISCHARGE SUMMARY

Doctors all develop their own style of documentation, but it can help to start with a template and update it over time. Have a look at some example discharge letters from your department so you can familiarise yourself with the structure.

One job of a discharge summary is to hand over care to the community, informing the GP of the key events of admission and how this affects the patient's ongoing care. Another role involves educating patients and their families and, in the event of a future admission, informing the admitting team of the circumstances of this hospital stay.

From the point of view of GPs with several discharge summaries on their desk, huge blocks of text can be unhelpful. If the hospital team instead breaks down the information into short paragraphs and bullet points, the salient information can be more easily absorbed. Using widely known abbreviations such as CXR for chest X-ray is acceptable, but avoid anything specialty-specific.

The details included may be dictated by individual context: if the patient is being transferred to another trust or to the care of a new GP, a more detailed letter would be appropriate.

AN EXAMPLE STRUCTURE

1. The opening sentence or two should describe the way the patient first presented. This is helpful if someone is readmitted with similar presentations as you can identify similarities and differences.

   Mrs Wright presented with a 2-day history of constant, severe, crushing central chest pain that was worse on exertion and radiated to her left jaw.

2. Details of initial examination and simple investigations. Patients will often talk to their GP about results of their admission so it can help if the GP knows what was tested and found. It also establishes a baseline from which the GP can compare other results.

   Examination on admission revealed tachycardia but nil else of note. An ECG showed sinus rhythm with T-wave inversion in the lateral leads. Serial troponin I was raised at 34 + 272. CXR and other bloods were unremarkable. An inpatient echocardiogram showed mild left ventricular dysfunction.

3. Address the diagnosis. Demonstrate how your examination and results have led to this.

   The patient was discussed with the cardiology team, who recommended conservative treatment as a non-ST-segment myocardial infarction (NSTEMI). She was started on aspirin 75 mg OD, ticagrelor 90 mg BD (for 12 months), ramipril 10 mg OD, bisoprolol 2.5 mg OD, and simvastatin 40 mg OD. Fondaparinux was given for three days whilst in hospital.

4. If anything else of note happened, you can mention it here. Highlight any medications that have been changed or stopped.

   During admission, the patient developed a prerenal AKI which has since resolved. As part of her management, ramipril has been reduced from 10 mg OD to 5 mg OD.

5. Finally, summarise the management plan. This is also a good place to mention any advanced care planning or escalation decisions that have been made.

   She is on all appropriate NSTEMI medication, and will be discharged with follow-up in cardiology clinic and further outpatient investigations, including a CT coronary angiogram and a repeat echocardiogram.

6. Other sections of the discharge letter may include input from other MDT members, such as occupational therapy/physiotherapy review.

   This patient was assessed by the ward physiotherapist, and was found to be mobilising at baseline with a stick.

7. It can be helpful to bullet point the key notes of the discharge plan at the end to consolidate your information.

   Plan on discharge:

   - Continue reduced dose of ramipril 5 mg OD and clopidogrel 75 mg with ticagrelor 90 mg BD (for 12 months)
   - Outpatient CT coronary angiogram: this has been requested
   - Follow-up with cardiology: this has been arranged
   - GP to repeat urea and electrolytes in 1 week to ensure renal function remains stable

A layout like this will convey essential information, and as you become more experienced you can tailor things.

FURTHER READING

Baile, W. F., et al. (2000). SPIKES – a six-step protocol for delivering bad news: application to the patient with cancer. *Oncologist*, *5*(4), 302–311.

Croskerry, P. (2013). *Critical thinking program*. Halifax: Dalhousie University.

Cutter, W. J., et al. (2011). Identifying and managing deprivation of liberty in adults in England and Wales. *BMJ*, *342*, c7323.

Kahneman, D. (2012). *Thinking, fast and slow*. London: Penguin.

Mental Capacity Act. (2005). *Code of practice*. Available at: www.gov.uk/government/uploads/system/uploads/attachment_data/file/497253/Mental-capacity-act-code-of-practice.pdf. [Accessed 10 January 2022].

Nicholson, T. R. J., Cutter, W., & Hotopf, M. (2008). Assessing mental capacity: the Mental Capacity Act. *British Medical Journal*, *336*, 322.

Resuscitation Council UK. (2017). *Decisions relating to cardiopulmonary resuscitation* (3rd ed.). Available at 20160123 Decisions Relating to CPR – 2016.pdf (resus.org.uk) (accessed 9 January 2022).

2 Data Interpretation

Content Outline

STATION 2.1: ARTERIAL BLOOD GAS INTERPRETATION

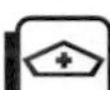

The Bleep Scenario

You are bleeped by a nurse on the respiratory ward. A 35 year old non-binary person is being treated for an acute exacerbation of asthma. His saturations have dropped to 84% on room air. Your fellow junior doctor has already started treatment when you arrive and you are asked to process and review the patient's arterial blood gas (ABG). The values are as follows: pH 7.29, $PaCO_2$ 4.0 kPa, PaO_2 7.0 kPa, HCO_3^- 24 mmol/L.

INITIAL THOUGHTS

An ABG is an excellent test to determine the oxygenation status and acid–base balance quickly. There are six key pieces of information: pH, PaO_2 (partial pressure of oxygen in arterial blood), $PaCO_2$ (partial pressure of carbon dioxide in arterial blood), bicarbonate, base excess and lactate.

COMPONENTS

pH

- The acidity/alkalinity of a solution is determined by the concentration of hydrogen ions.
- The pH of a normal arterial blood sample lies between 7.35 and 7.45, which is 36–44 nmol/L hydrogen ions (H^+), with an inverse relationship between pH and H^+ concentration.
- It is important to remember that small changes in pH represent large changes in hydrogen ion concentration.

PARTIAL PRESSURE OF OXYGEN

- Partial pressure is measured in kilopascals (kPa) and represents the contribution each gas makes to the total pressure of a mixture.
- The concentration of oxygen in inspired air is 21%, with a partial pressure of 21 kPa.
- As air passes towards the alveoli, the partial pressure of oxygen is reduced as a result of: (1) addition of water vapour; and (2) addition of CO_2 in the alveoli
- The partial pressure of oxygen in the alveoli is ~13 kPa, whereas the PaO_2 of arterial blood is lower than in the alveoli, therefore creating a gradient for gaseous exchange.
- In a healthy individual breathing room air, PaO_2 of an arterial sample should be >10 kPa.
- As a general rule, the PaO_2 for a given inspired concentration should be roughly 10 kPa less than the inspired concentration (%).
- For example, the inhalation of 40% oxygen should result in PaO_2 = 30 kPa.
- Oxygenation (i.e. arterial PaO_2) is determined by gaseous exchange and alveolar ventilation.

PARTIAL PRESSURE OF CARBON DIOXIDE

- $PaCO_2$ is the partial pressure of CO_2 in arterial blood and should be 4.7–6.0 kPa when oxygenating on room air in a healthy patient.
- CO_2 is an important waste product of metabolism. High levels of CO_2 imply inability of the lungs to adequately remove CO_2 from the blood: i.e. poor ventilation.
- In normal functioning, CO_2 is transported to the lungs bound on protein, haemoglobin or dissolved in plasma, where it reacts with water to form hydrogen ions and bicarbonate as per the bicarbonate buffer system equation:

$$CO_2 + H_2O \rightleftharpoons H_2CO_3 \rightleftharpoons HCO_3^- + H^+$$

BICARBONATE

- Bicarbonate is a base and is the principal buffer in the body.
- The lungs eliminate excess protons via $CO_2 + H_2O$, creating a bicarbonate deficit; the kidneys buffer any remaining H^+ ions and replace the bicarbonate

deficit (by excreting H^+ ions in urine and filtering and returning HCO_3^- to the plasma).

- The normal range of bicarbonate is 22–26 mmol/L.
- The bicarbonate buffer system responds slowly and can take many hours to days to produce additional bicarbonate to meet the increased acid load.

BASE EXCESS

- Base excess is a measure of the excess acid or base in the blood resulting from metabolic imbalance.
- It demonstrates the amount of acid or base that would need to be added to the blood sample to restore it to a normal pH.
- A base excess more negative than –2 mmol/L is suggestive of a metabolic acidosis, i.e. more base would need to be added to restore normal pH.
- A base excess greater than +2 mmol/L is indicative of a metabolic alkalosis, i.e. more acid would need to be added to restore normal pH.

Table 2.1 shows the range of normal values and Table 2.2 shows common patterns.

Table 2.1 Range of normal values

pH	7.35–7.45 kPa
PaO_2	11–13 kPa
$PaCO_2$	4.7–6.0 kPa
HCO_3^-	22–26 mEq/L
Base excess	–2 to +2 mmol/L
Lactate	0.5–1 mmol/L

LACTATE

- Lactate is produced as the end product of anaerobic metabolism
- Normal levels are 0.5-2.2 mmol/L
- It is mainly generated by skeletal muscles, the brain, the gut, red blood cells and the skin
- It is metabolised in the liver and by myocytes. The kidney also has a role in conditions of hyperlactataemia
- A raised lactate will be produced in any conditions which result in reduced oxygen supply to the body, or increased production or decreased removal of lactate
- In general the greater the lactate, the greater the severity of the condition
- Lactate levels can also be used as a marker of response to treatment

INTERPRETATION

1. How is the patient clinically?
    - A 'very low' PaO_2 in a patient who looks completely well, with no shortness of breath and has a normal O_2 saturations on pulse oximetry is likely secondary to a venous sample.
    - A 'normal'-range PaO_2 (i.e. 11–13 kPa) in a patient on high-flow oxygen is abnormal, as you would expect the patient to have a PaO_2 roughly 10 kPa less than the inspired concentration (%).
    - A patient with chronic obstructive pulmonary disease (COPD) will show signs of respiratory acidosis (i.e. raised CO_2) and compensatory metabolic alkalosis (i.e. raised HCO_3^-) with a normal pH; without a detailed history, this may be misinterpreted as a primary metabolic alkalosis with compensatory respiratory acidosis.

Table 2.2 Common ABG patterns

ABNORMALITY	SIGNIFICANT FINDINGS ON ABG	EXAMPLES
Respiratory acidosis, uncompensated Respiratory acidosis, partially compensated Respiratory acidosis, fully compensated	↑ $PaCO_2$, ↓ pH, normal HCO_3^- ↑ $PaCO_2$, ↓ pH, ↑ HCO_3^- ↑ $PaCO_2$, normal pH, ↑↑ HCO_3^-	Respiratory depression (e.g. opiates), asthma, COPD, over-oxygenation in oxygen sensitive patients, Guillain-Barre syndrome, OSA
Respiratory alkalosis, uncompensated Respiratory alkalosis, partially compensated Respiratory alkalosis, fully compensated	↓ $PaCO_2$, ↑ pH, normal HCO_3^- ↓ $PaCO_2$, ↑ pH, ↓ HCO_3^- ↓ $PaCO_2$, normal pH, ↓↓ HCO_3^-	Any cause of hyperventilation (anxiety, pain), excessive mechanical ventilation
Metabolic acidosis, uncompensated Metabolic acidosis, partially compensated Metabolic acidosis, fully compensated	Normal $PaCO_2$, ↓ pH, ↓ HCO_3^- ↓ $PaCO_2$, ↓ pH, ↓ HCO_3^- ↓ $PaCO_2$, normal pH, ↓↓ HCO_3^-	Loss of HCO_3^- from gut (diarrhoea), renal failure, lactic acidosis, ketoacidosis
Metabolic alkalosis, uncompensated Metabolic alkalosis, partially compensated Metabolic alkalosis, fully compensated	Normal $PaCO_2$, ↑ pH, ↑ HCO_3^- ↑ $PaCO_2$, ↑ pH, ↑ HCO_3^- ↑ $PaCO_2$, normal pH, ↑↑ HCO_3^-	Diuretics (loop, thiazide), loss of H+ from gut (vomiting), excess mineralocorticoids
Mixed acidosis	↑ $PaCO_2$, ↓ pH, ↓ HCO_3^-	Cardiac arrest, multi-organ failure
Mixed alkalosis	↓ $PaCO_2$, ↑ pH, ↑ HCO_3^-	Hyperemesis gravidarum, hyperventilation in COPD

2. What is the PaO_2?
   - When breathing room air, the PaO_2 should be 10.0–13.0 kPa.
   - When breathing supplemental oxygen, the PaO_2 should be ~10 kPa less than the inspired concentration (%); if there is a difference >10 between the inspired concentration and the concentration in the arterial sample, there is a defect in oxygenation.
   - Type 1 respiratory failure is caused by impaired gaseous exchange, resulting in a PaO_2 <8 kPa with normal or low arterial $PaCO_2$.
   - Type 2 respiratory failure is caused by alveolar hypoventilation, resulting in a PaO_2 <8 kPa and PaO_2 > 6 kPa.
3. What is the pH?
   - Is the patient acidaemic (pH<7.35) or alkalaemic (pH>7.45)?
   - In principle, the body never overcompensates; therefore the primary problem should be clear.
4. What is the $PaCO_2$?
   - If $PaCO_2$ is increased (>6.0 kPa) and pH is decreased, this suggests respiratory acidosis.
   - If $PaCO_2$ is decreased (<4.7 kPa) and pH is increased, this suggests respiratory alkalosis.
   - Look at step 5 to see if there is any metabolic abnormality as both can coexist, or there may be a degree of compensation.
5. What is the HCO_3^-?
   - If HCO_3^- is increased (>26 mEq/L) and pH is increased, this suggests metabolic alkalosis.
   - If HCO_3^- is decreased (<22 mEq/L) and pH is decreased, this suggests metabolic acidosis.
   - Remember to review the $PaCO_2$ to detect any respiratory compensation.
6. What is the base excess?
   - A high base excess (> +2 mmol/L) indicates a higher-than-normal amount of HCO_3^- in the blood; this can be caused by primary metabolic alkalosis or a compensated respiratory acidosis.
   - A low base excess (< –2 mmol/L) indicates a lower-than-normal amount of HCO_3^- in the blood; this can be caused by primary metabolic acidosis or a compensated respiratory alkalosis
7. What is the lactate?
   - A raised lactate can be attributed to several causes but is most commonly used as a marker of sepsis
   - Hyperlactataemia can be related to:
     - Reduced tissue oxygen delivery: seizures, severe asthma, cardiac arrest, regional ischaemia, severe anaemia and carbon monoxide poisoning
     - Underlying disease process: liver failure, sepsis, cancers, enzyme deficiencies
     - Drugs: metformin, adrenaline, beta-2 agonist

Clinical Scenarios

The patient in Scenario 1.1 has a respiratory acidosis, consistent with type 1 respiratory failure. Four other examples are described below:

1. You are asked to review a 59 year old man, with a background of COPD, who is complaining of worsening shortness of breath and increased sputum production. The ABG results ar as follows:
- pH: 7.15 (7.35–7.45)
- PO_2: 7.5 (10.0–13.0) kPa
- PCO_2: 7.8 (4.5–6.0) kPa
- HCO_3^-: 28 (22–26) mmol/L
- Base excess: +4 (–2 to +2) mmol/L

ABG Interpretation
- Type 2 respiratory failure and respiratory acidosis, with partial metabolic compensation.
- Acidosis is likely acute-on-chronic as patient normally retains CO_2 and likely has a chronically raised HCO_3^-

2. You review a 23 year old man who was found collapsed by his friend during a night out. ABG results are as follows:
- pH: 7.23 (7.35–7.45)
- PO_2: 12 (11–13) kPa
- PCO_2: 4.0 (4.5–6.0) kPa
- HCO_3^-: 13 (22–26) mmol/L
- Base excess: –14 (–2 to +2) mmol/L

ABG Interpretation
- Metabolic acidosis with respiratory compensation
- Causes of metabolic acidosis mnemonic: MUDPILES: Methanol, uraemia, diabetic ketoacidosis (DKA), propylene glycol, isoniazid, lactate, ethylene glycol, salicylates. Toxic ingestion ought to be considered here.

3. A 17 year old girl presents following a vasovagal episode during a school exam. At present, she reports feeling light-headed and short of breath. ABG results are as follows:
- pH: 7.49 (7.35–7.45)
- PO_2: 11.9 (11–13) kPa
- PCO_2: 3.9 (4.5–6.0) kPa
- HCO_3^-: 23 (22–26) mmol/L
- Base excess: +2 (–2 to +2) mmol/L

ABG Interpretation
- Respiratory alkalosis, uncompensated
- Most likely due to anxiety-induced hyperventilation

4. A 33 year old male presents with severe diarrhoea and vomiting after returning from his recent travels abroad. ABG results are as follows:
- pH 7.6 (7.35–7.45)
- PO_2: 11.5 (11–13) kPa
- PCO_2: 5.2 (4.5–6.0) kPa
- HCO_3^-: 30 (22–26) mmol/L
- Base excess: + 5 (–2 to + 2) mmol/L

ABG INTERPRETATION
- Metabolic alkalosis, uncompensated
- Most likely secondary to persistent diarrhoea and vomiting

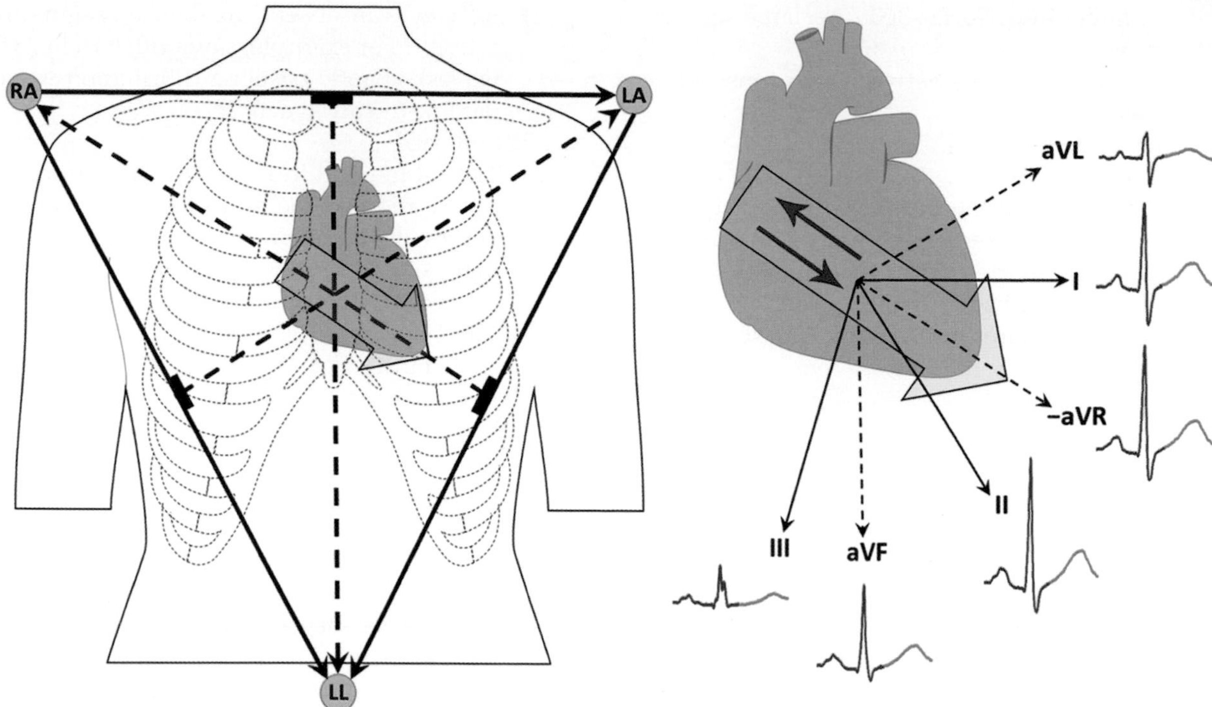

Fig. 2.1 The frontal electrocardiogram (ECG) leads. Left panel: using three extremity electrodes, right arm (RA), left arm (LA) and left leg (LL), a total of six dipolar leads can be constructed in the frontal plane. The solid black arrows constitute dipolar limb leads (I, II and III), and the dashed black arrows constitute augmented limb leads (aVR, aVL and aVF). Right panel: the waveform morphology in each frontal lead depends on the geometric angle between each lead and the averaged cardiac axis (large opaque arrow). Note that leads better aligned with the cardiac axis are more likely to have dominant waveform deflections. The colour of each ECG waveform morphology is mapped to either a depolarisation impulse (red arrow) or repolarisation impulse (blue arrow). (Source: El-Baz, A. and Suri, J.S. [2022]. *Cardiovascular and coronary artery imaging*. London: Academic Press.).

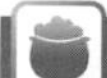 Clinical Tip

A normal $PaCO_2$ in a hypoxic asthmatic patient is a sign of exhaustion and the need for urgent intensive therapy unit review.

 Clinical Tip

A very low PaO_2 in a patient who looks completely well without dyspnoea and with normal O_2 saturations is likely a venous sample.

STATION 2.2: ECG INTERPRETATION

 The Bleep Scenario

You are bleeped by a nurse on the surgical admissions unit to review an electrocardiogram (ECG) for a patient, in preparation for an emergency laparotomy.

INITIAL THOUGHTS

As a junior doctor you will be asked to interpret ECGs on a regular basis. It is important you stay calm and have a structured approach.

Begin by checking the patient demographics and ECG calibrations. Then assess the rate, rhythm and axis before proceeding to assess the wave morphologies (Fig. 2.1) and segments of the ECG. Document your findings on the ECG and in the patient notes.

INTERPRETATION

1. **Demographic data**
   - Check the name, date of birth and hospital number.
   - Check the date and time the ECG was taken.
2. **Calibration**
   - Horizontal calibration: check the ECG paper is calibrated to 25 mm/s. Therefore a small square (1 mm) is 0.04 s or 40 ms, and a large square (5 mm) is 0.2 s or 200 ms.
   - The standard rhythm strip should be 10 s long.
   - Vertical calibration: this is indicated by the rectangular box on the ECG paper and 1 cm should equal 1 mV.
3. **Rate**
   - Regular rhythm,

     Method 1: count the number of large squares between two consecutive R waves and divide

this number into 300, i.e. 300 / no. large squares. Example:
- Two large squares between two consecutive R waves
- Rate = 300 / 2
- Rate = 150 bpm

Method 2: count the number of small squares between two consecutive R waves (the R–R interval) and divide this number into 1500, i.e. 1500 / no. small squares. Example:
- 10 small squares between two consecutive R waves
- Rate = 1500 / 10
- Rate = 150 bpm

- Irregular rhythm: on a standard rhythm strip (duration of 10 s), count all the R waves and multiply this number by 6, i.e. no. R waves × 6. Example:
  - 12 R waves on a 10-s rhythm strip
  - Rate = 12 × 6
  - Rate = 72 bpm

4. **Rhythm**
   - Rhythm is best interpreted from the lead that shows the P wave most clearly, usually lead II or V1.
   - Sinus rhythm: every P wave is followed by a QRS complex.
   - Regular versus irregular: mark four R waves on a piece of a paper and move the paper along the trace to see if the rhythm is regular (marks on paper match with subsequent R waves) or irregular (marks on paper do not match with subsequent R waves).
5. **Cardiac axis**
   - Cardiac axis indicates the direction of the wave of ventricular depolarisation.
   - Normal axis is between –30 and +90° and lead II has the most positive deflection (predominantly upwards) compared to leads I and III.
   - Simple method (that works in most cases):
     - If leads I and II are positive, the cardiac axis is normal.
     - If lead I is positive and lead II is negative (i.e. the leads are *'leaving'* each other), there is *left*-axis deviation.
     - If lead I is negative and lead II is positive (i.e. the leads are *'reaching'* to each other), there is *right*-axis deviation.
6. **P wave**
   - The P wave represents the transmission of excitation from the sinoatrial node through the atria.
   - P waves should be <0.12 s, represented by three small squares, with an amplitude of < 2.5 mm.
     - A tall P wave is called 'P pulmonale' and is suggestive of right atrial hypertrophy.
     - A broad, bifid P wave is 'P mitrale' and is suggestive of left atrial hypertrophy (usually due to mitral stenosis).
   - If P waves are absent, are there any signs of atrial activity? For example, sawtooth baseline (flutter waves), chaotic baseline (fibrillation waves) or flat line (no atrial activity).
7. **PR interval**
   - The PR interval indicates the time from the depolarisation of the sinus node to the onset of ventricular depolarisation via the atrioventricular node (AVN) and the bundle of His to the ventricular muscle.
   - The PR interval should be 120–200 ms, represented by 3–5 small squares.
     - **Shortened PR interval:**
       - The P wave is originating from somewhere closer to the AVN, or there is an accessory pathway.
     - **Prolonged PR interval:**
       - First-degree heart block: fixed, prolonged PR interval >200 ms.
       - Second-degree heart block (Mobitz type 1/ Wenckebach): PR interval slowly increases, followed by a dropped QRS complex.
       - Second-degree heart block (Mobitz type 2): fixed, prolonged PR interval but there are dropped QRS complexes, usually at a frequency of 2:1, 3:1 or 4:1.
       - Third-degree heart block: prolonged PR interval and complete dissociation between the P wave and the QRS complexes.
8. **QRS complex**
   - The QRS complex represents the transmission of excitation through the ventricles. A broad QRS complex may occur in the presence of bundle branch block or when depolarisation is initiated by a focus in the ventricular muscle.
   - Duration: QRS complexes should be ≤120 ms, represented by three small squares.
     - Broad complexes occur in the presence of bundle branch block, or when depolarisation is initiated by a focus in the ventricular muscle.
   - Height: QRS complexes should be ≤ 4 large squares.
     - Increased QRS height represents increased muscle mass, i.e. ventricular hypertrophy.
   - R-wave progression:
     - QRS complexes should progress from mostly negative in V1 (dominant S wave) to mostly positive in V6 (dominant R wave).
   - Morphology:
     - The presence of delta waves may indicate Wolff–Parkinson–White syndrome.
     - Q waves >40 ms (one small square) in width and >2 mm height are suggestive of established or previous myocardial infarction.
9. **ST segment**
   - The ST segment represents the interval between ventricular depolarisation and repolarisation and should be an isoelectric line between the

Table 2.3 Electrocardiogram (ECG) findings that can help to determine the territory affected in a myocardial infarction (MI)

TERRITORY OF MI	LEADS WITH ST ELEVATION	ARTERY INVOLVED
Anterior	V2–4, or left bundle branch block	Left anterior descending
Anteroseptal	V1–4	Left anterior descending
Anterolateral	V4–5, I, aVL	Left anterior descending or left circumflex
Lateral	I, aVL, V5–6	Left circumflex
Inferior	II, III, aVF	Right coronary
Posterior	Depression in V1–2	Right coronary or left circumflex

end of the S wave (the J point) and the beginning of the T wave.
- ST elevation is significant when it is greater than 1 mm in two or more contiguous limb leads or >2 mm in two or more chest leads; it is most commonly caused by acute full-thickness myocardial infarction (Table 2.3) or pericarditis.
- Horizontal ST depression of the ST segment with an upright T wave is usually a sign of ischaemia.

10. **T waves**
    - The T wave represents ventricular repolarisation and should be < 5 mm tall in limb leads and < 10 mm tall in precordial leads.
    - T-wave inversion is normal in leads III, aVR and V1; inversion in other leads may be seen in myocardial ischaemia and infarction, bundle branch block, ventricular hypertrophy and pulmonary embolism.
    - Peaked T waves are seen in the early stages of ST-segment myocardial infarction (STEMI) and in hyperkalaemia.
    - Flattened T waves are seen in cardiac ischaemia (if dynamic or in contiguous leads) and hypokalaemia.
11. **QT interval**
    - The QT interval represents the time taken for ventricular depolarisation and repolarisation and is normally ≤450 ms.
    - A prolonged QT interval may lead to polymorphic ventricular tachycardia (torsades de pointes), a potentially fatal arrhythmia.
    - Causes of a prolonged QT include drugs, electrolyte abnormalities (hypocalcaemia, hypomagnesaemia and hypokalaemia), hypothermia, certain disease states (e.g. intracranial haemorrhage) and prolonged QT genetic syndromes.

Clinical Tip

Wherever possible, compare the current ECG with a previous one so that new changes can be identified compared to pre-existing abnormalities.

Clinical Tip

Serial ECGs can be useful to detect dynamic changes suggestive of significant cardiac events.

STATION 2.3: BLOOD TEST INTERPRETATION

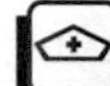
The Bleep Scenario

You are bleeped by an junior doctor colleague who has finished her shift for the day. You are asked to chase blood results for 3 patients on the elderly care ward.

INITIAL THOUGHTS

Being asked to 'chase bloods' is a common bleep scenario and is also a common scenario at handover. It is important to determine what you are looking for on the bloods and what management may be required if certain findings are evident. For example, if you are asked to chase a urea and electrolytes (U&E) test you should ask why this is required, i.e. is there a suspicion of acute kidney injury (AKI), or hyperkalaemia, or an upper gastrointestinal (GI) bleed? You should also ask what management might be indicated. For example, if there is suspicion of an upper GI bleed, what management has already been started, has the patient already been discussed with the gastroenterology team and what needs to happen next?

FULL BLOOD COUNT

The most common derangements on the full blood count affect the three cell lines from the bone marrow:
- Haemoglobin
- Leukocytes
- Platelets

LOW HAEMOGLOBIN (ANAEMIA)

If a patient is anaemic (defined by a cut-off of 130 g/L in men, 120 g/L in non-pregnant women, 110 g/L in pregnant women), you should consider the following:
- Is the patient symptomatic, or haemodynamically unstable?

Table 2.4 Platelet transfusion thresholds according to clinical scenarios

PATIENTS WITH THROMBOCYTOPENIA WHO ARE ACTIVELY BLEEDING	
Platelet count (×10⁹/L) transfusion threshold	*Clinical scenario*
<30	Clinically significant bleeding (WHO bleeding grade 2)
<100	Severe bleeding (WHO bleeding grades 3 and 4)
<100	Bleeding in critical sites (CNS, including eyes)
PATIENTS WHO ARE *NOT* BLEEDING AND/OR ARE NOT HAVING INVASIVE PROCEDURES OR SURGERY	
Platelet count (×10⁹/L) transfusion threshold	*Clinical scenario*
<10: prophylactic transfusion	Do *not* have any of the following: • Chronic bone marrow failure • Autoimmune thrombocytopenia • Heparin-induced thrombocytopenia • Thrombotic thrombocytopenic purpura
PATIENTS WHO ARE HAVING INVASIVE PROCEDURES OR SURGERY	
Platelet count (×10⁹/L) transfusion threshold	*Clinical scenario*
<50: prophylactic transfusion	To have invasive procedure / surgery
<75: prophylactic transfusion	To have invasive procedure / surgery with high-risk bleeding, taking into consideration: • Procedure patient will undergo • Cause of thrombocytopenia • Trend of platelet count • Coexisting causes of abnormal haemostasis
<100: prophylactic transfusion	Surgery in critical sites, such as the CNS (including the posterior segment of the eyes)
PATIENTS WHO DO NOT NEED ROUTINE PROPHYLACTIC TRANSFUSIONS	
• Chronic bone marrow failure • Autoimmune thrombocytopenia	• Heparin-induced thrombocytopenia • Thrombotic thrombocytopenic purpura • Low-risk procedure including central venous catheter insertion, bone marrow biopsy

CNS, central nervous system; WHO, World Health Organization.

- Previous haemoglobin readings – is the decrease acute or chronic?
- Mean corpuscular volume (MCV) – is the anaemia microcytic, normocytic or macrocytic?

As a standard, patients will usually require red blood cell transfusion if the haemoglobin levels drop below 70 g/L, or below 80 g/L if the patient is symptomatic or has additional clinical risk factors. Further information on the diagnosis and management of anaemia is covered in Chapter 12.

HIGH HAEMOGLOBIN (POLYCYTHAEMIA)

A high haemoglobin is suggestive of dehydration, secondary polycythaemia or polycythaemia vera. These patients will require haematology input and perhaps prophylactic low-molecular-weight heparin due to the increased risk of thrombosis.

LOW PLATELETS (THROMBOCYTOPENIA)

A low platelet count is a reading <150 × 10^9/L. Causes of a low platelet count include:

- Reduced platelet production (bone marrow failure): infections (particularly viral), drug-induced, leukaemia, aplastic anaemia, late-stage myelofibrosis, bone marrow infiltration (myeloma, metastatic disease), myelodysplasia, megaloblastic anaemia
- Increased platelet destruction: heparin-induced thrombocytopenia, idiopathic thrombocytopenic purpura, thrombotic thrombocytopenic purpura, hypersplenism, disseminated intravascular coagulation

See Table 2.4 for transfusion thresholds.

HIGH PLATELETS (THROMBOCYTOSIS)

A high platelet count is a reading >400 × 10^9/L. Causes of a high platelet count include:

- Reactive (secondary) thrombocytosis: infection, inflammation, malignancy, bleeding, pregnancy, post-splenectomy
- Primary haematological disorder: essential thrombocytosis, chronic myelogenous leukaemia, myelodysplasia, polycythaemia rubra vera

In some cases, haematology input may be required due to the increased risk of arterial and venous thrombosis and microvascular occlusion. If in doubt, contact the on call haematology team for advice.

WHITE CELL COUNT

The white cell count includes neutrophils, lymphocytes and eosinophils.

- Neutrophilia (>7.5 × 10^9/L): bacterial infection, inflammation, acute illness, malignancy, myeloid leukaemia, treatment with corticosteroids
- Neutropenia (<2.0 × 10^9/L): viral infection, sepsis, drugs (carbimazole, clozapine), bone marrow failure, postchemotherapy, splenomegaly, autoimmune disease, reduced B_{12}/folate.
- Lymphocytosis (>3.5 × 10^9/L): viral infection, inflammation, lymphocytic leukaemia, lymphoma, chronic infections
- Lymphopenia (<1.5 × 10^9/L): steroids, chemotherapy, malignancy, human immunodeficiency virus (HIV), autoimmune disease, bone marrow failure
- Eosinophilia (>0.5 × 10^9/L): allergic disorders, atopy, asthma, parasitic infection, hypereosinophilic syndrome, malignancy
- Eosinopenia (<0.01 × 10^9/L): rarely pathological but may be associated with acute bacterial infection, treatment with corticosteroids, physical stress

UREA AND ELECTROLYTES

The U&E test consists of sodium, potassium, urea and creatinine readings. The main risks when plasma electrolytes are dangerously abnormal are cardiac arrhythmias and central nervous system events, including seizures.

See Table 2.5 for common findings on U&E test results.

- Hyponatraemia (<135 mmol/L): this is a common cause of confusion among junior doctors. The most important step is to determine the volume status (hypovolaemia, euvolaemia, hypervolaemia). For patients with hyponatraemia, common initial investigations include serum cortisol, paired urine and serum osmolalities, urinary sodium and thyroid function tests.
- Hypernatraemia (<145 mmol/L): iatrogenic, fluid losses (diarrhoea, vomiting, burns), diabetes insipidus, DKA/hyperosmolar hyperglycaemic syndrome
- Hypokalaemia (<3.5 mmol/L): diuretics, endocrine causes (hyperadrenalism, hyperaldosteronism), renal tubular acidosis, vomiting/diarrhoea, hypomagnesaemia
- Hyperkalaemia (>5 mmol/L): renal failure, drugs, iatrogenic, adrenal insufficiency, DKA, rhabdomyolysis, artefactual (i.e. haemolysed blood sample)

A rise in urea and creatinine is suggestive of renal failure. A comparison with previous results will indicate if it is acute or chronic in nature. Other things to be aware of are:

- Decreased urea: malnutrition, liver disease, pregnancy

Table 2.5 Common urea and electrolyte result patterns

DISORDER	BLOOD RESULTS
Dehydration	• Increased urea and increased creatinine • Hypo/hypernatraemia
Kidney failure	• Increased urea and increased creatinine • Hyperkalaemia • Metabolic acidosis • In CKD: secondary / tertiary hyperparathyroidism, with possible calcium changes • Anaemia
Thiazide and loop diuretics	• Hyponatraemia, hyperkalaemia • Increased sodium bicarbonate • Increased urea
Addison's disease	• Hyperkalaemia and hyponatraemia
Cushing's syndrome	• Hypokalaemia, hypernatraemia • Increased sodium bicarbonate
Conn's syndrome	• Hypokalaemia • Increased sodium bicarbonate • Normal / increased sodium
Diabetes insipidus	• Hypernatraemia • Increased plasma osmolality • Decreased urine osmolality
SIADH	• Hyponatraemia • Decreased plasma osmolality • Increased urinary osmolality • Increased urinary sodium

CKD, chronic kidney disease; eGFR, estimated glomerular filtration rate; SIADH, syndrome of inappropriate antidiuretic hormone secretion.

- Increased urea: dehydration, AKI, chronic kidney disease (CKD), GI bleed, increased protein breakdown (surgery, trauma, infection, malignancy), high-protein diet, drugs
- Increased creatinine: AKI, CKD, high muscle mass, drugs

LIVER FUNCTION TESTS

Liver function tests are composed of measurements of bilirubin and liver enzymes, including aminotransferases, alkaline phosphatases and gamma-glutamyl transferase. These measurements are more indicative of liver cell damage than the liver 'function' itself. Some markers of hepatic call damage include serum albumin, prothrombin time and bilirubin levels. For this reason, these measures can reflect clinical outcome and are often included in prognostic scoring.

See Table 2.6 for common liver function test findings.

BILIRUBIN

Normal serum bilirubin is 3–17 µmol/L. Jaundice is usually clinically detectable at levels >40 µmol/L, although it may be harder to pick up on more pigmented skin.

Raised bilirubin levels may be the result of increased excretion or increased production. It is often useful to determine whether the raised bilirubin is unconjugated or conjugated. Of note, a rise in bilirubin often occurs earlier in the course of biliary disease than in liver parenchymal pathology. Further liver function tests will help identify the underlying cause. In the case of suspected haemolysis, follow-up with reticulocyte count, blood film, haptoglobin measurement and lactate dehydrogenase will give a clearer indication of the aetiology.

- Unconjugated hyperbilirubinaemia: haemolysis, impaired hepatic uptake (drugs, congestive cardiac failure), Gilbert's syndrome
- Conjugated hyperbilirubinaemia: hepatocellular injury, cholestasis

ALBUMIN

Albumin is a protein that is synthesised in the liver. It binds bilirubin, free fatty acids, calcium and some drugs.

- Hypoalbuminaemia: reduced synthesis (liver disease, acute-phase response, malabsorption, malnutrition, malignancy), increased loss (nephrotic syndrome, burns, protein-losing enteropathy), oedema
- Hyperalbuminaemia: suggestive of dehydration

ALT AND AST

Alanine aminotransferase (ALT) and aspartate aminotransferase (AST) are located in the cytoplasm of the hepatocyte. AST is also located in the hepatocyte mitochondria. ALT is considered more specific for liver damage as its presence outside the liver is relatively low. In contrast, AST also increases in myocardial infarction, skeletal muscle damage and haemolysis.

ALP

Alkaline phosphatase (ALP) is widely distributed; the main sites of production are the liver, GI tract, bone, placenta and kidney. ALP enzymes in the liver are sited in cell membranes of hepatic sinusoids and biliary canaliculi; therefore, ALP levels rise with intrahepatic and extrahepatic biliary obstruction and sinusoidal obstruction. ALP isoenzyme is a better test of isolate liver related ALP rises.

GGT

Gamma-glutamyltransferase (GGT) is a microsomal enzyme located predominantly in the hepatocytes and epithelial lining of the small bile ducts in the liver. An isolated elevation of GGT is relatively common and can occur when microsomal enzyme-inducing drugs have been ingested, e.g. alcohol.

Table 2.6 Common liver function test result patterns

DISORDER	LIVER FUNCTION TESTS
Prehepatic jaundice	• Increased bilirubin (unconjugated) • Haemolysis: low haemoglobin, high reticulocytes, low haptoglobins
Hepatic jaundice	• High bilirubin (mixed) • Increased ALT/AST • Increased GGT
Cholestatic jaundice	• Increased bilirubin (conjugated) • Raised ALP • Raised GGT
Hepatocellular damage	• Raised AST/ALT • Raised ALP and GGT
Liver failure	• Raised bilirubin • Prolonged PT • Deranged clotting • Low albumin
Alcoholism	• Increased GGT • Raised MCV • Thrombocytopenia
Pancreatitis	• Raised amylase • Hypocalcaemia • Hyperglycaemia • High CRP
HELLP (pregnancy)	• Increased AST/ALT • Increased GGT • Low haemoglobin and thrombocytopenia

ALP, alkaline phosphatase; ALT, alanine transaminase; AST, aspartate aminotransferase; CRP, C-reactive protein; GGT, gamma-glutamyltransferase; HELLP, haemolysis, elevated liver enzymes and low platelets; MCV, mean corpuscular volume; PT, prothrombin time.

Further tests as part of a liver screen may include the following:

- Viral screen: hepatitis A/B/C, Epstein–Barr virus, cytomegalovirus
- Antimitochondrial antibody (AMA)
- Anti-smooth-muscle antibody (ASMA)
- Anti-liver/kidney microsomal antibodies (anti-LKM)
- Antinuclear antibody (ANA)
- Perinuclear antineutrophil cytoplasmic antibody (p-ANCA)
- Immunoglobulins
- Alpha-1 antitrypsin
- Serum copper or ceruloplasmin
- Ferritin

Clinical Tip

Ensure regular monitoring for markers of liver dysfunction to help accurately determine the patients clinical progress.

FURTHER READING

Hampton, J. R. (2008). *The ECG made easy* (7th ed.). Edinburgh: Churchill Livingstone/Elsevier.

Longmore, M., et al. (2010). *Oxford handbook of clinical medicine* (8th ed.). Oxford: Oxford University Press.

NICE. (2015). *Blood transfusion*. NG24. Available at: www.nice.org.uk/guidance/ng24/chapter/recommendations. (Accessed 16 January 2022).

Nolan, J., et al. (2016). *Advanced life support book* (7th ed.). London: Resuscitation Council UK.

Raine, T., et al. (2011). *Oxford handbook for the foundation programme* (3rd ed.). Oxford: Oxford University Press.

Resuscitation Council UK. (2021). *Advanced life support book* (8th ed.). London: Resuscitation Council UK.

3 Prescribing

Content Outline

STATION 3.1: INTRAVENOUS FLUIDS

The Bleep Scenario

You are bleeped by a nurse on the acute medical unit (AMU) to review a 48 year old man being treated for sepsis secondary to community-acquired pneumonia. His blood pressure has dropped from 120/80 mmHg to 80/55 mmHg.

You are asked to prescribe intravenous (IV) fluids for resuscitation. The patient has no known drug allergies.

WHAT IS EXPECTED OF YOU?

As a junior doctor, you will be asked to prescribe IV fluids on an almost daily basis. Fluids may be prescribed for resuscitation, replacement or maintenance. It is important to consider the indication and the comorbidities of the patient. You should specify the type of fluid, volume, rate of infusion and whether any drugs are to be added.

Fig. 3.1 presents a flowchart of indications for IV fluids.

Whenever you assess a patient, use the ABCDE approach to determine if they are stable or unstable to help you select the most appropriate type of fluid they need and at what rate, i.e. maintenance, replacement or resuscitation.

COMMON SCENARIOS

RESUSCITATION (FIG. 3.2)

This form of fluid replacement is indicated in scenarios where a patient is in shock, for example hypovolaemic or septic shock. This may be evidenced by systolic blood pressure < 100 mmHg, heart rate >90 bpm, cool peripheries, prolonged capillary refill time, raised National Early Warning Score (NEWS), tachypnoea and reduced urine output.

A challenge of a 500-mL crystalloid bolus should be given, e.g. 0.9% sodium chloride or Hartmann's solution. You would not normally add electrolytes to these fluids as these should not be given quickly.

In a cardiac arrest scenario, fluids may also be given to help hypovolaemic shock. Once a patient is stable, then you can switch to the other methods of fluid replacement depending on the patient's clinical needs.

REPLACEMENT (FIG. 3.3)

Replacement fluids are prescribed in scenarios where a patient has lost fluid and/or electrolytes or their ability to maintain intravascular volume is impaired (Table 3.1).

Fluid balance (input and output) as well as electrolyte values should be monitored regularly, so that there is appropriate fluid and electrolyte replacement.

MAINTENANCE

Maintenance fluids are prescribed to ensure patients meet their daily requirements when they are not getting this orally; for example, if someone is nil by mouth before or after surgery. Maintenance fluid must include the appropriate electrolytes needed for nutrition.

- In an average person, daily requirements are:
  - 25–30 mL/kg water
  - 1 mmol/kg potassium
  - 50–100 g/day glucose (e.g. glucose 5% contains 50 g/1000 mL)
- In elderly patients or those with renal impairment / cardiac failure / risk of refeeding syndrome:
  - Consider reducing total fluid to 20–25 mL/kg/day
- In obese patients:
  - Consider using ideal body weight (IBW) – most patients do not need more than about 3 L/day as maintenance

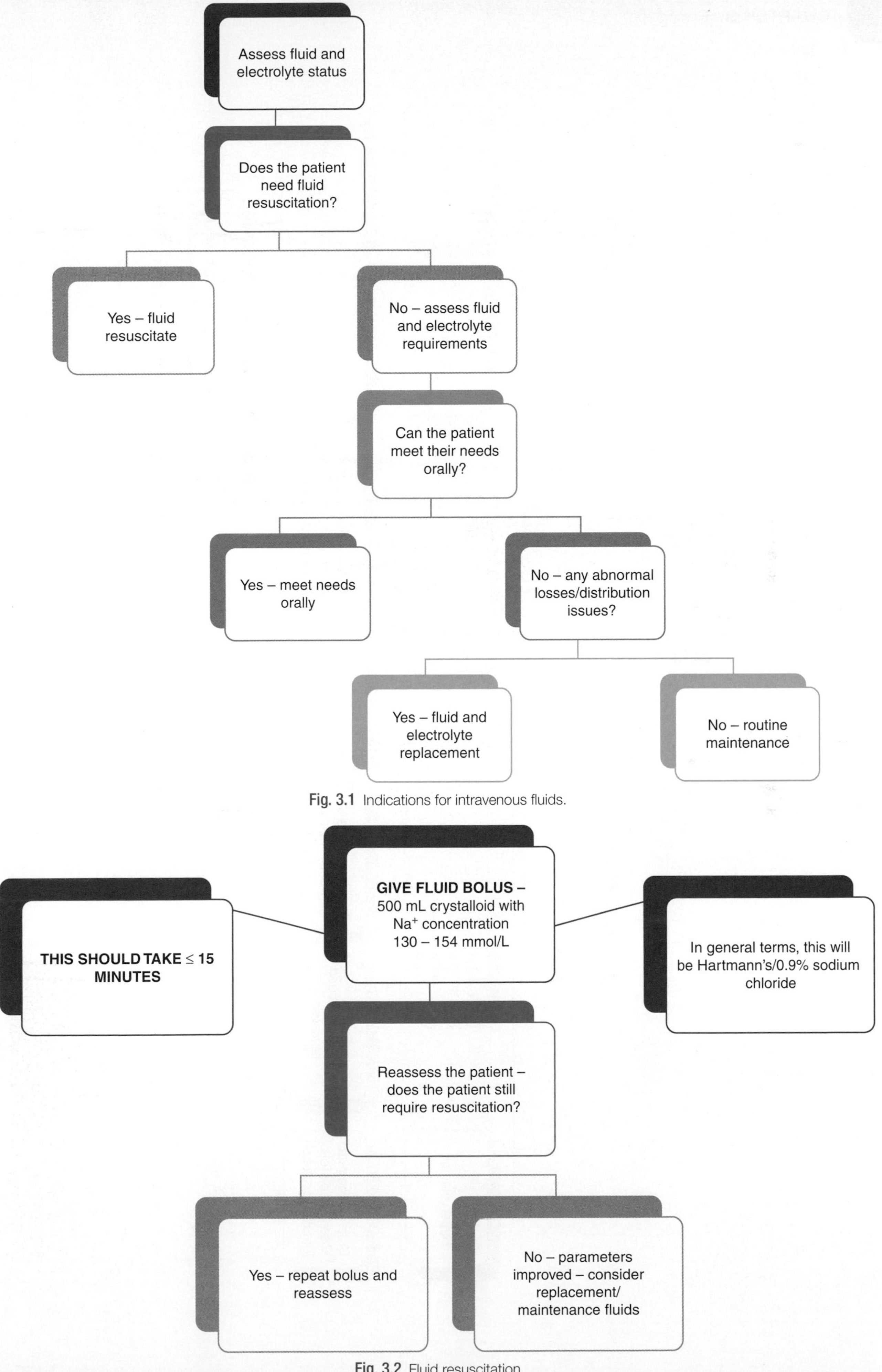

Fig. 3.1 Indications for intravenous fluids.

Fig. 3.2 Fluid resuscitation.

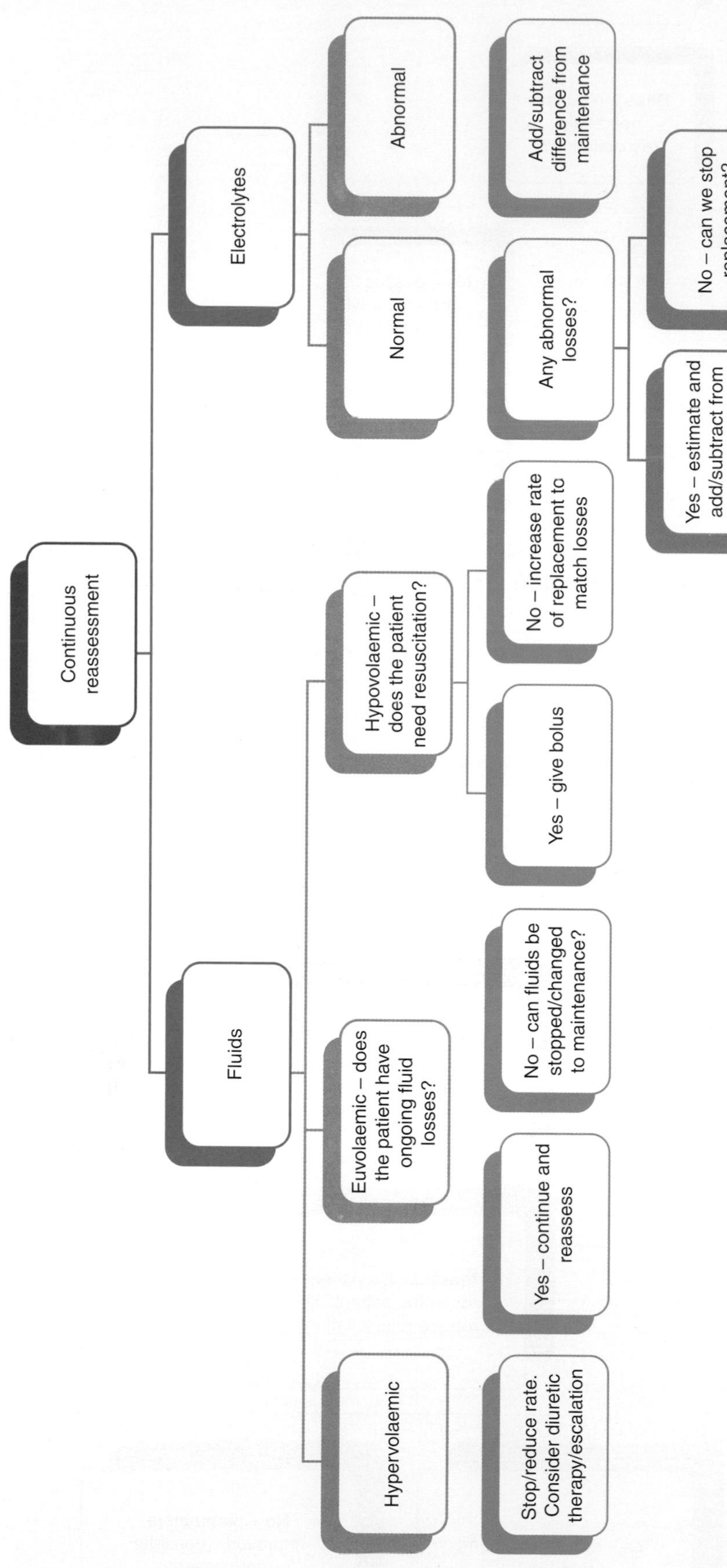

Fig. 3.3 Fluid replacement.

Table 3.1 Causes of fluid loss

EXCESS LOSSES	ABNORMAL REDISTRIBUTION	SPECIAL CIRCUMSTANCES

• Excess insensible losses
  • Fever
  • Hyperventilation
• Vomiting and diarrhoea
• Known outputs
  • Stoma
  • Fistula
  • NG tubes
• Drains in situ
  • Biliary
  • Pancreatic
• Polyuria
• Blood loss
  • Haematemesis/ melaena
  • Trauma
  • Postoperative
	• Severe sepsis
	  • Capillary leak
	• Gross oedema
	  • Heart failure
	  • Liver failure
	  • Renal failure
	  • Iatrogenic overload
	• Postoperative retention and redistribution
		• Cardiac failure
		• Renal failure
		• Malnourishment/refeeding
		• Patients with NG / PEG / TPN feeds (ask dietician for advice)

NG, nasogastric; PEG, percutaneous endoscopic gastrostomy; TPN, total parenteral nutrition.

An example of maintenance fluid is sodium chloride 0.18% / dextrose 4% with the addition of potassium as calculated according to the patient's daily requirements.

If a patient needs maintenance fluid for more than a few days, it may be better to use enteral routes instead of IV.

SUMMARY

- Ensure you prescribe the most appropriate fluids for the most appropriate indication, i.e. resuscitation, replacement, maintenance.
- Remember to check biochemical values regularly in patients on replacement fluids.
- Always review observations and clinical status along with inputs/outputs for any patient for whom you are prescribing IV fluids.
- Once the patient is able to meet their requirements orally, consider stopping IV fluids.

ESCALATION

If you are unsure about escalation, you can discuss with a senior member of your team. If it is an emergency – for example, a severely volume-depleted patient with tachycardia, hypotension and reduced urine output – you must alert the medical emergency/periarrest team.

STATION 3.2: ANALGESIA

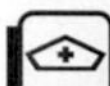 **The Bleep Scenario**

You are bleeped by a nurse on the general surgical ward. A 65 year old man underwent laparoscopic appendicectomy today and is now crying in pain. He has already tried paracetamol to no effect.

You are asked to prescribe stronger analgesia for him. He has no known drug allergies.

WHAT IS EXPECTED OF YOU?

As a junior doctor, the above scenario is very common. You will frequently be asked to prescribe pain relief, for example, for surgical patients, other inpatients or on discharge prescriptions. You will need to determine the cause of the patient's pain; for example, if a post-surgical patient (as in this scenario) is already on maximum pain relief, it may suggest that a complication has occurred and pain relief may mask a more serious problem. You should also determine the severity of the pain and what analgesia the patient is already receiving. Once you have done this, you can decide the most appropriate treatment.

THE WHO PAIN LADDER

The World Health Organization (WHO) pain ladder is a guide to how to increase pain relief (Table 3.2).

When using the pain ladder, you should consider the following before prescribing analgesia:

- Consider the cause of severity of the patient's pain and start at the most appropriate step, e.g. if a patient has an ankle fracture and is in severe pain, then you should commence analgesia at step 3 rather than attempting step 1 to see if the pain improves with paracetamol and non-steroidal anti-inflammatory drugs (NSAIDs).
- If the patient's pain is uncontrolled, avoid exchanging one drug for another of the same class/potency. For example, if the patient's pain is uncontrolled with codeine, switching to hydrocodone will offer no benefit; instead, you should move on to the next step.
- In general, the route of administration should be oral whenever possible. Common alternative routes (depending on the drug) include: topical, transdermal, subcutaneous (SC), intramuscular (IM) and IV. Surgical patients may have local analgesia, such as

Table 3.2 World Health Organization (WHO) pain ladder drugs

DRUG CLASS	EXAMPLES	SIDE EFFECTS	IMPORTANT CAUTIONS

Non-opioids	Paracetamol	Rare, but may include:
		• Rashes
		• Thombocytopenia
		• Neutropenia
		• Liver failure in overdose
			• Reduce dose in:
			  • Patients with body weight under 50 kg
			  • Those with risk factors for hepatocellular toxicity
			  • Patients taking enzyme-inducing antiepileptic medications

	NSAIDs (ibuprofen, naproxen, etoricoxib)	• Gastrointestinal toxicity
		• Renal impairment
		• Increased risk of cardiovascular events
		• Hypersensitivity reactions
		• Fluid retention
			• Avoid in patients with:
			  • Severe renal impairment
			  • Heart failure
			  • Liver failure
			  • Known NSAID hypersensitivity

Weak opioids	Codeine, dihydrocodeine, tramadol	• Common side effects: nausea, constipation, dizziness, drowsiness • Overdose can cause neurological and respiratory depression • Codeine and dihydrocodeine should never be given intravenously (severe anaphylactoid reaction)	• Reduce dose in elderly patients and those with renal and/or hepatic impairment • Epilepsy • Avoid in patients taking SSRIs, tricyclic antidepressants, antipsychotics and benzodiazepines
Strong opioids	Morphine, oxycodone, fentanyl, buprenorphine	• Common side effects: nausea and vomiting, constipation, drowsiness, confusion, itching, urinary retention, vertigo • Overdose can cause neurological and respiratory depression, bradycardia • Look out for pupillary constriction and reduced level of consciousness • Chronic use can lead to dependence, hypogonadism and adrenal suppression	• Reduce dose in elderly patients and those with renal and/or hepatic impairment • In patients with renal impairment, oxycodone can be used in preference to morphine • Avoid use with other sedating drugs • Morphine is contraindicated for head injury patients, comatose patients, in acute respiratory depression, raised ICP and where there is a risk of paralytic ileus

ICP, intracranial pressure; NSAIDs, non-steroidal anti-inflammatory drugs; SSRIs, selective serotonin reuptake inhibitors.

epidural, spinal or injections of local anaesthetic, sedation or general anaesthesia.

SPECIAL SCENARIOS: PALLIATIVE CARE

The focus of pain management in palliative care is to achieve pain control to avoid breakthrough pain. Drugs from the different classes of analgesia (Table 3.3) are used alone or in combination according to the type of pain and response to treatment. Analgesics are more effective in preventing pain and therefore they should be given regularly rather than as needed. As with all analgesia, you should use the WHO pain ladder to guide pain management and seek advice from your seniors and specialist teams (pain team, palliative care) if you are unsure. Of note, the patient may also require a syringe driver; the palliative care team will be able to help you determine when this is appropriate and how to prescribe.

You should also familiarise yourself with the trust's guideline regime for the anticipatory end-of-life medications. Note that the regime shown in Table 3.4 may vary; it is provided simply as an example. You will need to prescribe this regime on discharge summaries as well as hospital charts in cases where such patients are going to a hospice or home.

SUMMARY

- Prescribe analgesia according to the cause and severity of the patient's pain.
- Use the WHO pain ladder to guide appropriate analgesia prescriptions.
- Consider the patient's age, comorbidities, renal and hepatic function before prescribing opioid analgesia.
- The oral route should always be first-line unless there is a valid reason for using alternative routes (e.g. patient is nil by mouth or experiencing ongoing vomiting, oral trauma, dysphagia, etc.).
- In patients with complex pain or palliative care patients you should seek advice from specialist teams to guide management.

Table 3.3 **Palliative care prescribing considerations**

BONE METASTASES	NEUROPATHIC PAIN	GASTROINTESTINAL PAIN / COLIC
• Conventional analgesia (WHO ladder) • Bisphosphonates • Corticosteroids • Radiotherapy	• Conventional analgesia (WHO ladder) • Tricyclic antidepressants (amitriptyline) • Gabapentin/pregabalin • Ketamine • Corticosteroids • Nerve blocks/regional anaesthesia	• Conventional analgesia (WHO ladder) • Loperamide hydrochloride • Hyoscine hydrobromide • Hyoscine bromide • Glycopyrronium bromide • Domperidone • Metoclopramide

WHO, World Health Organization.

Table 3.4 **Example regime of anticipatory medications**

ANTICIPATORY MEDICATIONS	
Pain or breathlessness	• Morphine 2.5–5 mg SC hourly as needed
Anxiety or distress or agitation	• Midazolam 2.5–5 mg SC hourly as needed (maximum 60 mg daily)
Secretions	• Hyoscine butylbromide 20 mg SC 2-hourly (maximum 60 mg daily)
Nausea	• Levomepromazine 6.25 mg SC 6-hourly as needed (maximum 25 mg daily), or haloperidol 500 mcg SC 12=hourly as needed
Delirium or confusion	• Haloperidol 500 mcg SC twice daily as needed or levomepromazine 12.5 mg SC 2-hourly as needed

SC, subcutaneously.

STATION 3.3: ANTIEMETICS

The Bleep Scenario

You are bleeped by a nurse on AMU. A 23 year old woman has been admitted with severe vomiting. She has been reviewed by the surgical team, who suspect gastro-oesophageal reflux disease (GORD).

You are asked to prescribe antiemetics for her. She has no known drug allergies.

WHAT IS EXPECTED OF YOU?

As a junior doctor, you should be able to determine the most appropriate antiemetic for each patient. You will frequently be asked to prescribe antiemetics for a variety of patients, including surgical, postoperative and medical patients. You will need to determine the cause of the patient's nausea and vomiting and match the most appropriate antiemetic according to its mechanism of action.

A broad-spectrum antiemetic may be appropriate if the cause is unclear, and a combination may be needed to achieve symptom control. Special considerations are needed for certain patient groups, e.g. pregnant patients and patients with Parkinson's disease.

Remember that symptomatic patients will require IV / IM / SC / transdermal administration; however, once the vomiting has settled or the patient has nausea only, the oral route should be first-line.

MECHANISM OF VOMITING (FIGS 3.4 AND 3.5)

The vomiting centre in the medulla has many triggers. Visceral stimulation comes from the gastrointestinal (GI) tract, conducted by parasympathetic and sympathetic fibres, and is caused by direct visceral stimulation and/or distension. Inflammation, for example, in pancreatitis, can also trigger it, as well as gastroparesis. The chemoreceptor trigger zone is activated by drugs, hormones and toxins. Metabolic causes such as hyponatraemia, hypercalcaemia, pregnancy and diabetic ketoacidosis (DKA) also affect this pathway. Higher neurological inputs can be caused by emotion, smells, motion sickness, vertigo and the gag reflex.

The act of vomiting requires upper oesophageal sphincter relaxation, closure of the glottis, soft-palate elevation, contraction of the diaphragm and abdominal wall and relaxation of the lower oesophageal sphincter.

DIFFERENTIAL DIAGNOSIS

- Neurology: increased intracranial pressure, glaucoma, migraine, pain, emotional distress, noxious sights/smells

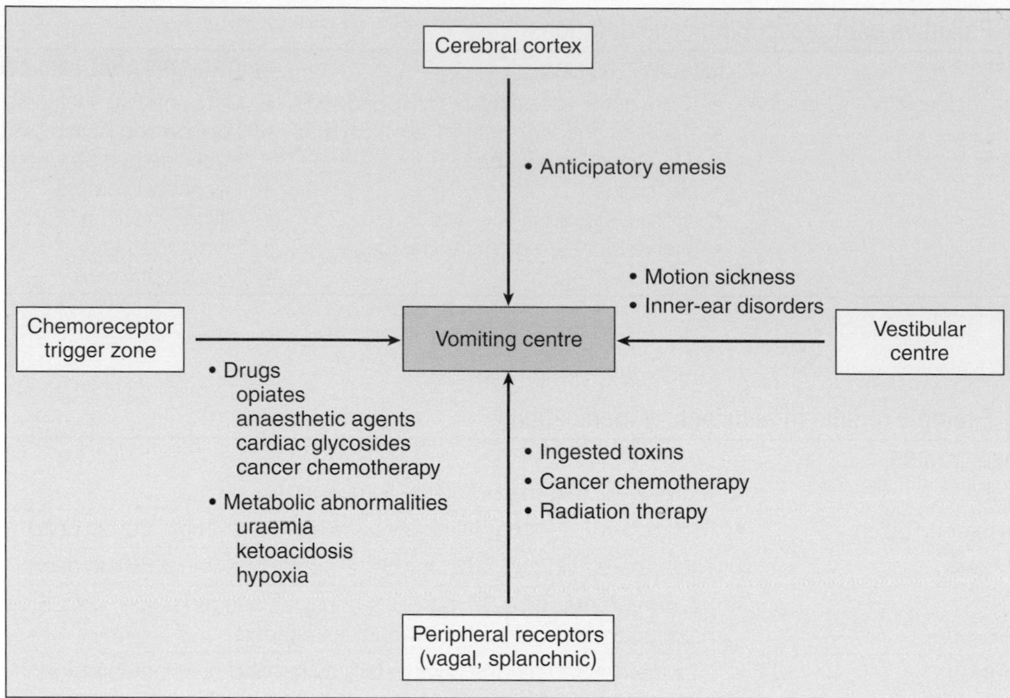

Fig. 3.4 Mechanisms of vomiting. (Source: Abeloff, M.D. et al. (2020) *Abeloff's clinical oncology*. Philadelphia, PA: Elsevier.)

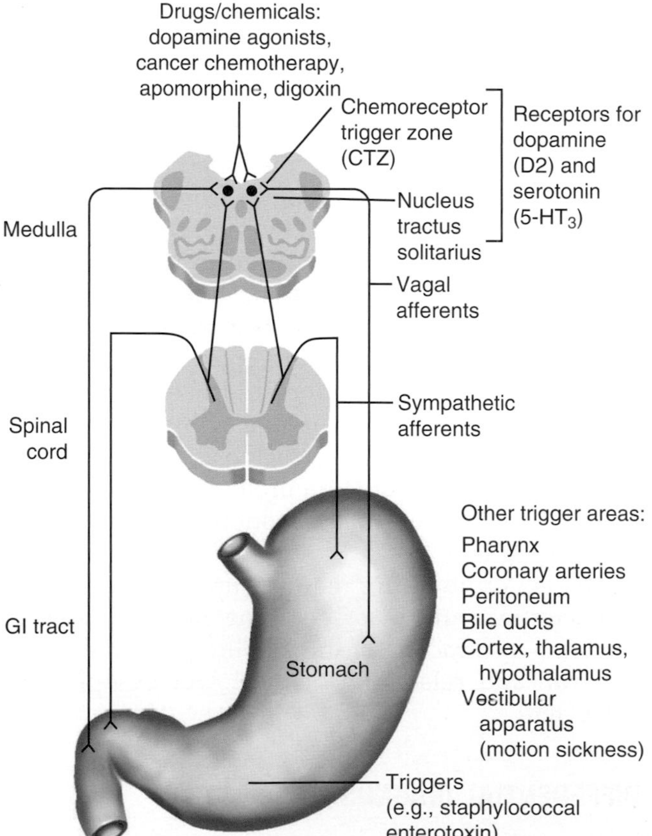

Fig. 3.5 Schematic representation of the proposed neural pathways that mediate vomiting. 5-HT, 5-hydroxytryptamine; GI, gastrointestinal. (Source: Feldman, M., Friedman, L.S. and Brandt, L.J. [Eds.]. [2021]. *Sleisenger and Fordtran's gastrointestinal and liver disease: pathophysiology, diagnosis, management*. Philadelphia, PA: Elsevier Health Sciences.)

- Infection: meningitis, urinary tract infection, sepsis, gastroenteritis
- Metabolic: DKA, metabolic acidosis
- Endocrine: adrenal insufficiency, pregnancy-related
- Drugs: chemotherapy, alcohol, opiates, anaesthetic agents
- Inner ear: motion sickness, labyrinthitis, benign paroxysmal positional vertigo
- Gastrointestinal: GORD, constipation, hepatitis, pancreatitis, biliary disorders

See Table 3.5 to learn more about the types of antiemetics and Fig. 3.6 to see how they work.

USE IN CHEMOTHERAPY

- In low-risk chemotherapy types, domperidone or metoclopramide are recommended following the chemotherapy.
- In moderate-risk types, dexamethasone plus domperidone or metoclopramide are used before and after.
- In high-risk types a 5HT-3 antagonist is combined with dexamethasone before chemotherapy, then dexamethasone plus domperidone or metoclopramide plus levomepromazine are used in combination afterwards.

SUMMARY

- Select the antiemetic based on the cause of the nausea or vomiting and the pharmacokinetic profile of the drug.

Table 3.5 Different types of antiemetics

DRUG CLASS AND MECHANISM OF ACTION	EXAMPLES	INDICATIONS	SIDE EFFECTS	IMPORTANT CAUTIONS
5-HT$_3$ antagonists Block 5-HT$_3$ receptors in CTZ and GI tract	Ondansetron	• Broad-spectrum • Particularly useful in general anaesthesia and in chemotherapy	• Dizziness, constipation, QT prolongation, serotonin syndrome	• Avoid in patients with long QT interval • Avoid in patients already taking drugs that prolong QT (antipsychotics, SSRIs, amiodarone, fluoroquinolones, macrolides)
H$_1$ receptor antagonists Block H$_1$ receptors in vomiting centre	Cyclizine, promethazine	• Broad-spectrum • Particularly useful in motion sickness or vertigo	• Drowsiness, dry mouth, with IV use: tachycardia, palpitation	• Avoid in patients with: hepatic encephalopathy; those susceptible to anticholinergic side effects (e.g. BPH)
Anticholinergics Block muscarinic receptors	Hyoscine	• Motion sickness	• Dry mouth, blurred vision, drowsiness, tachycardia, constipation, urinary retention	• Avoid in patients at risk of arrhythmias and those with angle closure glaucoma
Dopamine antagonists Block D$_2$ receptors in CTZ, also block histamine and muscarinic receptors	Chlorpromazine, prochlorperazine, haloperidol	• Cancer, radiation therapy, cytotoxic drugs, opioids, anaesthetic agents	• Drowsiness, hypotension, extrapyramidal symptoms	• Avoid in patients with liver/renal dysfunction, Parkinson's disease, cardiac failure and hypothyroidism
Dopamine antagonists Block D$_2$ receptors in CTZ and GI tract	Metoclopramide, domperidone	• Prokinetic agent	• Diarrhoea, sedation, QT prolongation, extrapyramidal symptoms (not domperidone, as it does not cross the BBB)	• Avoid in children and young adults • Contraindicated in intestinal obstruction and intra-abdominal perforation • Contraindicated in patients taking dopaminergic agents for Parkinson's disease
Corticosteroids Potentiate effect of 5-HT$_3$ antagonists, suppress inflammation and prostaglandin production	Dexamethasone	• Chemotherapy, raised ICP	• Sleep disturbances, hyperactivity, poor glucose control	• Avoid in children and the elderly

BBB, blood–brain barrier; BPH, benign prostatic hyperplasia; CTZ, chemoreceptor trigger zone; GI, gastrointestinal; ICP, intracranial pressure; IV, intravenous; SSRIs, selective serotonin reuptake inhibitors.

- Adjust doses according to response and beware of potential side effects.
- Do not prescribe two drugs that work on the same receptor – for example, domperidone and metoclopramide – as you will not get additional benefit but there will be an increased risk of side effects.
- Palliative care teams or oncology teams should be contacted for end-of-life/cancer patients whose vomiting cannot be managed easily.
- Antiemetic failure is defined as prolonged and distressing nausea, or two or more episodes of vomiting in 24 hours, in which case a new antiemetic should be tried.

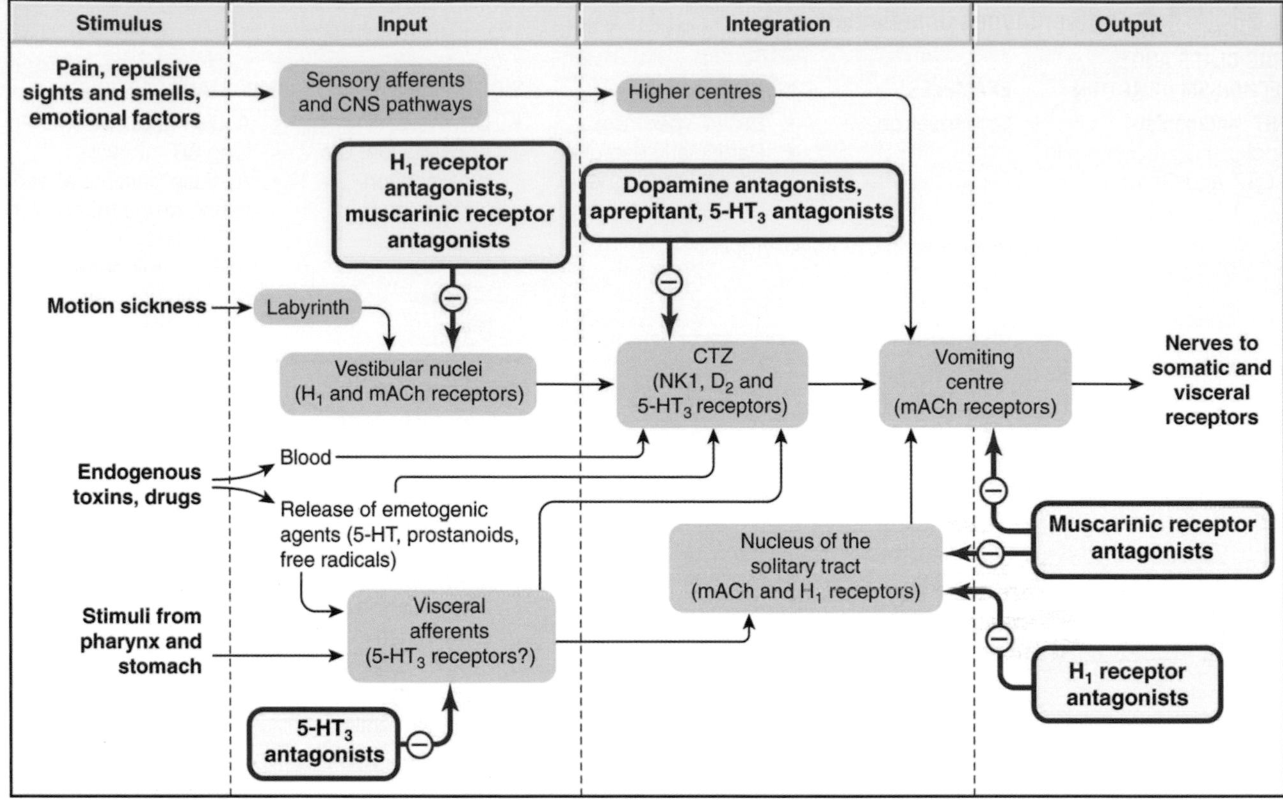

Fig. 3.6 Sites targeted by the different groups of antiemetics. CNS, central nervous system; CTZ, chemoreceptor trigger zone; mACh, muscarinic acetylcholine; NK1, neurokinin-1. (Source: Rang, H. P., Dale, M. M., Ritter, J. M., Flower, R. J., & Henderson, G. [2011]. *Rang & Dale's pharmacology.* Elsevier.)

STATION 3.4: BLOOD TRANSFUSION

The Bleep Scenario

You are bleeped by the on call biochemist. A 68 year old man's haemoglobin on preoperative bloods has been reported as 57 g/L.

You are asked to prescribe a blood transfusion for him. He has no known drug allergies.

WHAT IS EXPECTED OF YOU?

Prescribing blood products is a common occurrence in the acute hospital setting. However, it is widely recognised that a number of risks are associated with this therapy and patients should not be exposed unnecessarily to blood components.

As part of your hospital induction, you should receive training on prescribing blood products. This section covers common indications and products you will encounter.

PRESCRIBING AND ADMINISTERING BLOOD PRODUCTS

Always remember to prescribe the right blood, to the right patient, at the right time and in the right place. Checks are important because 1 in 13,000 blood components are given to the wrong patients.

When prescribing blood products (Table 3.6), remember to state:

- What you are prescribing, e.g. red blood cells
- How many units, e.g. 1 unit
- The duration of the transfusion, e.g. 3 hours

If you are prescribing more than 1 unit, prescribe them individually to avoid confusion and waste.

A complete set of observations must be taken at the following times:

- Before the transfusion starts (no more than 1 hour before the start of the transfusion)
- 15 minutes after the transfusion started
- 1 hour after the transfusion started
- At completion (within 1 hour of completion)

SPECIAL SCENARIOS

ALTERNATIVES TO BLOOD TRANSFUSION

Some patients may object to blood transfusion (e.g. patients of the Jehovah's Witness faith) but are accepting of other blood products. There may be other scenarios where you can consider the following alternatives:

- Intraoperative cell salvage: used in elective or emergency surgery where there is high blood loss or major haemorrhage
- Postoperative cell salvage and reinfusion
- Tranexamic acid can be given orally or intravenously. It is proven to reduce mortality in traumatic bleeds and has benefits in surgery or obstetric emergencies as well as GI bleeds

Table 3.6 Common blood products and indications

PRODUCT	INDICATIONS(S)	DOSE	RATE OF INFUSION
Packed red cells	• Anaemia (symptomatic, or Hb ≤70 g/L) • Major haemorrhage • DIC	1 unit: 300–330 mL	2–4 hours
Platelets	• Therapeutic: thrombocytopenia and clinically significant bleeding • Prophylactic: thrombocytopenia and undergoing invasive procedure / surgery • Major haemorrhage • DIC	1 dose: 50–200 mL	30 minutes
Fresh frozen plasma	• Clinically significant bleeding and deranged clotting • Major haemorrhage • DIC	1 dose: 200–300 mL	30 minutes
Cryoprecipitate	• Clinically significant bleeding and low fibrinogen • Major haemorrhage • DIC	1 dose: typically, 2 units of pooled cryoprecipitate	Stat
Prothrombin complex concentrate	• Emergency reversal of warfarin in patients with severe bleeding, or head injury with suspected intracerebral haemorrhage	25–50 units/kg	Stat

DIC, disseminated intravascular coagulation; Hb, haemoglobin.

Table 3.7 Transfusion reactions (acute and delayed)

REACTION	SIGNS/SYMPTOMS	TREATMENT
Acute		
Non-haemolytic febrile transfusion reaction	Slow rising temperature (>1°C)	• Stop transfusion and review patient • Consider transfusing at slower rate • Give paracetamol
Allergic reaction	Urticaria, pruritus, rarely anaphylaxis	• Stop transfusion and review patient • Antihistamines • Adrenalin in anaphylaxis
Haemolytic transfusion reaction	Fever, chills, pain at infusion site, nausea/vomiting, hypotension, oliguria	• Stop transfusion and review patient • Supportive care • IV fluids ± diuretics
Transfusion-related acute lung injury (TRALI)	Dyspnoea, hypoxaemia, bilateral chest infiltrates	• Stop transfusion • Control airway • Urgent senior help • Give oxygen • Some patients may neeed NIV/mechanical ventilation
Transfusion-associated circulatory overload	Dyspnoea, oedema	• Diuretics • Slow transfusion
Delayed		
Delayed transfusion reaction	5–10 days posttransfusion, fever, falling Hb, jaundice, haemoglobinuria	• Supportive care
Graft-versus-host disease	Rash, elevated LFTs, pancytopenia	• Immunosupression • Prevention: irradiated products in at-risk patient groups

IV, intravenous; LFTs, liver function tests.

- Erythropoiesis-stimulating agents such as erythropoietin
- Parenteral iron infusions (Ferinject): also suitable for patients who do not tolerate oral iron

MAJOR HAEMORRHAGE

In any major haemorrhage, it is important to recognise it as quickly as possible, to get immediate senior help and send urgent blood samples.

You must activate (with senior advice) the major haemorrhage or major obstetric haemorrhage protocol, so that the lab will prioritise your patient and you can get appropriate help (for example, the anaesthetist will attend and consultant haematologists will be made aware).

TRANSFUSION REACTIONS (TABLE 3.7)

Adverse reactions must be reported to Serious Hazards of Transfusion (SHOT) in the UK.

In any suspected transfusion reaction:

- Stop (or in some cases slow) the transfusion.
- Assess the patient (rapid clinical assessment).
- Check patient identification and blood compatibility label.
- Inspect the blood product (turbidity, clots, discoloration).
- Contact the laboratory and on call haematologist for advice.

SUMMARY

- Ensure you have the right products for the right patient and prescribe them correctly.
- Familiarise yourself with local protocols on the transfusion of blood products.
- Call for help early in cases of major haemorrhage.
- O-negative blood can be used in emergencies if you do not know the patient's blood group or have a recent group-and-save sample.
- Irradiated products may be needed if the patient is at risk of transfusion-associated graft-versus-host disease.
- Always seek the advice of the on call haematology registrar or consultant if you are unsure.

STATION 3.5: GENTAMICIN

The Bleep Scenario

You are bleeped to urgently clerk a patient on AMU. An 82 year old woman has presented with symptoms consistent with urosepsis.

As per hospital protocol, you need to prescribe gentamicin for the patient. She has no known drug allergies.

DEFINITION

Gentamicin is a bactericidal aminoglycoside antibiotic given intravenously and requires monitoring due to risk of toxicity.

WHAT IS EXPECTED OF YOU?

As a junior doctor in a hospital setting, prescribing gentamicin and adjusting its dose according to gentamicin levels form common bleep scenarios. It is important to get this right to ensure it is therapeutic and prevent toxicity. Gentamicin is an aminoglycoside with bactericidal activity and acts by inhibiting protein synthesis. It is effective against Gram-negative aerobic bacteria, staphylococci and mycobacteria (Table 3.8).

Treatment duration will depend on the indication but should be as short as possible to limit toxicity. If gentamicin is required beyond 48 hours, make sure the patient is on the correct antibiotic (for example, with culture results or microbiology advice) and ideally it should not be continued beyond 7 days.

Table 3.8 Common indications for gentamicin

Common indications for gentamicin
Pyelonephritis and complicated UTIs
Biliary and other intra-abdominal sepsis
HACEK or Gram-positive endocarditis
Pneumonia (in hospital)
Listeria meningitis and other CNS infections
Severe sepsis

CNS, central nervous system; HACEK, *Haemophilus*, *Aggregatibacter* (previously *Actinobacillus*), *Cardiobacterium, Eikenella, Kingella*; UTIs, urinary tract infections.

Most trusts have a protocol for gentamicin administration to which you should refer. If in doubt about dosages/calculations, always seek advice from microbiology or pharmacy.

DOSE CALCULATIONS

ONCE-DAILY DOSING

Once-daily administration of gentamicin in adults is less toxic and more convenient than multiple daily dosing. The initial dose of gentamicin is calculated according to the patient's actual body weight (ABW) and renal function.

Note that some trusts will advise against a once-daily dosing regime if the creatinine clearance is less than 20 mL/minute. See below for guidance on multiple daily dosing regimens.

1. Calculate the patient's body weight:

   If the patient is >20% above their IBW, or has a body mass index (BMI) >30 kg/m^2, the dose should be prescribed according to the patient's IBW to avoid toxicity.

   - IBW male (kg) = 50 + (2.3 × number of inches above 5 feet in height) OR 22 × (height in meters)^2
   - IBW female (kg) = 45.5 + (2.3 × number of inches above 5 feet in height) OR 22 × (height in meters – 10 cm)^2

2. Calculate the patient's renal function:

   Use creatinine clearance rather than estimated glomerular filtration rate. You can use the Cockcroft and Gault's equation below (available as an app in most trusts).

$$\text{Estimated creatinine clearance}\left(\frac{\text{mL}}{\text{minutes}}\right) = (140 - \text{age}) \times \text{weight} \times \text{constant}$$

$$\text{Age in years, weight in kg (use IBW as needed),}\\ \text{constant} = 1.23 \text{ for men; } 1.04 \text{ for women}$$

3. Prescribe dose according to ABW/ IBW and renal function (Table 3.9):

   Note that some trusts use the corrected body weight to prescribe for obese patients. Always follow your trust's guidelines:

$$\text{CBW} = \text{IBW} + 0.4\,(\text{ABW} - \text{IBW})$$

Table 3.9 Possible dosing of gentamicin according to creatinine clearance

CREATININE CLEARANCE >30 ML/MINUTE	CREATININE CLEARANCE <30 ML/MINUTE
Give gentamicin 5 mg/kg according to actual or ideal body weight as appropriate	Give gentamicin 3 mg/kg according to actual or ideal body weight as appropriate
Maximum dose 480 mg every 24 hours	Maximum dose 320 mg every 24 hours

Table 3.10 Scenarios when multiple daily dosing might be used

CREATININE CLEARANCE <10 ML/MINUTE	CREATININE CLEARANCE 10–20 ML/MINUTE	CREATININE CLEARANCE 20–50 ML/MINUTE
Dose: 80 mg (reduce to 60 mg if patient weight <60 kg) Frequency: every 48 hours	Dose: 80 mg (reduce to 60 mg if patient weight <60 kg) Frequency: every 24 hours	Dose: 80 mg (reduce to 60 mg if patient weight <60 kg) Frequency: every 12 hours

In an emergency, if the on call pharmacist is unavailable, or the patient's renal function is unknown, prescribe a stat dose of 3 mg/kg up to a maximum of 320 mg and check serum levels after 24 hours.

MULTIPLE DAILY DOSING

Multiple daily dosing can be used in renal impairment, for endocarditis or in pregnancy (Table 3.10). It may also be advised in elderly patients.

MONITORING

Aminoglycosides accumulate in renal tubular epithelial cells and in cochlear and vestibular hair cells. Monitoring of plasma concentrations (Table 3.11) with careful dose adjustment (Table 3.12) is essential to prevent nephrotoxicity and ototoxicity.

All trough levels should be taken within 60 minutes prior to the next scheduled gentamicin dose.

Note that some trusts use the Hartford nomogram (Fig. 3.7) to guide the frequency of gentamicin dosing according to the gentamicin concentration and the time the measurement was taken.

Table 3.12 Monitoring trough levels of gentamicin on standard regime (guidelines may vary)

IF TROUGH LEVEL <1 MG/L	IF TROUGH LEVEL >1 MG/L
• Next dose can be safely given	• Check sample was taken pre-dose and within 1 hour of next dose being due • If sample taken too early, then repeat at the correct time whenever possible • Withhold next dose • Repeat trough serum level at appropriate interval • Discuss with on call microbiologist / pharmacist for advice on changes to the dose and / or dosing interval

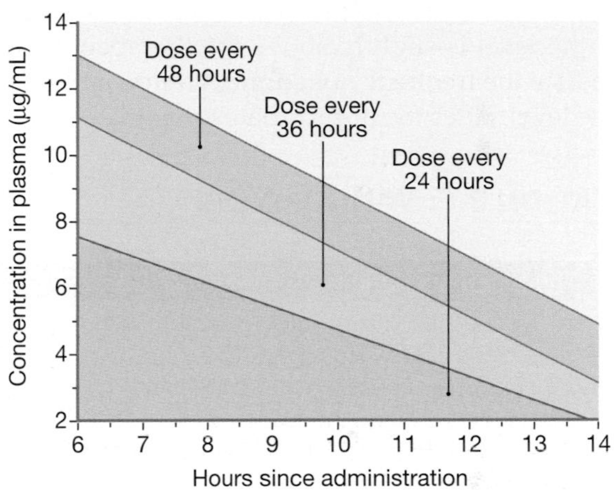

Fig. 3.7 Hartford nomogram. (Source: Ralston, S.H. et al. (Eds.) (2018) *Davidson's principles and practice of medicine*. Edinburgh: Elsevier.)

IMPORTANT CONSIDERATIONS (TABLE 3.13)

Patients also require daily monitoring of renal function plus regular monitoring of the full blood count, liver function and fluid balance. Some trusts also advise audiology referrals after 7 days of gentamicin.

Table 3.11 Possible monitoring of gentamicin dosing according to creatinine clearance

PATIENTS WITH CREATININE CLEARANCE <30 ML/MINUTE	PATIENTS WITH CREATININE CLEARANCE >30 ML/MINUTE
• Check the trough gentamicin level before the second dose • Do not administer the second dose until the assay result is known	• Check the trough gentamicin level before the second or (if necessary) third dose • The second dose can be given without the need for an assay result • If a level was not sent before the second dose, do not administer the third dose until the assay result is known
• Recheck trough gentamicin level before every dose if the gentamicin is high, or renal function is changing	• Recheck trough gentamicin level every 2 or 3 days (i.e. before fourth or fifth dose) in patients with gentamicin levels within the therapeutic range and stable renal function

Table 3.13 Important considerations when prescribing gentamicin

SIDE EFFECTS	IMPORTANT CAUTIONS	IMPORTANT INTERACTIONS
• Nephrotoxicity • Ototoxicity • Hypersensitivity reactions • Nausea and vomiting • Myasthenia-like syndrome	Avoid in the following patient groups: • Myasthenia gravis • Pregnancy • Hypersensitivity Use with caution in the following patient groups: • Liver failure • Acute kidney injury • Chronic kidney disease	• Increased nephrotoxicity with NSAIDS, ciclosporin, vancomycin and cephalosporins • Increased ototoxicity with loop diuretics • Gentamicin increases effects of muscle relaxants (e.g. suxamethonium, vecuronium)

NSAIDs, non-steroidal anti-inflammatory drugs.

SUMMARY

- Familiarise yourself with the gentamicin dosing calculations and monitoring regime used in your trust.
- If the level of gentamicin is in the toxic range, discuss this with the on call microbiologist or pharmacist.
- If the level is slightly above the therapeutic range, reduce the frequency of administration and recheck the levels after the appropriate interval.

STATION 3.6: VANCOMYCIN

The Bleep Scenario

You are bleeped by the on call microbiologist. A 76 year old man on the elderly care ward has tested positive for *Clostridium difficile*. The patient is currently nil by mouth as per the speech and language team.

You are asked to prescribe vancomycin for him. He has no known drug allergies.

DEFINITION

Vancomycin is a glycopeptide bactericidal antibiotic used for Gram-positive infections and given intravenously.

WHAT IS EXPECTED OF YOU?

As a junior doctor, you will likely prescribe vancomycin less frequently compared to other antibiotics. You should know that it is a glycopeptide antibiotic which requires careful dosing and monitoring. Vancomycin acts against aerobic and anaerobic Gram-positive bacteria, including methicillin-resistant *Staphylococcus aureus* (MRSA). It is commonly given in combination with other antibiotics.

Common indications:

- Surgical prophylaxis
- Dialysis-associated peritonitis
- *C. difficile* colitis
- Skin and soft-tissue infections
- Bone/joint infections
- Pneumonia
- Infective endocarditis
- Meningitis
- Bacteraemia secondary to infections listed above

Treatment duration will depend on the indication. Longer doses of 4–6 weeks are used for necrotising skin infections, bone and joint infections and endocarditis.

Most trusts have a protocol for vancomycin administration to which you should refer. If in doubt about dosages or calculations, always seek pharmacy advice.

DOSE CALCULATIONS – IV USE

Vancomycin dosing should be based on body weight and creatinine clearance. Subsequent doses should be based on the therapeutic concentration and renal function.

Patients are given one loading dose followed by maintenance dosing according to age, sex, body weight and creatinine clearance.

Patients on the intensive care unit may receive continuous IV infusions. This should be prescribed and administered under specialist supervision only.

LOADING DOSE

The loading dose is based on the patient's body weight (Table 3.14).

If a patient is critically ill, a loading dose of 25–30 mg/kg can be given; however, you should seek senior advice for this decision. Normal doses are 15–20 mg/kg every 8–12 hours (maximum 2 g per dose).

MAINTENANCE DOSE

Vancomycin is eliminated almost completely unchanged in the urine, therefore renal function is the most important factor in determining the maintenance dose. The maintenance dose is given 12, 24 or 48 hours after the initial loading dose.

Table 3.14 Possible loading doses of vancomycin according to body weight

WEIGHT	LOADING DOSE	INFUSION TIME
<60 kg	1000 mg	2 hours
60–90 kg	1500 mg	3 hours
>90 kg	2000 mg	4 hours

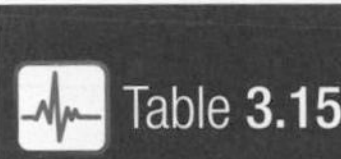

Table 3.15 Possible maintenance doses of vancomycin according to creatinine clearance

CREATININE CLEARANCE (ML/MINUTE)	DOSE INTERVAL	MAINTENANCE DOSE	INFUSION TIME
<20	48 hours	500 mg	1 hour
20–29	24 hours	500 mg	1 hour
30–39	24 hours	750 mg	1.5 hours
40–54	12 hours	500 mg	1 hour
55–74	12 hours	750 mg	1.5 hours
75–89	12 hours	1000 mg	2 hours
90–110	12 hours	1250 mg	2.5 hours
>110	12 hours	1500 mg	3 hours

Calculate the patient's creatinine clearance from age, sex, body weight and serum creatinine (Cockcroft and Gault). Your trust may have an app or calculator that you can readily access to calculate the correct dosing regimen for your patient (Table 3.15).

MONITORING

IV vancomycin has a narrow therapeutic index and regular monitoring is required. Pre-dose vancomycin levels are used to ensure therapeutic levels are reached and nephrotoxicity is minimised (Table 3.16).

- All levels should be taken within 60 minutes prior to the next scheduled dose.
- Trough vancomycin concentrations should be 10–20 mg/L (Table 3.17 and Fig. 3.8) *For Staphylococcus aureus* infections and deep-seated infections (i.e. infective endocarditis, osteomyelitis) the target range is often higher (15–20 mg/L).

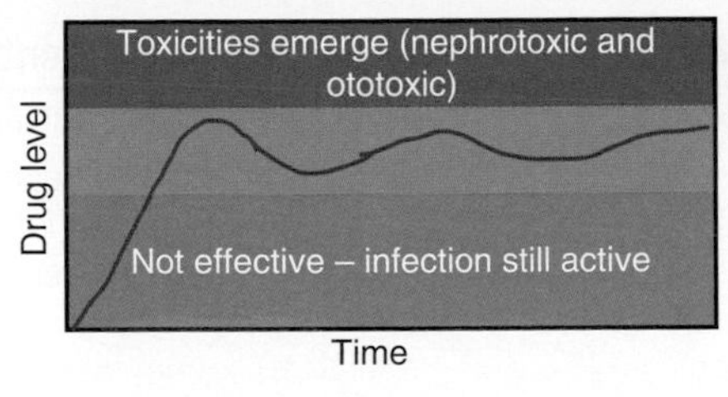

Fig. 3.8 Dosing and monitoring vancomycin. (Source: Guerra, A. (2022) *Pharmacology made simple*. Elsevier.)

IMPORTANT CONSIDERATIONS (TABLE 3.18)

Patients also require daily monitoring of renal function plus regular monitoring of the full blood count, and liver function.

DOSE CALCULATIONS – ORAL USE

Oral vancomycin is typically used in the treatment of *C. difficile* infection (CDI) where direct gut action is required.

- Recommended dose for the first episode of non-severe CDI: 125 mg every 6 hours for 10 days
- Recommended dose for severe CDI: 500 mg every 6 hours for 10 days
- In patients with multiple recurrences, consideration may be given to 10 days of standard treatment followed by tapering the dose (e.g. gradually decreasing dose until 125 mg/day) or a pulse regimen (e.g. 125–500 mg/day every 2–3 days for at least 3 weeks)
- The maximum daily dose is 2 g
- Oral dosing does not usually require therapeutic monitoring (with the exception of inflammatory bowel disease patients)

Table 3.16 Possible monitoring of vancomycin

48-hourly dosing	12-hourly dosing	24-hourly dosing
• Check vancomycin level after 48 hours, before the first maintenance dose is given • Recheck trough vancomycin level before every dose	• Check vancomycin level before the third or fourth dose • Recheck trough level every 48–72 hours once vancomycin level within therapeutic range	• Check vancomycin level before the second or third dose • Recheck trough level every 48–72 hours once vancomycin level within therapeutic range

Table 3.17 Potential actions if trough vancomycin concentrations are not in the target range

IF TROUGH LEVEL >20 MG/L	IF TROUGH LEVEL <10 MG/L
• Check sample was taken pre-dose and within 1 hour of the next dose being due • Withhold next dose • Contact a senior (consultant, on call microbiologist or pharmacist) for further advice	• Check sample was taken pre-dose and within 1 hour of the next dose being due • Check the drug chart to see if any doses have been missed; if they have, then recheck trough levels once two consecutive doses have been given • If Increase dose of vancomycin e.g. by 10% with advice from senior (consultant, on call microbiologist or pharmacist):

Table 3.18 Important considerations when prescribing vancomycin

SIDE EFFECTS	IMPORTANT CAUTIONS	IMPORTANT INTERACTIONS
• Nephrotoxicity • Ototoxicity • Blood disorders (neutropenia, thrombocytopenia) • Thrombophlebitis • Anaphylactoid reactions, including red-man syndrome	• History of hearing impairment • Avoid rapid infusions • Caution in renal impairment and elderly	• Increased nephrotoxicity with ciclosporin and aminoglycosides • Increased ototoxicity with loop diuretics • Increased risk of blood disorders if used with other drugs causing neutropenia/ agranulocytosis • Vancomycin increases effects of muscle relaxants (e.g. suxamethonium, vecuronium)

SUMMARY

- Patients on vancomycin require monitoring and dose adjustments as per renal function.
- Be aware of risks for ototoxicity and nephrotoxicity.
- Seek advice from seniors if you are uncertain on how to prescribe or monitor vancomycin.

STATION 3.7: INSULIN

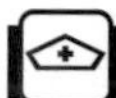

The Bleep Scenario

You are bleeped by a nurse on the surgical assessment unit. A 45 year old woman with type 1 diabetes has been admitted with suspected cholecystitis.

You are asked to prescribe her regular insulin. She has no known drug allergies.

DEFINITION

Synthetic insulin is administered as a treatment for type 1 diabetes and some patients with type 2 diabetes.

WHAT IS EXPECTED OF YOU?

As a junior doctor you will be asked to prescribe insulin in a variety of circumstances. Examples include:

- Prescribing a patient's regular insulin regimen in insulin-dependent diabetic patients
- Reviewing insulin doses in cases of hyper- or hypoglycaemia. Note that adjustments should be based on readings from the previous 48 hours with adjustments of 10–20% only
- Prescribing a sliding scale (variable-rate intravenous insulin infusion or VRIII) for patients who are having surgery or have poor control of their blood sugar, e.g. sepsis, ileus – in these cases, the nurses adjust the rate of infusion based on the patient's blood sugar
- Prescribing a fixed-rate insulin infusion for patients being treated for diabetic ketoacidosis

Remember that you are not a specialist and therefore you are not expected to initiate insulin or decide on treatment regimens for diabetic patients (Table 3.19 and Fig. 3.9). You may also encounter patients on an insulin pump, in which case you should always refer to the diabetes team (Table 3.20).

COMMON SCENARIOS

PRESCRIBING REGULAR INSULIN

Ask the patient for as much detail as you can on their insulin prescription. Patients may take long-, short- or medium-acting insulins or a mixture of them. You will need to prescribe the type of insulin they take, what time(s) they take it and how many units they take. Insulin should be prescribed by brand name.

CHANGES IN REQUIREMENTS

Patients who have DKA, are septic, on steroids, have pancreatitis or are dehydrated will have increased insulin requirements. Those who have reduced calorie intake, poor renal function or excessive alcohol intake may need less insulin than normal.

HYPOGLYCAEMIA (CAPILLARY BLOOD GLUCOSE < 4.0 MMOL/L)

Patients on a sulphonylurea or insulin are at risk of hypoglycaemia, especially in the context of an acute kidney injury or reduced oral intake.

- If the patient is alert, 15–20 g of quick-acting carbohydrate is recommended (e.g. 150–200 mL of orange juice), then recheck the blood sugar in 10–15 minutes and repeat if needed (up to three times).
- If the patient is confused, uncooperative or aggressive but still able to swallow, then proceed with two tubes of Glucogel.
- If the patient is unable to swallow, proceed with IM glucagon 1 mg or IV glucose 10% 250 mL.
- In cases of severe hypoglycaemia where the patient is unconscious, follow an ABCDE approach and treat with IV glucose – refer to Station 9.3: Hypoglycemia.
- Note that frequent episodes of hypoglycaemia can impair the patient's ability to detect them and lead to hypoglycaemic unawareness.

ESCALATION

For cases of severe or difficult-to-treat hypoglycaemia, always seek senior assistance and involve the diabetes

Table 3.19 Types of insulin

TYPE OF INSULIN	USE(S)	EXAMPLES	FEATURES
Rapid-acting	• Usually taken before meals as part of a basal bolus regime in patients with type 1 diabetes	• NovoRapid (insulin aspart) • Apidra (insulin glulisine) • Humalog (insulin lispro)	Onset: immediate Peak: 1–3 hours Duration: 2–5 hours
Short-acting	• Used in intravenous insulin regimes, or form the quick-acting component of mixed insulins	• Hypurin bovine neutral • Hypurin porcine neutral • Actrapid • Humulin S • Insuman Rapid	Onset: 30–60 minutes Peak: 1–3 hours Duration: 6–12 hours
Intermediate-acting	• Used once or twice daily in patients with type 2 diabetes patients to supplement oral agents or reduce morning glucose levels	• Hypurin Bovine Isophane • Hypurin Porcine Isophane • Insulatard • Humulin I • Insuman Basal	Onset: Up to 2 hours Peak: 4–12 hours Duration: up to 24 hours
Long-acting	• Form part of a basal bolus regime in patients with type 1 diabetes • Used in patients with type 2 diabetes where insulin is added to their oral agents	• Lantus (insulin glargine) • Levemir (insulin detemir) • Tresiba (insulin degludec)	Onset: 1–4 hours Peak: flat profile Duration: up to 24 hours (up to 48 hours for Tresiba)
Biphasic / mixed insulin	• May be used in patients with type 2 or type 1 diabetes (where a basal bolus regime is inappropriate) • Typically administered twice daily	• Humulin M3 • Humalog Mix 50 • Humalog Mix 25 • Novomix 30	Onset: 30–60 minutes Peak: 1–12 hours Duration: Up to 24 hours

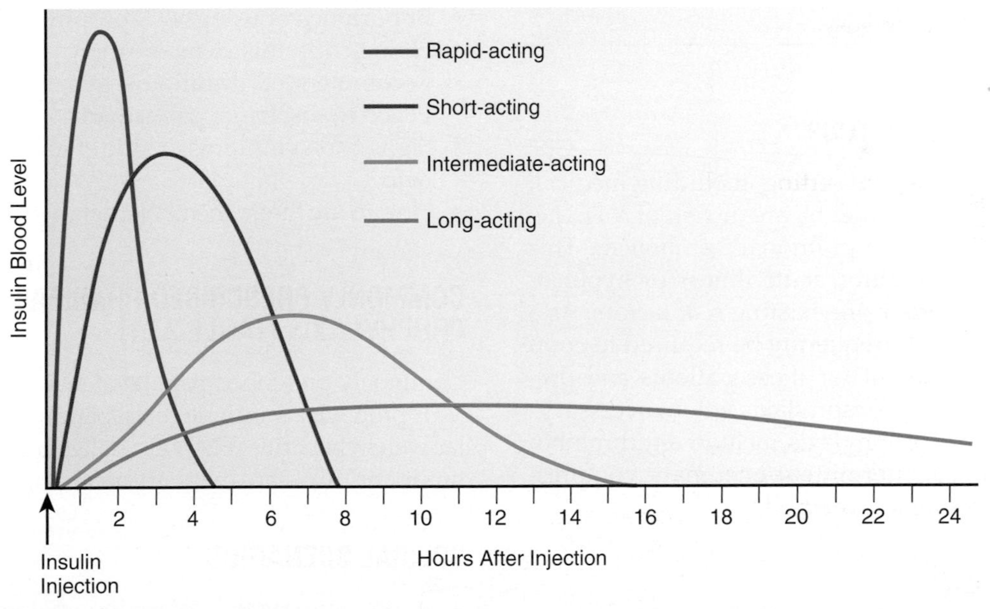

Fig. 3.9 Types of insulin and their effect. (Source: Burchum, J. and Rosenthal, L.D. [2022]. *Lehne's pharmacology for nursing care*. St Louis, MO: Elsevier.)

Table 3.20 Common mistakes when prescribing insulin

PRESCRIBING	ADMINISTRATION	INSUFFICIENT KNOWLEDGE
• Incorrect dose(s) • Incorrect type of insulin prescribed • Incorrect timing • Incorrect frequency • Use of abbreviations for units	• Route/dose • Incorrect syringe • Omitted or delayed administration	• Errors in dose alteration • Use of VRIII • Treatment of diabetic emergencies (DKA, HHS, hypoglycaemia)

DKA, diabetic ketoacidosis; HHS, hyperosmolar hyperglycaemic syndrome; VRIII, variable-rate intravenous insulin infusion.

team. Severe hypoglycaemia is a medical emergency and can be fatal.

SUMMARY

- Do not forget insulin as part of your admission clerking or prescriptions. Most hospitals have separate charts for insulin prescriptions.
- If you initiate treatment that is likely to result in poor blood sugar control or if your patient is going to be starved, ensure you prescribe a VRIII.
- When a fixed regime is started for DKA, ensure you monitor the patient regularly with biochemical markers to adjust and stop the regime at the correct time.
- Find out how to contact your hospital's diabetic specialist teams.

STATION 3.8: VTE PROPHYLAXIS

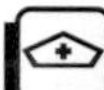

The Bleep Scenario

You are bleeped by a nurse on the surgical assessment unit. A 28 year old woman has been admitted and her venous thromboembolism (VTE) prophylaxis has not yet been completed.

You are asked to prescribe appropriate VTE prophylaxis. She has no known drug allergies.

WHAT IS EXPECTED OF YOU?

All patients in the hospital setting, including medical, surgical and obstetric patients, are at risk of VTE, i.e. deep-vein thrombosis or pulmonary embolism. This is due to reduced mobility, acute illness or hypercoagulable state and other pre-existing risk factors. As a junior doctor, you will frequently be required to complete the risk assessment for these patients and prescribe appropriate VTE prophylaxis where necessary.

Methods of VTE prophylaxis include antithromboembolism stockings, intermittent pneumatic compression and pharmacological methods.

RISK ASSESSMENT

All patients should have a documented risk assessment on a validated tool on admission or by first consultant review. The decision to use pharmacological methods should be based on a balance of individual's risk of VTE versus their bleeding risk. If recommended, VTE prophylaxis should be administered as soon as possible, within 14 hours of admission.

A reassessment should be made at consultant review or if the clinical condition changes.

Patients already on antiplatelets may still need pharmacological methods if the risk of VTE outweighs the risk of bleeding. If pharmacological prophylaxis is contraindicated, mechanical options can be used.

IMPORTANT CONTRAINDICATIONS TO PHARMACOLOGICAL PROPHYLAXIS

- Active bleeding
- Concomitant anticoagulants
- Thrombocytopenia, or previous heparin-induced thrombocytopenia
- Platelets <75 × 10^9/L
- Active GI ulcer or risk of GI haemorrhage
- Acquired liver failure
- Uncontrolled systolic hypertension (>230 mmHg)
- Untreated inherited bleeding disorder
- Bacterial endocarditis

  Note: severe peripheral vascular disease is a contraindication to mechanical VTE prophylaxis

COMMUNICATION WITH PATIENTS AND FAMILY/CARERS

You should inform the patient and their family or carers (if appropriate) about the necessity of a risk assessment, the risks and consequences of VTE, importance of prophylaxis and side effects, correct use of prophylaxis and how to reduce risk, i.e. keeping well hydrated, exercising and keeping mobile.

Patients should be given both verbal and written information that explains the following:

- Importance of using VTE prophylaxis
- How to administer medication
- Recommended duration – this should also be conveyed in discharge paperwork
- Signs and symptoms of side effects and how to seek help
- How to use thromboembolic deterrent stockings (TEDS)

COMMONLY PRESCRIBED PHARMACOLOGICAL VTE PROPHYLAXIS (TABLE 3.21)

Commonly prescribed parenteral anticoagulants used for VTE prophylaxis include fondaparinux and low-molecular-weight heparins (LMWHs: dalteparin, enoxaparin and tinzaparin). Dosages may vary according to local protocols.

SPECIAL SCENARIOS

- Acute myocardial infarction: patients already on anticoagulation (fondaparinux) do not usually need additional pharmacological VTE prophylaxis.
- Elective hip/knee replacements: direct oral anticoagulants (DOACs) may be used instead of LMWH/unfractionated heparin. Rivaroxaban is preferred (although apixaban/dabigatran can also be used).
- Renal impairment: LMWH/unfractionated heparin should be used (doses may need to be adjusted).
- Palliative care: if used, LMWH/fondaparinux should be suspended in the last days of life.
- Anaesthesia: time the administration of LMWH for regional anaesthesia so that patients are not at increased risk of epidural haematoma.

Table 3.21 Possible examples of venous thromboembolism (VTE) prophylaxis

LMWH	VTE PROPHYLAXIS (MEDICAL)	VTE PROPHYLAXIS (SURGICAL)
Dalteparin Avoid if CrCl < 30 mL/minute	5000 units daily	If moderate risk, 2500 units 1–2 hours before surgery then daily. If high risk 5000 units the evening before surgery, then daily (or 2500 units 1–2 hours before surgery and 8–12 hours after then 5000 units daily)
Enoxaparin Dose reduction if CrCl < 30	40 mg daily	20 mg 2 hours before then daily for medium-risk surgery and 40 mg 12 hours before then daily for high-risk surgery (e.g. orthopaedic surgery)
Tinzaparin Avoid if CrCl < 20 mL/minute	4500 units daily	3500 units 2 hours before surgery then daily (general surgery) 4500 units 12 hours before surgery then daily (orthopaedic surgery)
Fondaparinux Dose reduction if CrCl < 30 mL/minute	2.5 mg once daily	2.5 mg 6 hours after surgery then once daily Used for patients having abdominal, bariatric, thoracic or cardiac surgery or those with lower-limb immobilisation or fragility fractures of the pelvis, hip or proximal femur

CrCl, creatinine clearance; LMWH, low-molecular-weight heparin.
N.B.: Doses may also need adjusting according to the weight of the patient (as well as renal function), e.g. if they weigh less than 50 kg or above 100 kg.

- Spinal injury: give either TEDS or IPC on admission and reassess their risk 24 hours later; give pharmacological prophylaxis if the patient is not due for surgery in the next 1–2 days or start after surgery.
- Extended VTE prophylaxis for cancer patients: 28 days of pharmacological VTE prophylaxis should be considered for cancer patients who have had major abdominal surgery, e.g. colorectal cancer resection.

SUMMARY

- Thromboprophylaxis is hugely important in maintaining safety amongst patients admitted to hospital; pulmonary embolism remains the leading cause of preventable in-hospital death.
- The risk of VTE depends on medical versus surgical admission and the type of surgery.
- Every patient should have a VTE risk assessment at admission or by first consultant review.
- Pharmacological options for VTE include fondaparinux and LMWH.
- Mechanical options for VTE include TEDS and IPC.

STATION 3.9: WARFARIN

The Bleep Scenario

You are bleeped by a nurse on the elderly care ward. An 82 year old woman is being initiated on warfarin following a new diagnosis of atrial fibrillation. Her international normalised ratio (INR) has just come back as 1.5.

You are asked to prescribe the next dose of warfarin. She has no known drug allergies.

DEFINITION

Warfarin is an anticoagulant used to reduce the risk of thrombosis in specific settings and requires monitoring to ensure it is being taken at safe doses.

WHAT IS EXPECTED OF YOU?

Warfarin (a vitamin K antagonist) is an anticoagulant used to reduce the risk of thrombosis in patients with certain conditions, including atrial fibrillation, heart valve replacements or previous VTE.

Prescribing warfarin is a job you will frequently encounter in various scenarios, such as initiation of warfarin or restarting it following surgery. If a patient has previously been on warfarin, you will be able to find their dosing regimen from their yellow book.

Absolute contraindications to warfarin include previous haemorrhagic stroke, significant bleeding, being within 2 days postpartum, bleeding disorders or being within 3 days of major surgery with bleeding risks.

COMMON SCENARIOS

INITIATING WARFARIN

The initiation of warfarin depends upon the indication and certain patient factors. 'Fast' initiation is used if the presence of a clot is suspected whereas 'slow' initiation can be used if there is no suspicion of a clot.

Warfarin is usually started at a dose of 5–10 mg, and the dose is adjusted according to the patient's INR on day 3. For atrial fibrillation, warfarin can be started at 1–2 mg per day as a rapid effect is not needed.

If an immediate anticoagulant effect is needed (for example, in treatment of deep-vein thrombosis or pulmonary embolism), you will also need to prescribe heparin or treatment dose LMWH until the INR is within therapeutic range. Risk factors (for increased risk of bleeding): elderly, liver disease, renal impairment, low body weight, cardiac failure, frequent falls.

Table 3.22 Target ranges

TARGET INR 2.5 (2.0–3.0)	TARGET INR 3.0 (2.5–3.5)	TARGET INR 3.5 (3.0–4.0)
• Mitral stenosis or regurgitation (in patients with AF, history of embolism, a left atrial thrombus or an enlarged left atrium) • AF • Cardioversion • Dilated cardiomyopathy • Treatment of DVT / PE • Bioprosthetic heart valves • Antiphospholipid syndrome • Acute arterial embolism leading to embolectomy • Myocardial infarction	• Mechanical aortic valves	• Recurrent DVT or PE in patients currently receiving anticoagulation and with an INR above 2 • Mechanical mitral valves

AF, atrial fibrillation; DVT, deep-vein thrombosis; INR, international normalised ratio; PE, pulmonary embolism.

Table 3.23 How to manage a raised international normalised ratio (INR) based on the clinical scenario

INR	ACTION
Major bleeding	• Stop warfarin • Give vitamin K 5 mg IV • Give either dried prothrombin complex (Beriplex/Octaplex) or fresh frozen plasma (seek advice from seniors or haematology team)
Minor bleeding, INR >8.0	• Stop warfarin • Give vitamin K 1–3 mg IV • Repeat vitamin K if INR still too high after 24 hours • Restart warfarin when INR <5.0
Minor bleeding, INR 5.0–8.0	• Stop warfarin • Give vitamin K 1–3 mg IV • Restart warfarin when INR <5.0
No bleeding, INR >8.0	• Stop warfarin • Give vitamin K 1–5 mg PO • Repeat vitamin K if INR still too high after 24 hours • Restart warfarin when INR <5.0
No bleeding, INR 5.0–8.0	• Withhold one or two doses of warfarin • Reduce subsequent maintenance dose (seek advice from seniors or haematology team)
Unexpected bleeding at therapeutic levels	• Investigate for any underlying cause, e.g. unsuspected renal or gastrointestinal tract pathology

IV, intravenous; PO, orally.

- If no risk factors, prescribe 10 mg (days 1 and 2), 5 mg (day 3).
- If one risk factor, prescribe 7 mg/day for 3 days.
- If two or more risk factors, prescribe 5 mg/day for 3 days.
- Measure INR on day 3.

If the patient is likely to be non-compliant with INR monitoring, you may prefer to use a DOAC such as rivaroxaban, dabigatran or apixaban. Choice of agent is not a junior decision, but it is important to be aware of the other options.

PREPARING FOR SURGERY AND RESTARTING WARFARIN

Warfarin should be stopped 5 days before surgery and the target INR before surgery is <1.5.

If warfarin has been stopped before surgery and you are asked to restart, ensure the surgical team is happy for warfarin to be restarted (for example, if the patient is actively bleeding or may need to go back to theatre).

Warfarin can normally be restarted on the same day or the next day. If this is the case, you may also need to prescribe LMWH with the patient's usual dose of warfarin (unless a different plan has been made by the anticoagulation clinic in advance) until the INR is back within therapeutic range (Table 3.22).

REVERSAL OF WARFARIN

The management of a raised INR depends on both INR level and whether or not the patient is bleeding (Tables 3.23–3.25).

Table 3.24 Common durations of treatment

INDICATION	DURATION
Distal DVT with known precipitant	Continue for 6 weeks
Proximal DVT/PE with known precipitant	Continue for 3 months
Unprovoked DVT/PE	Continue for 6 months
Recurrent DVT/PE	Lifelong
Atrial fibrillation	Lifelong

DVT, deep-vein thrombosis; PE, pulmonary embolism.

Table 3.25 Important interactions

CYTOCHROME P450 INHIBITORS (INCREASE INR)	CYTOCHROME P450 INDUCERS (REDUCE INR)
Quinolones	Rifampicin
Selective serotonin reuptake inhibitors	Barbiturates such as Phenobarbitol
Grapefruit juice / alcohol	Carbamazepine
Macrolides	Phenytoin
Azole antifungals	Griseofulvin
Protease inhibitor	St John's wort
Omeprazole	
Amiodarone	
Sodium valproate	
Metronidazole	

INR, international normalised ratio.

ESCALATION

Most hospitals will have a protocol for warfarin prescribing to which you should have access. If unsure, you can discuss with the anticoagulation clinic, a senior member of your team or a haematologist/cardiologist depending on the scenario.

SUMMARY

- Ensure you know the patient's target range and indication for warfarin.
- Consider whether the patient needs LMWH in addition to warfarin until their INR is within range.
- Don't forget to prescribe the warfarin on the drug chart and (if possible) try and prescribe it in advance for the weekend (unless it would not be safe).
- If unsure, refer to the patient's yellow book or ask for help.

FURTHER READING

Blackburn, J., & Spencer, R. (2015). Postoperative nausea and vomiting. *Anaesthesia & Intensive Care Medicine*, *16*(9), 452–456.

EMC. (2021). *Vancomycin 1g powder for solution for infusion*. Available at: www.medicines.org.uk/emc/product/6255/smpc. [Accessed 9 January 2022].

Garraghan, F., & Fallon, R. (2015). Gentamicin: Dose regimens and monitoring. *Pharmaceutical Journal*. Available at: www.pharmaceutical-journal.com/learning/learning-article/gentamicin-dose-regimens-and-monitoring/20069096.article. [Accessed 17 January 2022].

Hunt, B. J., et al. (2015). A practical guideline for the haematological management of major haemorrhage. *British Journal of Haematology*, *170*, 788–803.

Joint Formulary Committee. *British National Formulary* (online). London: BMJ Group and Pharmaceutical Press.

Kumar, A., & Kumar, A. (2013). Antiemetics: A review. *International Journal of Pharmaceutical Sciences and Research*, *4*(1), 113–123.

NHS Scotland. (2020). *Scotting palliative care guidelines: Anticipatory prescribing*. Available at: www.palliativecareguidelines.scot.nhs.uk/guidelines/pain/Anticipatory-Prescribing.aspx. [Accessed 9 January 2022].

NICE. (2013). *Algorithms for IV fluid therapy in adults*. Available at: www.nice.org.uk/guidance/cg174/resources/intravenous-fluid-therapy-in-adults-in-hospital-algorithm-poster-set-191627821. [Accessed 9 January 2022].

NICE. (2020). *Analgesia – mild-to-moderate pain*. Available at: https://cks.nice.org.uk/analgesia-mild-to-moderate-pain#!scenario:4. [Accessed 9 January 2022].

NICE. (2021). *Anticoagulation – oral: Scenario: Warfarin*. Available at: https://cks.nice.org.uk/anticoagulation-oral#!scenario:4. [Accessed 9 January 2022].

NICE. (2021). *BNF gentamicin*. Available at: https://bnf.nice.org.uk/drug/gentamicin.html. [Accessed 9 January 2022].

NICE. (2021). *BNF morphine*. Available at: https://bnf.nice.org.uk/drug/morphine.html. [Accessed 9 January 2022].

NICE. (2021). *BNF vancomycin*. Available at: https://bnf.nice.org.uk/drug/vancomycin.html. [Accessed 9 January 2022].

NICE. (2021). *Type 1 diabetes in adults: Diagnosis and management*. Available at: www.nice.org.uk/guidance/ng17. [Accessed 9 January 2022].

NICE. (2021). *Type 2 diabetes in adults: Management*. Available at: www.nice.org.uk/guidance/ng28. [Accessed 9 January 2022].

Norton, D., et al. (2014). Adverse effects of transfusion. In *Handbook of transfusion medicine* Available at: www.transfusionguidelines.org/transfusion-handbook/5-adverse-effects-of-transfusion. [Accessed 9 January 2022].

Rang, H. P., et al. (2011). *Rang and Dale's pharmacology* (7th ed.). Edinburgh: Elsevier Health Sciences, p. 366.

Routhier, N., & Tagalakis, V. (2021). Venous thromboembolism (VTE) prophylaxis. Symptoms, diagnosis and treatment. *BMJ Best Practice*. [Accessed 9 January 2022].

Western Sussex Hospitals NHS. (2014). Example of an insulin prescribing chart. Available at: www.diabetologists-abcd.org.uk/JBDS/Highly-commended_Chart_WS.pdf. [Accessed 9 January 2022].

Radiology

4

Content Outline

STATION 4.1: THE CHEST X-RAY

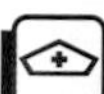

The Bleep Scenario

You are asked to review a 84 year old man who has been admitted to the ward with suspected pneumonia, with a CURB-65 score of 4. He has been commenced on appropriate intravenous (IV) antibiotics but his chest X-ray has not been reviewed.

INITIAL THOUGHTS

This man has been admitted and treated for pneumonia. However, his chest X-ray has only just been performed. You should review the chest X-ray urgently to ensure that the imaging fits with his current diagnosis and management plan. It may be helpful to compare images with previous imaging if available to identify new changes. You may need to reassess the patient if the imaging does not fit the working diagnosis.

INDICATIONS FOR A CHEST X-RAY

ACUTE

- Infection: pneumonia
- Chest pain: pneumothorax, aortic dissection
- Haemoptysis: suspected pulmonary embolism, malignancy, tuberculosis
- Acute dyspnoea: decompensated heart failure, pleural effusion, pulmonary oedema
- Trauma: pneumothorax, haemothorax, rib fractures

CHRONIC

- Follow-up imaging
- Chronic dyspnoea: heart failure, pleural effusion, interstitial lung disease, emphysema
- Other systemic illnesses that may have chest involvement

MISCELLANEOUS

- Checking the position of nasogastric tubes, endotracheal tubes and peripherally inserted central catheter (PICC) lines
- Perioperative and postoperative monitoring
- Monitoring in intensive care

REQUESTING RADIOLOGICAL IMAGING

WHAT TO INCLUDE

- Patient details
- Current observations (this will allow the radiologist to vet the urgency of the scan)
- Symptoms and examination findings
- Suspected diagnosis

WHAT NOT TO DO

- Write one diagnosis and a question mark to indicate query.
- Give no information on the history, diagnosis or observations.

DISCUSSING RADIOLOGICAL IMAGING WITH A RADIOLOGIST

When you discuss a scan with a radiologist your task is to attempt to convince them to take immediate action in order to accept your scan request, if it is required urgently. Remember, they have a long list of patients to prioritise, so it's in your best interest to make the conversation impactful and provide them with all the information that is required to make a safe and effective decision.

WHAT TO INCLUDE

- Patient's age
- Suspected diagnosis
- Observations

- Any significant risk factors in the past medical history that may escalate the speed in which the scan may be performed.

WHAT NOT TO DO

Do not attempt to discuss the scan without having a clear idea of why it is required urgently. This is a mistake that is often made, and can result in stressful interactions between the junior doctor and the radiologist. Ensure you have the relevant medical history of the patient and have information like recent blood results and imaging available as the radiologist may request these details as well.

INTERPRETING THE CHEST X-RAY

The following steps can be used to structure your interpretation of a chest radiograph.

STEP 1: ENSURING THE CHEST X-RAY IS APPROPRIATE FOR INTERPRETATION

1. Confirm patient details (name, date of birth, nhs number and address).
2. Assess image quality:
   - The medial aspect of each clavicle should be an equal distance from the spinous processes.
   - The spinous processes should be in a straight line with the vertebral bodies of the spine.
   - The lung apices, 5–6 anterior ribs and costophrenic angles should all be easily visible.
   - The edges of the ribs should be visible.
3. Projection:
   - Is this an anteroposterior (AP) or posteroanterior (PA) view? Usually, if it is an AP view, it will be labelled at the top.
4. Exposure:
   - The left hemidiaphragm should be visible.
   - Vertebrae should be visible behind the heart.

STEP 2: INTERPRETATION

1. Airway:
   - Assess for tracheal deviation.
   - Assess to see if the carina is visible.
   - Hilar structures:
     - The hilum consists of pulmonary vasculature, major bronchi and the lymph nodes.
     - The size of the hilum varies between individuals, but as a general rule, hilar asymmetry may indicate underlying malignancy.
2. Breathing:
   - Divide the lungs into three zones and assess them for lung pathology.
   - Inspect the pleura: these are generally not visible on a normal chest X-ray, but may become apparent with pleural thickening, for instance, in the case of mesothelioma.
3. Cardiac assessment:
   - Inspect the heart – in a normal patient, this would occupy no greater a ratio than 50% of the thoracic width.
4. Diaphragm:
   - Look at the diaphragm and costophrenic angles. You may also be able to see the gastric bubble or evidence of subdiaphragmatic air, i.e. pneumoperitoneum in cases of perforation.
5. Other features:
   - Lines/electrocardiogram (ECG) electrodes/permanent pacemaker.
6. Compare with previous imaging.

VIEWS OF THE CHEST X-RAY

There are many angles at which a chest X-ray could be performed, but the three main views are PA, AP and lateral (Fig. 4.1).

THE TECHNICALITIES

The Posteroanterior View

- The PA view is performed when the patient is standing, upon full inspiration.
- The PA view allows clear visualisation of the mediastinal cavity, the lungs, great vessels and bony cavities (Fig. 4.2).

The Anteroposterior View

- The AP view is often used for patients who are acutely ill and are therefore difficult to transport to the chest X-ray machine. These views are often done by portable X-ray.
- Because the AP view is technically challenging, it is inferior to the PA view in terms of interpretation:
  - The heart appears larger (the cardiothoracic ratio is approximately 50%).
  - The scapulae are not retracted, and therefore appear more prominent.

The Lateral View

- The patient is erect, and the image is taken from the left lateral position.
- The lateral view is a useful adjunct to the PA view as it provides greater coverage of the thoracic area. This becomes particularly useful in the context of visualising the size of lung lesions.

On reviewing the chest X-ray, you find the image (Fig. 4.3) confirms the diagnosis of pneumonia as it shows consolidation. You can now proceed with clinical reassessment of the patient, knowing the imaging confirms the suspected diagnosis.

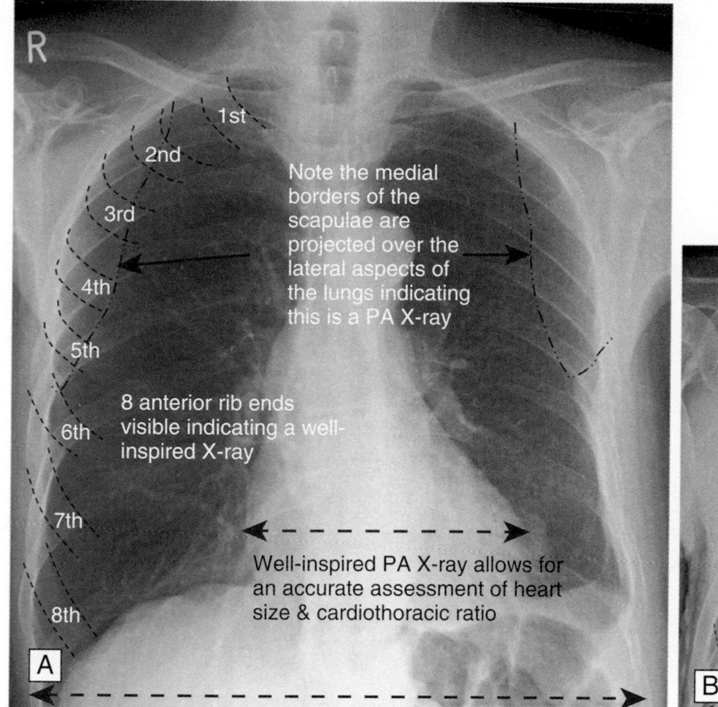

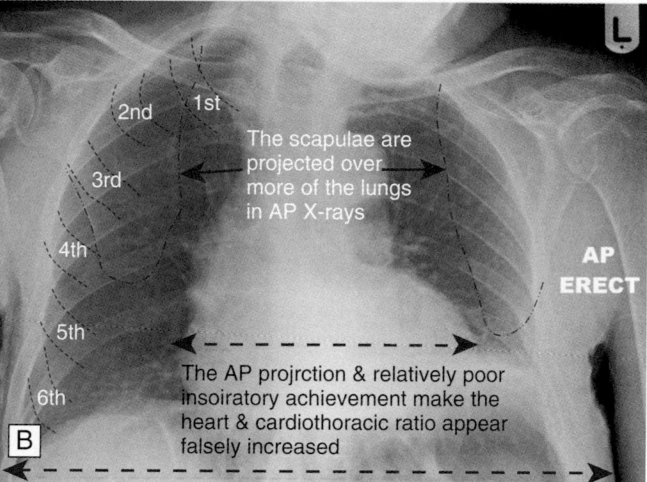

Fig. 4.1 These two chest X-rays are from the same patient. (A) A well-inspired posteroanterior (PA) chest X-ray. (B) A less well (but still adequately)-inspired anteroposterior (AP) X-ray. Notice the dramatic effect of the projection and degree of inspiration on the apparent heart size. Also note the amount of the scapulae which is projected over the lungs in each projection.

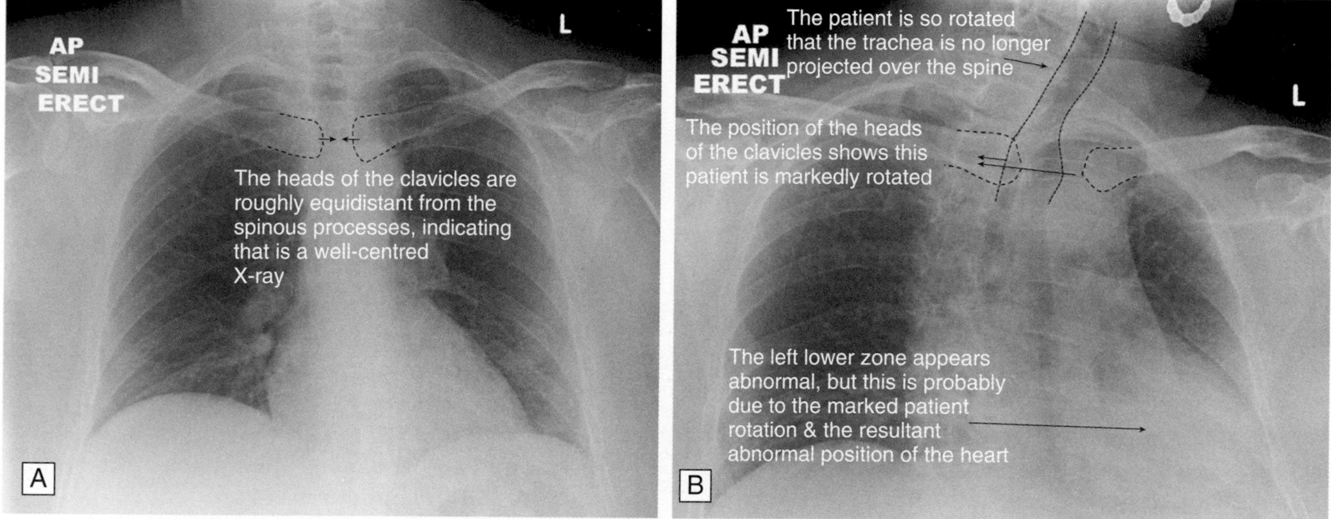

Fig. 4.2 These two X-rays are from the same patient. (A) The patient is well centred. (B) The patient is markedly rotated, which has resulted in apparent left lower zone consolidation. This appearance is, however, probably caused by the abnormally positioned cardiac shadow, and a repeat X-ray with the patient well centred should be obtained. AP, anteroposterior.

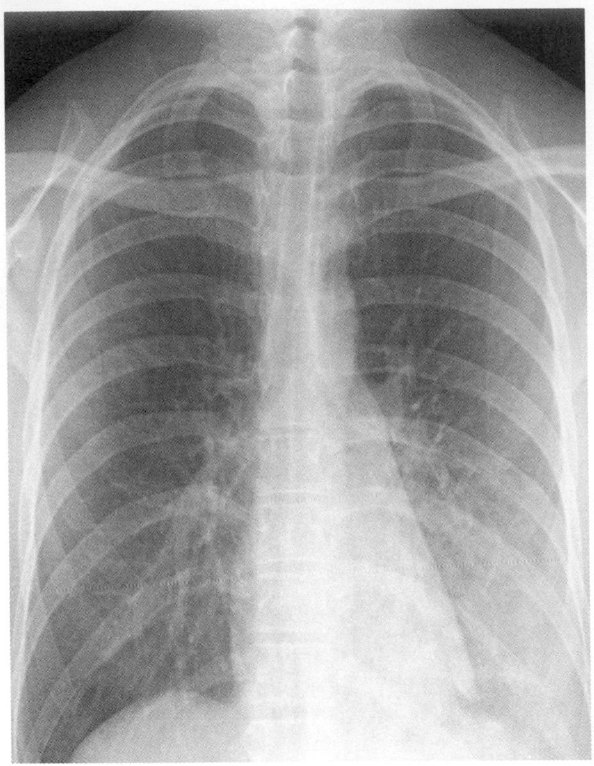

Fig. 4.3 An example of pneumonia.

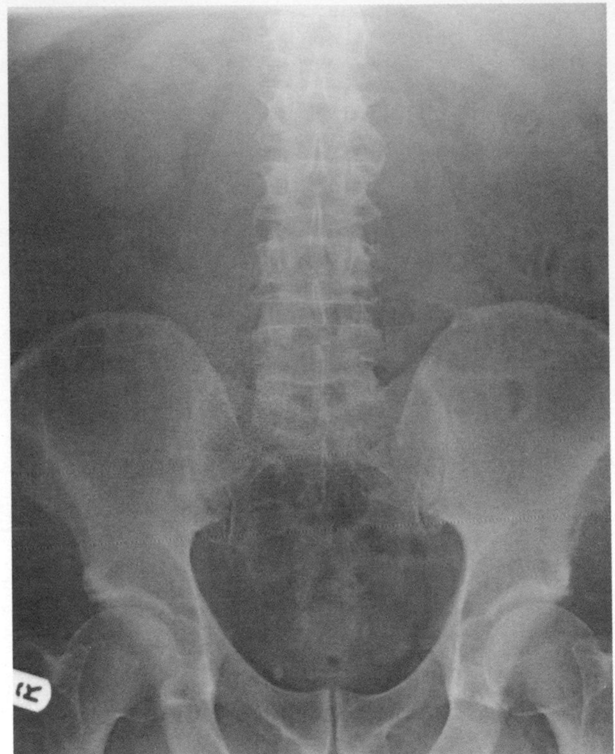

Fig. 4.4 A normal abdominal X-ray.

STATION 4.2: THE ABDOMINAL X-RAY

 The Bleep Scenario

You are asked to review an abdominal X-ray of an 86 year old man on the ward who has not passed stools for the past 3 days. This is a concern that he might have bowel obstruction.

INITIAL THOUGHTS

It is clear that the patient is suffering from constipation. What needs to be determined is if there is evidence of serious pathology such as obstruction. A review of the patient's drug chart and documented intake should be done. You should consider the abdominal imaging alongside the clinical picture; if the imaging is concerning, you should review the patient.

INDICATIONS FOR THE ABDOMINAL X-RAY

Considering these will help guide you more efficiently to a diagnosis. Note that abdominal X-rays are being used increasingly less frequently in favour of CT scans.

- Clinical symptoms of bowel obstruction
- Bowel ischaemia
- Acute exacerbation of inflammatory bowel disease (e.g. toxic megacolon)
- Foreign body ingestion
- Suspected perforation

INTERPRETING THE ABDOMINAL X-RAY

STEP 1: ENSURING THE ABDOMINAL X-RAY IS APPROPRIATE FOR INTERPRETATION

1. Confirm patient details (name, date of birth, NHS number and address).
2. Assess image quality:
   - The whole of the abdomen should be visible, from the diaphragm to the symphysis pubis and inguinal orifices
3. Projection:
   - Abdominal X-rays are often taken in the anterior–posterior supine projection.

THE STOMACH

- You can sometimes visualise the stomach in the left upper quadrant of the abdomen.
- The lowest point of the stomach crosses the midline.

THE SMALL BOWEL

- The small bowel stretches from the duodenum to the terminal ileum and is centrally placed in the abdomen.

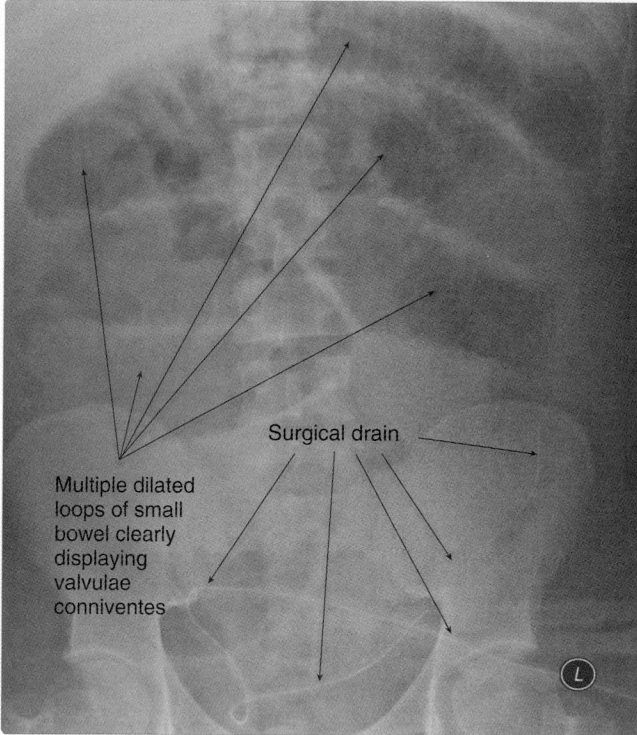

Fig. 4.5 Abdominal X-ray demonstrates small-bowel obstruction.

- The thin mucosal folds in the small intestine are called valvulae conniventes. These folds cross the full circumference of the small bowel.
- In the event of small-bowel obstruction, the valvulae conniventes appear more prominent and in conjunction with dilated loops of bowel are diagnostic of this condition (Fig. 4.5).
- Gas and air are of a lower density than in the other abdominal structures, so will appear dark on the X-ray.
- When analysing the abdominal X-ray, it is imperative to know the upper limits of diameter for the small and large bowels:
  - 3 cm for the small bowel
  - 6 cm for the large bowel
  - 9 cm for the caecum.

THE LARGE BOWEL

- In general, the large bowel tends to be quite clearly visualised.
- The longitudinal muscles of the large intestine are called taenia coli and, together with the circular muscles, form folds called haustrations.
- The caecum is the largest part of the large intestine. You can often visualise faeces here (Fig. 4.6).

On reviewing the abdominal X-ray, you find the image (Fig. 4.5) conthe diagnosis of small bowel obstruction. You can now proceed with clinical reassessment of the patient, knowing the imaging confirms the suspected diagnosis.

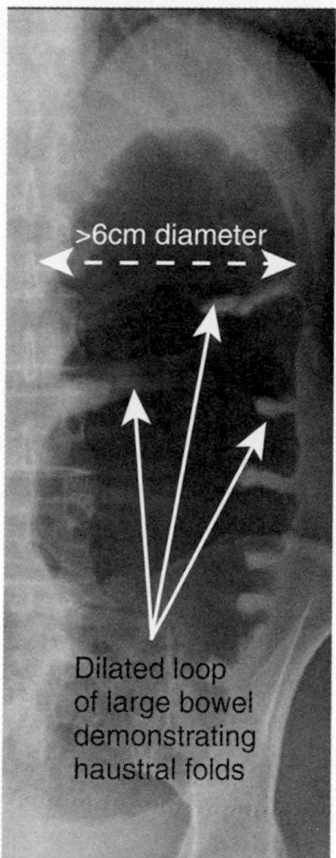

Fig. 4.6 An example of large bowel obstruction.

STATION 4.3: THE CT HEAD

The Bleep Scenario

An 18 year old man has presented to accident and emergency after a traumatic fall from his motorcycle. He appears confused and is mumbling. His eyes open spontaneously and he is able to obey commands. His observations are otherwise stable. A computed tomography (CT) head has been performed due to the confusion. You are asked to review the imaging.

INITIAL THOUGHTS

From the history, you can be fairly certain that this patient has acquired a traumatic head injury. From a radiological standpoint, the main consideration would be whether or not he requires an urgent CT head.

INDICATIONS FOR A CT HEAD

INDICATIONS FOR IMMEDIATE CT HEAD IN ACUTE HEAD INJURY

- Glasgow Coma Scale (GCS) <13
- GCS <15 at 2 hours after injury
- Suspected open or depressed skull fracture
- Signs of a basal skull fracture
- Posttraumatic seizure
- Focal neurological deficit
- More than one episode of vomiting after head injury

INDICATIONS FOR CT HEAD WITHIN 8 HOURS (ASSUMING THAT NONE OF THE ABOVE CRITERIA WERE PRESENT)

- Age >65 years
- History of bleeding or clotting disorder

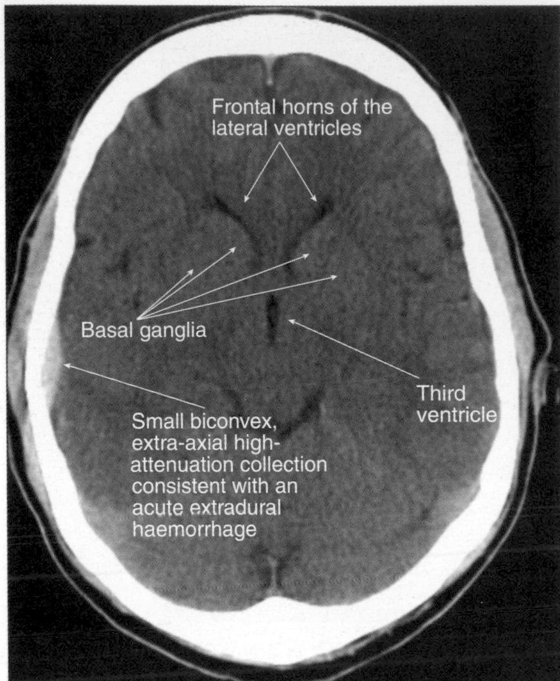

Fig. 4.7 Acute extradural haemorrhage.

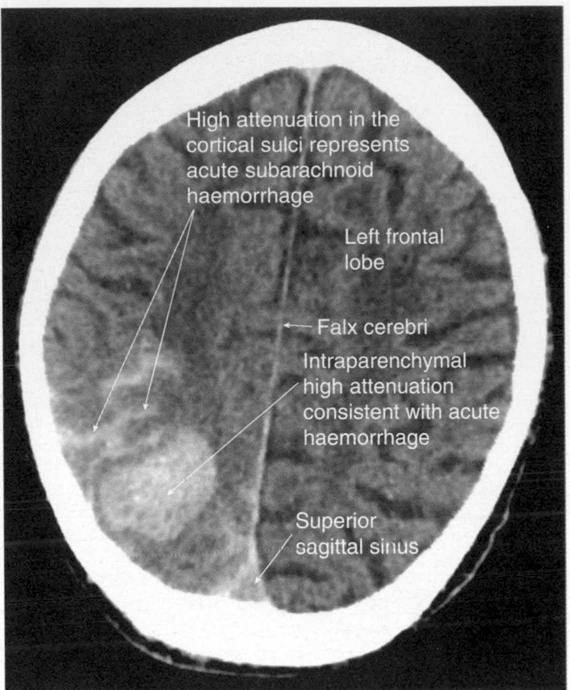

Fig. 4.8 Acute subarachnoid haemorrhage.

- A dangerous mechanism of injury present
- More than 30 minutes of retrograde amnesia of events immediately before the head injury

OTHER INDICATIONS

- Any history or examination findings indicating raised intracranial pressure
- Meningitis
- Encephalitis
- Cerebral infarction

INTERPRETING THE CT HEAD

Using a systematic approach for interpretation of the CT head will allow you to feel more confident and comprehensive in your assessment (Figs 4.7 and 4.8).

ASSESS THE BONY STRUCTURES

- Check for any signs of fractures.
- Oedematous soft tissue and air in the mastoid and paranasal sinuses may be indications of a concurrent fracture.

EXTRA-AXIAL/OUTSIDE THE BRAIN

- Assess for any signs of bleeding: extradural, subdural or epidural haematoma.
- Inspect the cisterns.

INTRA-AXIAL/WITHIN THE BRAIN TISSUE

- Check for symmetry in the cerebral tissue.
- Intraparenchymal haemorrhage or intraventricular haemorrhage.
- Assess for hypodensity (oedema, infarction and air) and hyperdensity (blood or calcification).
- Look for tumours and abscesses.

ASSESS THE VENTRICLES

- Assess for signs of haemorrhage in the ventricles.
- Assess for midline shift.

On reviewing the CT, you find the image (Fig. 4.7) confirms the diagnosis of extradural haemorrhage. You can now procteed with clinical reassessment of the patient, knowing the imaging confirms the suspected diagnosis.

- Remember CT heads will be reported by a radiologist, but you should get into the habit of looking at them to help with decision making for patients and you can ask seniors within your own team for help too.
- Other examples of pathological findings can be seen in Fig. 4.9.

In the remaining tables, we have summarised investigations you might be asked to undertake within each specialty.

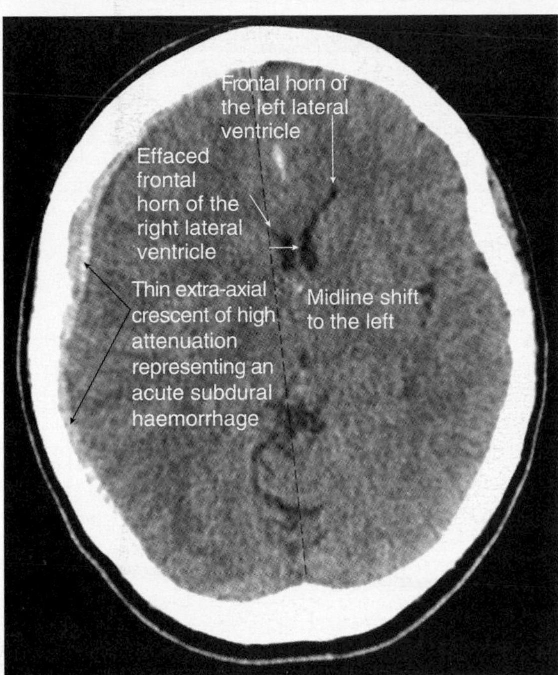

Fig. 4.9 Acute subdural haemorrhage.

Cardiology

Chest X-ray
Indications: suspected heart failure

Echocardiogram
Indications: valvular problems, determining the ejection fraction and visualising the cardiac chambers in case of thrombosis

Angiogram
Indications: visualisation of the coronary arteries and therapeutic action if necessary

Stress echocardiogram
Indications: suspected coronary disease

Cardiac magnetic resonance imaging (MRI)
Indications: this test is used for pathologies that require detailed imaging of the cardiac muscle, e.g. cardiomyopathy, atrial myxoma, cardiac myocarditis

Respiratory

Chest X-ray
To visualise the lungs in any respiratory pathology

Computed tomography pulmonary angiogram (CTPA)
The diagnosis of pulmonary embolism

Computed tomography of the thorax, abdomen and pelvis (CT TAP)
Visualisation of suspected malignancy or abscess

High-resolution computed tomography (HRCT)
For enhanced visualisation of the lung tissue in interstitial lung disease and bronchiectasis

Gastroenterology

Abdominal X-ray
To visualise the abdominal cavity in certain clinical presentations such as suspected bowel ischaemia or obstruction

Abdominal ultrasound
To visualise the liver and biliary tree, especially in the context of ascites and hepatic failure

Endoscopy
Visualisation of the upper gastrointestinal tract

Colonoscopy
Visualisation of the lower gastrointestinal tract

Computed tomography of the thorax, abdomen and pelvis (CT TAP)
Visualisation of suspected malignancy or abscess

Neurology

Computed tomography (CT) head
First-line imaging modality for cerebral infarction

Magnetic resonance imaging (MRI) with diffusion-weighted imaging
Gold-standard imaging for cerebral infarction; generally performed in addition to the CT head for clearer visualisation of the cerebral tissue

Carotid Doppler ultrasound
To be requested for all patients presenting with a suspected diagnosis of transient ischaemic attack or stroke

Renal Medicine

Abdominal X-ray
To visualise the renal tract and potential obstructive pathology

Renal ultrasound
To visualise the renal tract and any abnormalities

Computed tomography of the thorax, abdomen and pelvis (CT TAP)
If suspecting renal cell carcinoma

Radionuclide scanning
For detailed visualisation of multiple pathologies

Renal angiography
To visualise the renal vessels in the case of suspected vascular abnormalities

General Surgery

Abdominal X-ray
For suspicion of an abdominal mass or obstruction

Abdominal ultrasound
For visualisation of the biliary tree

Computed tomography (CT) abdomen
In the case of an abscess, suspected malignancy or for further visualisation of the abdominal structures

Magnetic resonance cholangiopancreatography (MRCP)
For detailed imaging of the biliary tree

Endoscopic retrograde cholangiopancreatography (ERCP)
For therapeutic benefit in biliary obstruction

Endoscopy

Colonoscopy

Vascular Surgery

Duplex ultrasound
The first-line investigation for peripheral vascular disease

Angiography
Gold-standard imaging and therapeutic modality for peripheral vascular disease

CT angiogram
Second-line imaging investigation for peripheral vascular disease when detailed imaging is required before proceeding to further intervention

Magnetic resonance angiogram
If further detail past the point of the computed tomography (CT) scan is required

Urology

X-ray of the kidneys, ureters and bladder (XR KUB)
To ascertain the presence of a ureteric stone

Computed tomography (CT) KUB
As a second line to the X-ray commonly used in the case of renal colic

Intravenous pyelogram
To view the ureteric tree in detail

Micturating cystourethrogram
To visualise the bladder on micturition in patients with voiding difficulties

Abdominal ultrasound

Transrectal ultrasound with prostate biopsy

Otolaryngology and Maxillofacial Surgery

X-ray of the skull
To visualise the skull and paranasal sinuses

X-ray of the orbit
In the case of orbital trauma

Orthopantomogram (OPG)
For visualisation of the jaws and teeth in maxillofacial trauma)

Ultrasound neck/thyroid/ salivary glands
For detailed tissue anatomy of these structures

CT head and neck
For visualisation of the tissue in depth
or CT facial bones alongside CT head
In cases of trauma

Magnetic resonance imaging (MRI) head and neck
For further visualisation of the tissue in depth at a level greater than computed tomography (CT)

Fine-needle aspiration (FNA) biopsy under ultrasound guidance
In suspected malignancy of thyroid, parathyroid or salivary glands

Positron emission tomography (PET) scan
For assessment of glucose uptake in suspected malignancy

FURTHER READING

Dick, E. (2000). Chest X rays made easy. *BMJ*, *321*, 0009316.

Marcus, A., Marcus, H., & Kirollos, R. (2013). Interpreting head computed tomography scans. *British Medical Journal*, *346*, f871.

NICE. (2014). *Algorithm for head injury*. Available at: www.nice.org.uk/guidance/cg176/resources/imaging-algorithm-pdf-498950893. [Accessed 9 January 2022].

Pezzotti, W. (2014). Chest X-ray interpretation. *Nursing*, *44*(1), 40–47.

Royal College of Radiologists. (2016). *Indications for plain abdominal films from the emergency department*. Available at: www.rcr.ac.uk/audit/indications-plain-abdominal-films-emergency-department. [Accessed 9 January 2022].

Wong, J. J., & Curtis, J. (2012). Interpreting the chest radiograph. *British Medical Journal*, *344*, e988.

Wong, J., Patel, L., & Curtis, J. (2012). Interpreting abdominal radiographs. *British Medical Journal*, *345*, e5375.

Recognition and Assessment of the Acutely Unwell Patient

5

Content Outline

STATION 5.1: ASSESSMENT AND RESUSCITATION

The Bleep Scenario

A 47 year old woman has been admitted this morning to the medical ward with pneumonia, and started on IV antibiotics. She has increasingly become more short of breath, and now has saturations of 80% despite being on a high flow oxygen mask. You are asked to review her urgently.

One of the most daunting aspects of going on call for the first time is dealing with critically ill patients. There are fewer staff overnight and your seniors may not always be able to come to your assistance immediately.

The National Early Warning Score (NEWS) is used as a prompt for the nursing staff to escalate to a doctor; however, these can be falsely reassuring, especially in otherwise fit and well young adults. On the other hand, a high NEWS does not always mean the patient is critically unwell, as you may have a man with chronic obstructive pulmonary disease (COPD) who normally tolerates lower oxygen saturation, has a high respiratory rate and is always on oxygen. NEWS-2 is now widely used as a result, and this takes into account patients such as the COPD patient.

In addition, if the patient is critically unwell, you are unlikely to get a full history from them. So, it is paramount that you follow a systematic approach whenever you are asked to review a patient. Following the ABCDE system, described below, will help you recognise any critically ill patient and formulate a management plan. You can tailor your ABCDE assessment based on your patient.

It is important to assess each component thoroughly and manage problems as you identify them.

A – AIRWAY

You know the airway is patent and safe when the patient is talking in full sentences with ease. Listen for added noise. Is there stridor? Is the patient gurgling? Is he snoring? All these signs suggest that the airway may be compromised.

Manoeuvres such as a chin lift or a jaw thrust are useful. In addition, simple airway adjuncts such as a nasopharyngeal or oropharyngeal airway can be tried, with the former being better tolerated in conscious patients. If your patient is tolerating an oropharyngeal airway, his Glasgow Coma Scale (GCS) score is unlikely to be normal.

If, despite the simple manoeuvres and adjuncts, the airway is obstructed, call the crash team (dial 2222), as you will get a team with members capable of managing the airway quickly. Apply 15 L/minute oxygen via a non-rebreather (NRB) mask if the patient is breathing adequately or assist ventilation with a self-inflating bag and mask, or a supraglottic airway, if respiratory effort is poor.

Cervical spine immobilisation is crucial, if cervical spine injury is suspected, before airway manipulation.

B – BREATHING

Ventilation and oxygenation are key once you have addressed the airway. Assessing the patient from the end of the bed will give you a good idea of the work of breathing. What is the respiratory rate? Is there pursed-lip breathing? Is the patient using accessory neck and abdominal muscles? All these suggest increased work of breathing, with an increased respiratory rate being a sensitive marker of critical illness.

Place a pulse oximeter on the patient and monitor the oxygen saturations. A target of 94–98% is recommended in patients who do not have irreversible obstructive or severe restrictive lung disease.

Oxygen at 15 L/minute through an NRB should give a fraction of inspired oxygen (FiO_2) of 0.6–0.8, so if the patient has low oxygen saturations despite having three to four times the amount of oxygen in room air (0.21), you must escalate to a senior as additional non-invasive or invasive ventilation may be beneficial.

Importantly, a thorough respiratory exam is vital. An arterial blood gas (ABG) must be done to assess the adequacy of gas exchange and a portable chest X-ray (CXR) may help to diagnose the pathology.

C – CIRCULATION

Yet again, end-of-bed observations can give you a good idea. Is the patient pale? Clammy? Does he look dry or peripherally shut down? Assess hydration status as part of your circulation assessment. Monitor the urine output and assess the fluid balance. Have a feel of the patient's hands, check the capillary refill time, blood pressure, heart rate and auscultate the heart. If there are signs of shock, do a straight-leg raise and assess fluid responsiveness. Consider, giving a fluid bolus. If so, you can always repeat the bolus if the patient is fluid-responsive. However, be cautious in patients with heart failure as they may develop pulmonary oedema. Fluid loading in non-fluid-responsive patients is like an overdose.

Get intravenous (IV) access via a large-bore cannula and take blood samples, particularly full blood count (FBC) and urea and electrolytes (U&Es). A venous gas at this point will give you immediate results to guide your treatment. If there is no response to fluids and the blood pressure remains low, involve the critical care team early to assess the suitability for vasopressors. If you suspect a bleed, get a group-and-save sample and call for help early. A cross-matched sample should be available within 40 minutes and every department will have access to emergency O-negative blood if you need blood before that.

Get an electrocardiogram (ECG) to exclude arrhythmias and cardiac ischaemia. Altered mental state may also be due to impaired circulation.

D – DISABILITY

The neurological status of a patient can explain problems you notice with the airway, breathing or circulation. Assessing the GCS or checking AVPU (alert, verbal, pain, unresponsive) is essential. In addition, check the pupils are equal and reactive. Unequal or fixed pupils on examination may warrant a computed tomography (CT) head. Pinpoint pupils are often, but not always, suggestive of opiate toxicity, thus may also warrant a CT head. A full neurological exam may be necessary based on your patient's presentation. As always, check the glucose and temperature.

E – EXPOSURE

Exposing the patient may reveal the cause of altered ABCD. There may be blood or melaena under the sheets or there may be an extensive purpuric or urticarial rash. Examine the abdomen and calves. Call the surgical team if the abdomen is peritonitic.

Input from the specialist teams early will help with overall patient care. Escalation to critical care may be necessary based on your ABCDE assessment. However, it may not always be in the best interest of the patient.

STATION 5.2: CARDIAC ARREST

The Bleep Scenario

A cardiac arrest call is put out whilst you are on your medical on call. You run to the scene. 'Adult cardiac arrest, ward 22. Adult cardiac arrest, ward 22.'

DEFINITION

Cardiac arrest is the abrupt loss of heart function in a person who may or may not have diagnosed heart disease.

INITIAL THOUGHTS

As a member of the crash team, you should head over to ward 22 immediately. You may be the first person to arrive there. Think about how to give CPR, what else you can do as part of the team and how to ask for help. On your way there, think through the steps of the BLS or ALS protocols you are familiar with.

ASSESSMENT AND RESUSCITATION

Check for any danger before approaching the patient. If you are the first person to arrive, check for a response and signs of life. If the patient is unresponsive with no signs of life or without normal respiratory effort for up to 10 seconds, declare a cardiac arrest and start cardiopulmonary resuscitation (CPR) based on the algorithm shown in Fig. 5.1. CPR must be at a rate of 100–120 compressions per minute at a depth of 5–6 cm. Defibrillator pads must be attached as soon as possible with minimal disruption to CPR. A self-inflating bag valve mask should be used to deliver breaths until a definitive airway is established. Once a 2-minutes cycle of CPR has been completed, pause for a rhythm check.

Rhythm recognition is of the utmost importance but most modern defibrillators can be switched to automated mode to help interpret the rhythm and prompt giving a shock. The Resuscitation Council

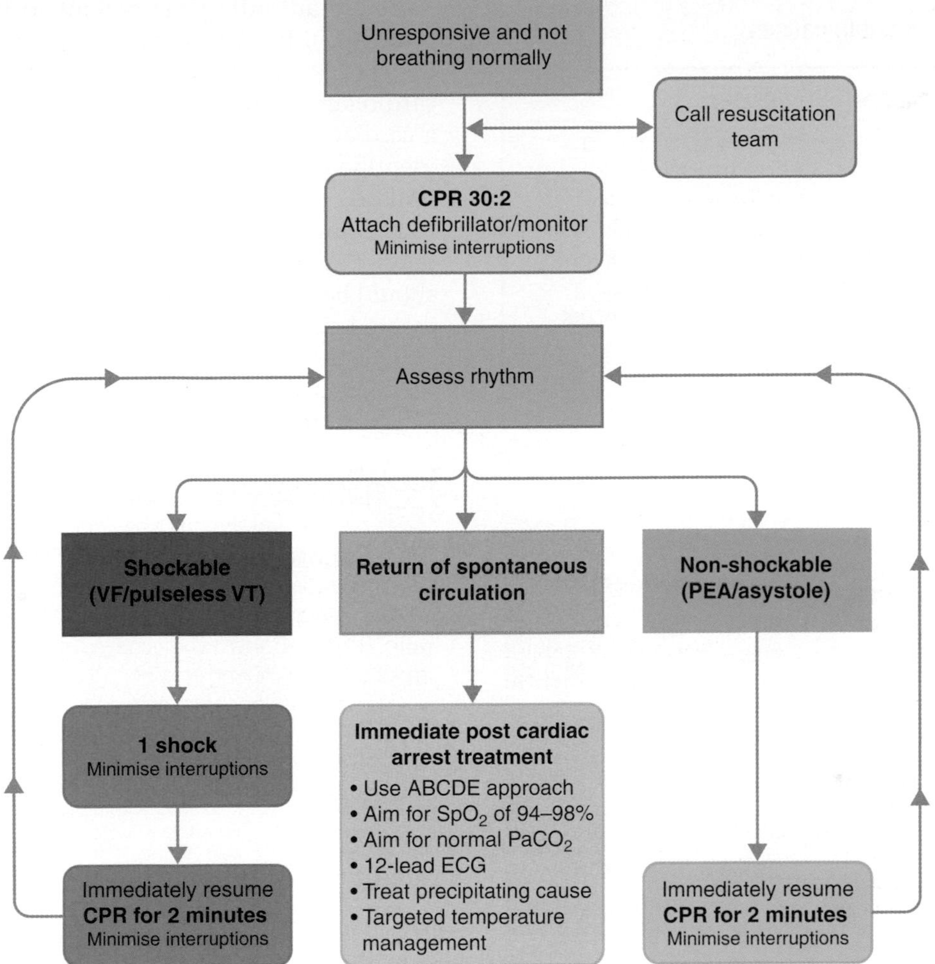

Fig. 5.1 Advanced Life Support algorithm. CPR, cardiopulmonary resuscitation; ECG, electrocardiogram; PEA, pulseless electrical activity; VF, ventricular fibrillation; VT, ventricular tachycardia. (Source: Resuscitation Council UK (2021) *Advanced life support 2021 guidelines*. Available at: https://www.resus.org.uk/library/2021-resuscitation-guidelines/adult-advanced-life-support-guidelines).

UK (RC UK) suggests ALS-trained staff should use the manual mode. Energy levels for biphasic shocking, for patients in ventricular fibrillation (VF) and pulseless ventricular tachycardia (pVT), must be set at 150 Joules for an adult.

Once more members of the crash team have arrived, roles must be assigned based on experience and expertise. This does not mean the consultant is always the leader of the cardiac arrest team. There may be members within the team who deal with these scenarios more frequently and so wish to take the lead. Commonly, the anaesthetic team takes charge of the airway and may lead the team.

Once a supraglottic airway or an endotracheal tube is inserted, uninterrupted CPR can be commenced. However, with supraglottic airways, there may be a risk of aspiration, so inserting a suction catheter via the port provided may be beneficial. Teamwork is essential during CPR. Rotating staff doing chest compressions every 2 minutes reduces ineffective compressions.

Delegating members of the team to obtain IV or intraosseous access, take blood samples, administer drugs (Box 5.1) and keep track of time is vital. IV adrenaline 1 mg (10 mL of 1:10,000) must be given as soon as possible in pulseless electrical activity (PEA) and asystole. In cases of VF and pVT, 1 mg adrenaline is given after the third shock along with IV amiodarone 300 mg. If there are sufficient team members available, a scribe, noting time and events, will help with documentation later on.

Box 5.1 During cardiopulmonary resuscitation (CPR)

- Ensure high-quality chest compressions
- Minimise interruptions to compressions
- Give oxygen
- Use waveform capnography
- Carry out continuous compressions when advanced airway is in place
- Create vascular access (intravenous or intraosseous)
- Give adrenaline every 3–5 minutes
- Give amiodarone after three and five shocks (shockable rhythms)

Box 5.2 Treat reversible causes

TREAT REVERSIBLE CAUSES	CONSIDER
• Hypoxia • Hypovolaemia • Hypo-/hyperkalaemia/ metabolic • Hypothermia • Thrombosis – coronary or pulmonary • Tension pneumothorax • Tamponade – cardiac • Toxins	• Ultrasound imaging • Mechanical chest compression to facilitate transfer/treatment • Coronary angiography and percutaneous coronary intervention • Extracorporeal cardiopulmonary resuscitation

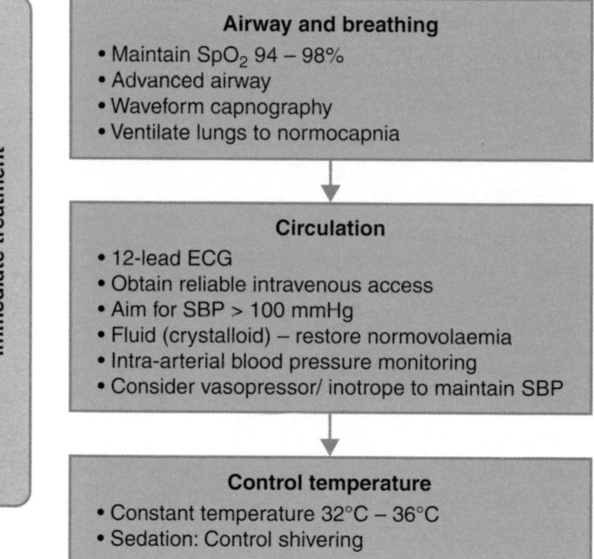

Fig. 5.2 Adult post resuscitation care. (Source: Resuscitation Council UK (2021) *Advanced life support 2021 guidelines.* Available at: https://www.resus.org.uk/sites/default/files/2021-04/Adult%20Post%20Resuscitation%20Care%20Algorithm%202021.pdf).

Once the initial management has begun, it is important to get the background of the patient and consider the reversible causes (Box 5.2). Ultrasound imaging may not always be possible due to the lack of availability of equipment or staff adequately trained to image and interpret the images.

ESCALATION

If there is a return of spontaneous circulation, a decision about the next step in management must be made. RC UK has guidelines on postarrest management (Fig. 5.2). Maintaining oxygenation is paramount and this may be via an endotracheal tube if respiratory effort is insufficient. Capnography must be attached and the anaesthetic team may insert an arterial line for invasive blood pressure monitoring and start peripheral vasopressors.

Before admitting the patient to the intensive care unit (ICU), RC UK suggests identifying the cause of the cardiac arrest. Discussion with the interventional cardiology team is essential if there is ST elevation or a cardiac cause is suspected. If a non-cardiac cause is identified, then the patient must be managed and optimised on ICU.

It is important that the cardiac arrest team have a debrief at the earliest opportunity. The patient's family should be informed and all the events should be documented clearly in the patient's notes.

STATION 5.3: RESPIRATORY FAILURE

The Bleep Scenario

A 35 year old woman has been admitted to the general medical ward with peripheral weakness and difficulty breathing. She has dropped her oxygen saturations despite being on 4 litres of oxygen via nasal cannula. She has been diagnosed with Guillain–Barré syndrome (GBS) and has been commenced on immunoglobulins.

Her current observations are: heart rate (HR) 96 bpm, blood pressure (BP) 110/70 mmHg, respiratory rate (RR) 28 breaths per minute, SpO_2 85% on 4 L oxygen and temperature 37°C. You are asked to review her.

DEFINITION

Respiratory failure refers to inadequate gas exchange by the respiratory system.

INITIAL THOUGHTS

This patient has GBS: ascending paralysis can progress to affect the respiratory muscles. As a consequence, respiratory effort may become suboptimal. She is normally otherwise fit and well, so there should be no reason for her to have oxygen saturations lower than normal.

Risk factors for respiratory failure include respiratory pathology, cardiac failure, hypercoagulable states, trauma, infection, drug toxicity or musculoskeletal disorders.

DIFFERENTIAL DIAGNOSIS

- Respiratory: pneumonia, exacerbation of COPD, pulmonary embolism, atelectasis, pulmonary fibrosis or pulmonary oedema
- Musculoskeletal: neuromuscular or skeletal disorders
- Systemic: drug toxicity, botulism

INITIAL INSTRUCTIONS OVER PHONE

Ask the referrer to switch the patient to 15 L/minute oxygen via an NRB mask and request that the patient is sat upright to see if this helps with breathing. In addition, ask if they obtain IV access and take bloods.

ASSESSMENT AND RESUSCITATION

- End-of-bed assessment: the patient appears to be in respiratory distress with laboured breathing.
- Airway: patent; the patient is struggling to complete her sentences.
- Breathing: RR 28, shallow breaths. SpO_2 89% on 15 L/minute oxygen via an NRB mask. On auscultation, there is reduced air entry throughout. Percussion is resonant.
  - Call for help immediately: dial 2222.
  - Check the patient's forced vital capacity (FVC).
  - ABG: pH 7.26, PCO_2 9.5 kPa, PPO_2 7.0 kPa, HCO_3^- 25 mmol/L (type 2 respiratory failure).
- Circulation: HR 96 bpm, regular. BP 110/70 mmHg, heart sounds (HS) I + II + 0. Jugular venous pressure (JVP) is normal. Capillary refill time (CRT) 2 s.
- Disability: GCS 15/15, pupils equal and reactive to light (PEARL), temperature 37°C, capillary blood glucose (CBG) 8 mmol/L. Reduced power, compared to normal, noted in all four limbs.
- Exposure: abdomen is soft and non-tender. Normal bowel sounds. Calves are unremarkable.

INITIAL INVESTIGATIONS

- Haematology: FBC (inflammation)
- Biochemistry: U&Es and C-reactive protein (CRP: inflammation)
- Microbiology: blood cultures, stool sample and urine dip (infection)
- Radiology: portable CXR (cardiorespiratory pathology)

MAKING A DIAGNOSIS

Type 1 respiratory failure refers to a low arterial oxygen partial pressure ($PaO_2 < 8$ kPa), whilst type 2 refers to low oxygen and high carbon dioxide partial pressures ($PaCO_2 > 6$ kPa) in arterial blood. Broadly speaking, type 1 failure is due to disease that damages lung tissue and type 2 is due to inadequate alveolar ventilation from other causes. However, there may be considerable overlap.

Respiratory failure may present with dyspnoea, tachypnoea, agitation, cyanosis, signs of airway obstruction or confusion progressing to feeble respiratory efforts and unconsciousness

MANAGEMENT

Oxygen saturations of 87% on high-flow oxygen is alarming and you must call for help immediately. This may include dialling 2222 and calling the Emergency Medical Response Team (EMRT).

This patient has GBS and is therefore more likely to have type 2 respiratory failure, as shown on her ABG. Her oxygenation isn't improving despite having a NRB mask that can deliver FiO_2 of 0.6–0.8. Non-invasive ventilation should be tried before intubation whenever possible. This patient will require bilevel positive airway pressure ventilation to remove the carbon dioxide. Continuous positive airway pressure (CPAP) ventilation would have been suitable if there was type 1 respiratory failure.

 **Clinical Tip**

A chest x-ray is mandatory, if not already done, before starting non-invasive or mechanical ventilation as pneumothoraces can worsen.

Type 2 respiratory failure can also be seen in a chronic carbon dioxide retainer. These patients often compensate for a high carbon dioxide by having higher than normal bicarbonate levels. As long as the pH is between 7.35 and 7.45, such patients with high carbon dioxide readings do not require bilevel ventilation, and controlled oxygen therapy on the ward may be sufficient. However, GBS can rapidly progress; a FVC of less than 15 mL/kg or less than 30% predicted or a rising PCO_2 on ABG is often a strong indicator for mechanical ventilation.

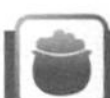 **Clinical Tip**

Serial FVC readings are recommended in GBS to monitor progression of weakness of respiratory muscles.

ESCALATION

An ABG result suggestive of type 1 or type 2 respiratory failure requires escalation. Contact your medical registrar first. The critical care team should also be informed if there is rapidly reducing FVC/forced expiratory volume in 1 s (FEV_1), bulbar dysfunction, evolving pneumonia or respiratory failure.

STATION 5.4: HAEMORRHAGE

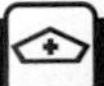 **The Bleep Scenario**

A 40 year old man has been admitted to the gastroenterology ward with haematemesis, tachycardia and hypotension. The patient had an endoscopy last week that showed multiple gastric and duodenal ulcers.

His observations are: HR 120 bpm, BP 84/50 mmHg, RR 28 breaths per minute, SpO_2 93% on room air and temperature 37.6°C. You are asked to review him.

DEFINITION

A haemorrhage is an escape of blood from a ruptured blood vessel.

INITIAL THOUGHTS

The most important step of any ongoing bleeding is to stop the bleeding at its source. However, before definitive endoscopic or surgical management, optimally resuscitating the patient is paramount.

DIFFERENTIAL DIAGNOSIS

- Gastrointestinal: peptic ulcer disease, oesophageal varices, Mallory–Weiss tear or Boerhaave's syndrome
- Haematological: coagulopathy, thrombocytopenia

INITIAL INSTRUCTIONS OVER PHONE

Ask the referrer to consider supplementary oxygen, obtain IV access with two large-bore cannulae, take bloods, commence fluid resuscitation and check if there is cross-matched blood for this patient.

ASSESSMENT AND RESUSCITATION

- End-of-bed assessment: the patient looks pale and clammy. He is drowsy but rousable.
- Airway: patent.
- Breathing: RR 30 breaths per minute, SpO_2 93% on room air. On auscultation, there are vesicular breath sounds with good air entry bilaterally.
  - Administer 15 L/minute oxygen via an NRB mask. Aim for oxygen saturations of 94–98%.
- Circulation: his hands are clammy. CRT > 3 s. HR 120 bpm, regular. BP 80/60 mmHg, JVP normal, HS I + II + 0.
  - Administer 500 mL crystalloid fluids stat to resuscitate the patient.
- Disability: GCS 14/15 (E3V5M6), PEARL, temperature 37°C, CBG 8.4 mmol/L.
- Exposure: abdomen is tense and generally tender. Normal bowel sounds. No other source of bleeding was identified.

 Clinical Tip

The severity of the patient's bleeding can be estimated based on their vital signs, mental status and urine output. This patient is likely to have had a significant bleed, losing at least 30% of their circulatory volume.

INITIAL INVESTIGATIONS

- Haematology: FBC or venous blood gas (to determine haemoglobin levels), coagulation screen (to check any dysfunction in the clotting cascade), cross-match 4 units of blood (in preparation for transfusion)
- Biochemistry: U&Es (electrolyte imbalance)

MAKING A DIAGNOSIS

There are many definitions of major haemorrhage. Here are a few:

- Loss of more than one blood volume within 24 hours (around 70 mL/kg, >5 L in a 70-kg adult)
- 50% of total blood volume lost in less than 3 hours
- Bleeding in excess of 150 mL/minute

In haemodynamically stable patients, the patient's history will assist in identifying the likely source of bleed.

- Peptic ulcer disease (non-steroidal anti-inflammatory drug use, *Helicobacter pylori* infection, smoking, personal or family history of peptic ulcer disease)
- Oesophageal varices (history of alcohol abuse, cirrhosis, hepatitis B or C infection, signs of decompensated cirrhosis – jaundice, encephalopathy, ascites)
- Mallory–Weiss tear or Boerhaave's syndrome (history of retching or vomiting)

The patient will also demonstrate non-specific signs of haemorrhage, e.g. light-headedness, fatigue or signs of hypotensive shock.

MANAGEMENT

Call for help early and put out a major haemorrhage call. This patient is critically unwell, unstable and deteriorating. He has gone from anxious to drowsy, suggesting further bleeding from the time of the bleep. Blood transfusion may not always be required, and studies have shown that resuscitation with crystalloids is sufficient in up to 30% of circulatory volume loss. However, resuscitation with blood is essential in patients who are symptomatic and have lost 30% or more of their blood volume, even if the baseline haemoglobin is normal. Ensure the major haemorrhage pathway is activated and contact the lab, to ensure you have 4 units cross-matched for your patient. O-negative blood can be given until cross-matched packed red cells are available. The patient should be catheterised, and urine output monitored.

In actively bleeding patients, platelet transfusion can be offered if the platelet count is less than 100×10^9/L. However, discussion with the haematologist is advised. Fresh frozen plasma is useful in these cases when the prothrombin time (or international normalised ratio) or activated partial thromboplastin time is greater than 1.5 times normal. If a patient's fibrinogen level remains less than 1.5 g/L despite fresh frozen plasma use, offer cryoprecipitate as well. Prothrombin complex concentrate is vital in actively bleeding warfarinised patients. Speak to the on call haematologist for guidance.

 Clinical Tip

Thromboelastography (TEG) machines help with diagnosing any clotting abnormalities and guide delivery of fresh frozen plasma, cryoprecipitate and platelets. TEG has also been shown to reduce the use of blood products in major haemorrhages.

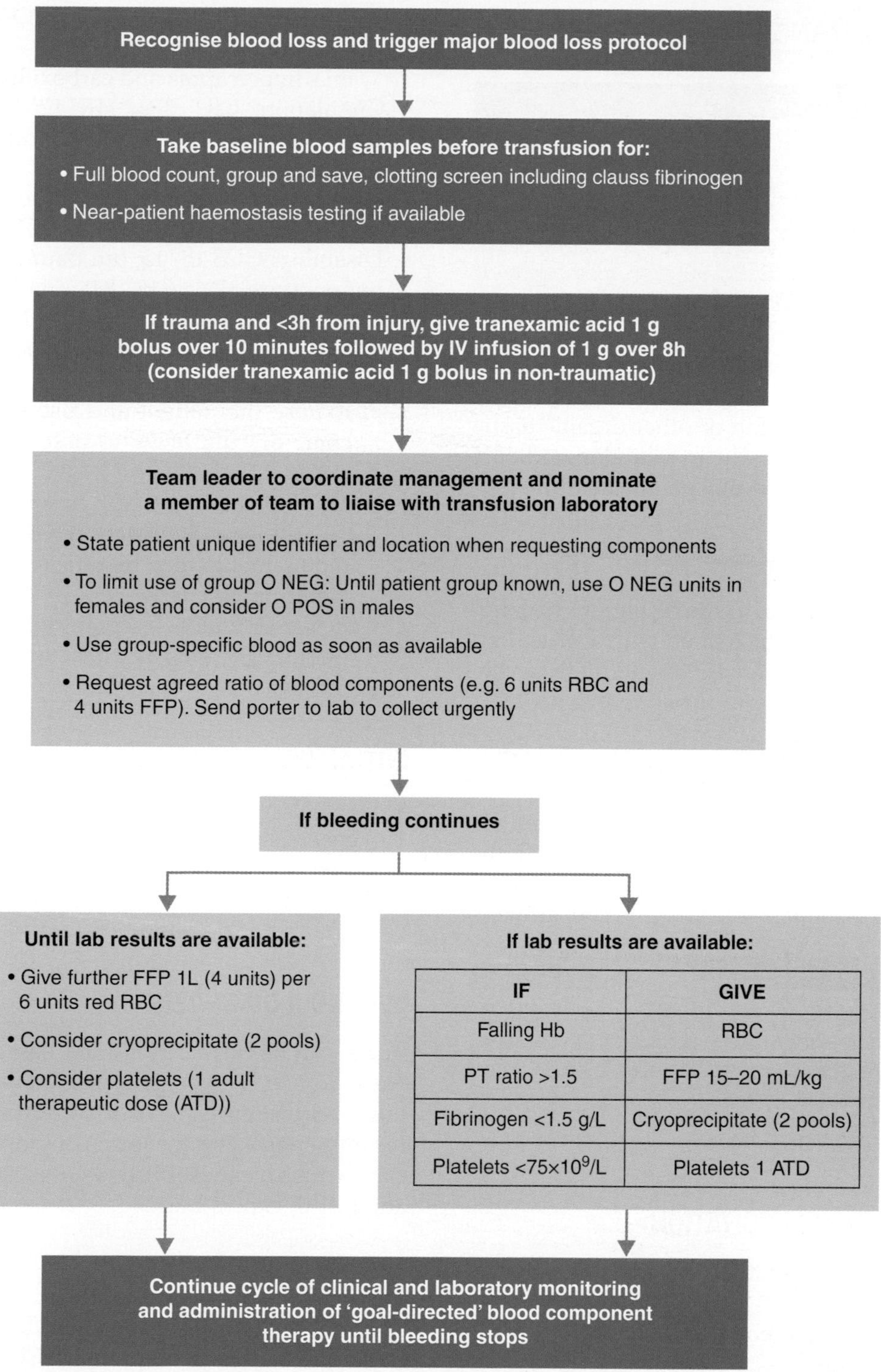

Fig. 5.3 Example of a major haemorrhage protocol. FFP, fresh frozen plasma; Hb, haemoglobin; IV, intravenous; PT, prothrombin time; RBC, Red blood cells. (Available at: https://www.transfusionguidelines.org/transfusion-handbook/7-effective-transfusion-in-surgery-and-critical-care/7-3-transfusion-management-of-major-haemorrhage).

ESCALATION

Dial 2222 and put out a major haemorrhage call if not already done. Assign roles and follow the major haemorrhage protocol (Fig. 5.3). It is essential you know your trust's policy on instigating the major haemorrhage protocol. The call will ensure you have extra pairs of hands available, and roles can be given based on expertise. The anaesthetic or critical care team, on call endoscopist and general surgeons must be informed.

STATION 5.5: BURNS

 The Bleep Scenario

A 30 year old man has arrived at the emergency department after tripping over and landing on a hot barbecue. He has burns all over his body after the barbecue fell on him. Paramedics say he is normally fit and well.

His observations are: HR 120 bpm, BP 105/50 mmHg, RR 28 breaths per minute, SpO_2 90% on room air and temperature 37°C. You are asked to assess him immediately.

DEFINITION

A burn is an injury to the skin or other organic tissue primarily caused by heat or due to radiation, radioactivity, electricity, friction or contact with chemicals.

INITIAL THOUGHTS

Reviewing a patient with burns can be highly challenging. Burns patients should be treated with a structured approach, like trauma patients. Patients with severe burns will need to be transferred to specialist units.

INITIAL INSTRUCTIONS OVER PHONE

Ask the referrer to commence 15 L/minute oxygen via a NRB mask, start running cold or tepid water over the burn and put out an adult trauma call to get the anaesthetic, surgical and orthopaedic teams in the department.

 Clinical Tip

Whilst the rule of 9s is important to guide your fluid replacement, stick to a sequential ABCDE approach. Getting distracted by the burns can lead to you missing other injuries. Assess the patient based on Advanced Trauma Life Support principles.

ASSESSMENT AND RESUSCITATION

- End-of-bed assessment: the patient is in obvious pain.
- Airway: patent; the patient is talking to you, but his voice sounds hoarse.
  - Look for airway oedema, change of voice, singed hairs, visible soot or facial burns.
  - If any of the above is present, the threshold to intubate must be low.
  - Inspect the neck for swelling and keep the cervical spine immobilised until injury is excluded.
  - Laboured breathing and burns greater than 50% body surface area (BSA) should also be considered for intubation.
- Breathing: RR 30 breaths per minute, SpO_2 93% on 15 L/minute oxygen via an NRB mask. Persistent coughing and an extensive wheeze are noted on auscultation.
  - ABG: pH 7.35, PO_2 8.5 kPa, PCO_2 6.0 kPa, HCO_3^- 20 mmol/L, lactate 2.2 mmol/L – look for hypoxaemia, hypercapnia and carboxyhaemoglobinaemia.
- Circulation: CRT 3 s. HR 125 bpm, regular. BP 109/50 mmHg. HS I + II + 0. No arrhythmias on cardiac monitor.
  - Insert two large-bore cannulae over unburnt skin, if possible, and start warmed fluid resuscitation.
- Disability: GCS 15/15, but pain is an issue. PEARL, temperature 37°C, CBG 8.0 mmol/L.
- Exposure: burns are noted on his torso, abdomen and back. No other injuries are identified on primary survey.
  - Expose the patient and use a Lund & Browder chart or rule of 9s to assess the extent of the burns.
  - The Mersey burns app is widely used by many practitioners. Calculations of burn size and fluid requirements may be quicker with the app than paper-based charts.
  - It is essential to keep the patient warm. Hypothermia is independently associated with worse mortality.

INITIAL INVESTIGATIONS

- Haematology: FBC (inflammation)
- Biochemistry: U&Es (electrolyte imbalances and acute kidney injury) and CRP (inflammation)
- Radiology: CXR to check for smoke inhalation, consolidation or pneumothorax

MAKING A DIAGNOSIS

Burns can be further classified based on the depth of tissue injury. Previously classified as first-, second- or third-degree burns, the British Burns Association now recommends using the terms epidermal burn, superficial partial-thickness burn, deep partial-thickness burn and full-thickness burn.

MANAGEMENT

The threshold for intubation should be low if there are any signs of airway compromise. Coughing and wheezing are suggestive of smoke inhalation and airway irritation. Salbutamol or adrenaline nebulisers will help with bronchodilation and starting the patient on steroids may reduce progression of airway inflammation. Ventilatory support will be necessary if there is airway compromise or laboured breathing. Cardiac support may be required, especially if there has been a sharp rise in serum potassium.

Get your senior to insert a central line if IV access is difficult but use the intraosseous approach if you need urgent vascular access: it is quicker and has fewer complications. IV fluid replacement is required if burns are greater than 15% BSA or 10% with smoke inhalation.

Parkland formula (volume of fluid to be replaced = 4 mL × weight in kg × percentage of total BSA burnt) is widely used, with half the volume given in the first 8 hours and the remaining half given over 16 hours.

Close monitoring of electrolytes is essential and nutrition is vital to help with wound healing. Pain must also be controlled. Full-thickness burns are often painless but for mixed burns multimodal analgesia, following the World Health Organization pain ladder, must be given as pain can severely compromise breathing.

Once the extent of the burns is assessed, covering the burnt skin with sterile cling film or plastic minimises further fluid loss and risk of infection. Commence broad-spectrum antibiotics as per local guidelines.

Eschars or circumferential burns can act as a restrictive non-compliant tourniquet. As swelling increases with leaking of extracellular fluid, compartment pressures may increase. Thus escharotomies, decompression therapies and debridement have a role too.

ESCALATION

Regardless of your seniority, you will not be expected to manage a major burns patient alone. A trauma call should get all the necessary personnel. Escalation to critical care will always be required if there is airway or breathing compromise, or more than 20% estimated burns surface area. Based on the extent of the burn, care may have to be transferred to a specialist burns unit.

STATION 5.6: ANAPHYLAXIS

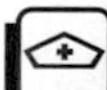 **The Bleep Scenario**

A 55 year old man has been admitted this morning to the medical ward with cellulitis. He has suddenly become short of breath, following the drug round. He is normally fit and well.

His observations are: HR 120 bpm, BP 100/60 mmHg, RR 25 breaths per minute, SpO_2 90% on room air and temperature 37.8°C. You are asked to review him urgently.

DEFINITION

Anaphylaxis is a severe and potentially life-threatening reaction to an allergen.

INITIAL THOUGHTS

Sudden-onset shortness of breath after a drug round may lead you towards anaphylaxis, but other causes of acute shortness of breath must be considered. If the patient is unresponsive and not breathing normally, a 2222 crash call should be put out immediately and ALS started. In a responsive patient, stick with an ABCDE approach, keeping in mind that the situation may change rapidly.

Risk factors for anaphylaxis include history of atopy or asthma, exposure to common sensitisers and previous episodes of anaphylaxis.

DIFFERENTIAL DIAGNOSIS

- Systemic: anaphylaxis
- Cardiology: acute myocardial infarction, acute left ventricular failure or acute pulmonary oedema
- Respiratory: pulmonary emboli or pneumothorax

INITIAL INSTRUCTIONS OVER PHONE

Ask the referrer to stop any new drug infusions, commence the patient on 15 L/minute oxygen via a NRB mask, obtain IV access and start IV fluids for resuscitation as required.

ASSESSMENT AND RESUSCITATION

- End-of-bed assessment: the patient appears sweaty and clammy.
- Airway: the patient is struggling to complete sentences and you hear stridor:
  - Inspect the airway as there may be gross swelling.
  - Dial 2222 and put out a crash call.
  - Ask for the crash trolley with emergency drugs.
- Breathing: the patient appears cyanosed. RR 35 breaths per minute. SpO_2 86% on 15 L/minute via a NRB mask. On auscultation, widespread wheeze is audible.
  - Adrenaline 0.5 mg intramuscularly (IM) (0.5 mL 1:1000 adrenaline) should be given immediately if you think this is anaphylaxis.
- Circulation: the patient's hands feel sweaty and clammy. CRT < 2 s. HR 120 bpm, regular. BP 86/40 mmHg. HS I + II + 0.
  - Continue fluid resuscitation as appropriate, e.g. 500 mL 0.9% sodium chloride stat.
  - Adrenaline 0.5 mg IM can be repeated at 5 minutes if the patient is no better.
- Disability: he is very distressed. GCS 14/15 (E4V5M6), PEARL, temperature 37.5°C, CBG 7.4 mmol/L.
- Exposure: there is swelling of the patient's eyes, lips and neck. An urticarial rash is noted. Calves and abdomen are soft and non-tender.

INITIAL INVESTIGATIONS

- Haematology: FBC (inflammation)
- Biochemistry: U&Es (electrolyte imbalances and acute kidney injury) and CRP (inflammation)
- Radiology: CXR (pneumothorax, consolidation, pneumonia)
- Immunology: Anaphylaxis can often be diagnosed clinically. However, mast cell tryptase levels support a diagnosis.

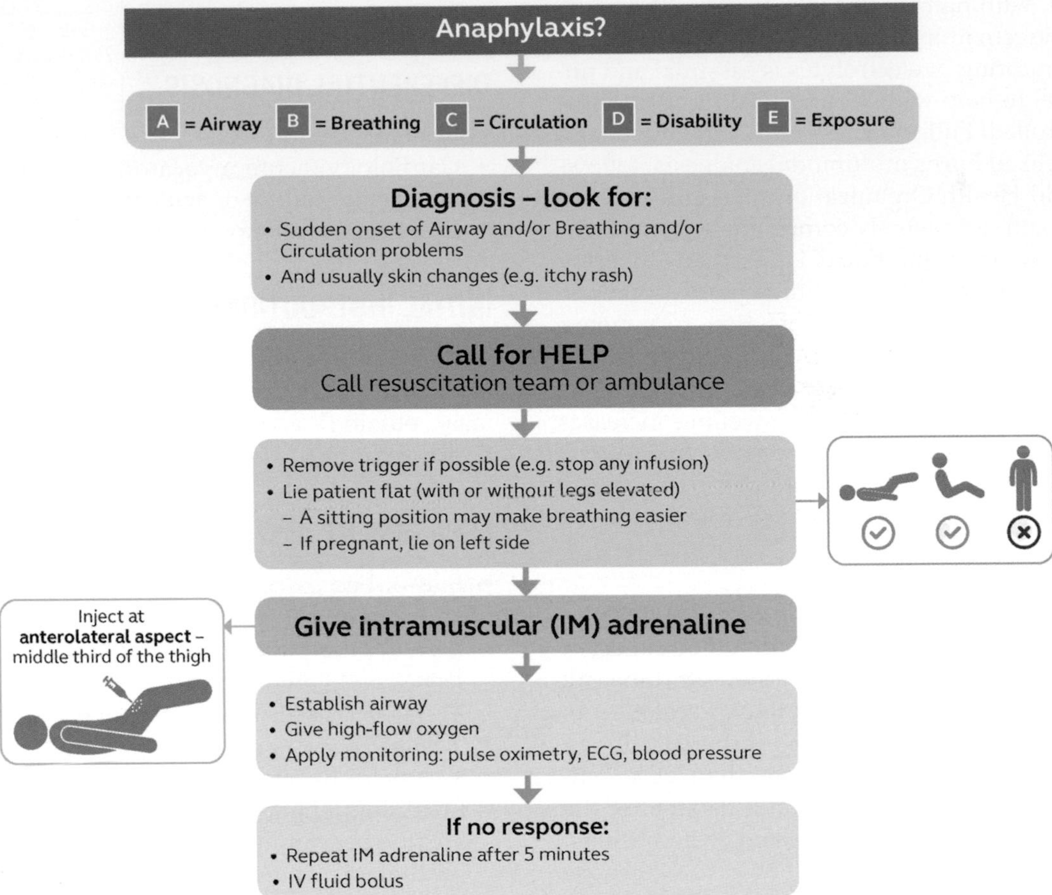

Fig. 5.4 Management of anaphylaxis. (Source: Copyright © Resuscitation Council (UK).)

MAKING A DIAGNOSIS

- Symptoms: acute-onset shortness of breath, confusion, agitation, pruritus, nausea, vomiting, diarrhoea, abdominal pain or cramps
- Signs: stridor, wheeze, laboured breathing, hypotension or urticaria

MANAGEMENT

Adrenaline, oxygen and volume replacement are the key components to managing anaphylaxis. Avoid colloids for fluid resuscitation. IM administration is the most common route on a ward. An adult dose of IM adrenaline is 500 mcg (0.5 mg). In situations with continuous cardiac monitoring, such as in the ICU, a trained individual may administer 50 mcg adrenaline (0.5 mL of 1:10,000 adrenaline) IV. Adrenaline can be repeated and IV or intraosseous doses should be titrated to response.

RC UK guidelines for anaphylaxis management are summarised in Fig. 5.4.

Anaphylaxis is characterised by vast mast cell and basophil degranulation. There is a surge in histamine release, amongst other inflammatory agents that cause swelling of the airway, bronchoconstriction and extensive vasodilation. Mast cell tryptase levels must be tested as per RC UK recommendations, given below:

- First sample – as soon as possible but not at the expense of resuscitation
- Second sample – 1–2 hours after the onset of symptoms
- Third sample – either at 24 hours or in a follow-up allergy clinic. The purpose of this sample is to get a baseline tryptase level

Identifying the causative agent is the next priority to ensure it does not happen again. Whilst in hospital, any new drugs started must be stopped and an alternative must be started if necessary. Referral to a specialist allergy or immunology centre, followed by a letter to the patient's general practitioner, is mandatory.

ESCALATION

Always call for help early. Put out a crash call – this will bring more people to the scene, who can look after the airway and commence the secondary management. This patient has a compromised airway and it is vital you call for an anaesthetist to maintain the airway.

Involvement of the critical care team is advised as the patient can be closely monitored for a secondary attack that may occur within 24 hours.

STATION 5.7: SEPSIS

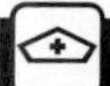

The Bleep Scenario

A 75 year old man has been admitted to the orthogeriatric ward following revision of his hip replacement 5 days ago. He is now confused and spiking a temperature. He is otherwise fit and well.

His observations are: HR 115 bpm, BP 90/50 mmHg, RR 24 breaths per minute, SpO_2 89% on room air and a temperature of 38.5°C. You are asked to review him.

DEFINITION

Sepsis is a life threatening condition that arises when the body's response to infection injures its own tissue.

INITIAL THOUGHTS

Pyrexia, hypotension and tachycardia in a patient who has been in hospital for 5 days postoperatively are strongly suggestive of sepsis. This elderly man has had a revision of his hip replacement. His mobility is likely to be reduced and he is also likely to have a catheter – both risk factors for an infection.

Other risk factors include old age, immunocompromise, diabetes, IV drug misuse, alcohol dependence, indwelling lines and breach of skin integrity.

DIFFERENTIAL DIAGNOSIS

- Respiratory: pulmonary embolism, pneumonia
- Metabolic: diabetic ketoacidosis, hypoglycemia
- Cardiology: myocardial infarction
- Systemic: hypovolaemia (e.g. due to diuretics, dehydration, haemorrhage), sepsis

INITIAL INSTRUCTIONS OVER PHONE

Ask the nurse to start 15 L/minute oxygen via a NRB mask, to obtain IV access, take bloods and start IV fluids for resuscitation as required.

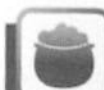

Clinical Tip

Your assessment should ensure that the confusion is not due to a neurological cause or fall on the ward.

ASSESSMENT AND RESUSCITATION

- End-of-bed assessment: the patient appears to be agitated.
- Airway: patent.
- Breathing: RR 26 breaths per minute, SpO_2 93% on 15 L/minute oxygen via an NRB mask, On auscultation, there are left-sided basal crackles.
    - ABG: pH 7.30, PO_2 8.0 kPa, PCO_2 5.5 kPa, HCO_3^- 20 mmol/L, lactate 3.0 mmol/L, glucose 8 mmol/L.
- Circulation: his hands are sweaty and clammy. CRT 3 s, HR 120 bpm, irregular. BP 83/40 mmHg, HS I + II + 0, JVP normal.
    - Administer 250 mL of crystalloid fluids stat to resuscitate the patient.
    - 12-lead ECG: fast atrial fibrillation (this is common with sepsis).
- Disability: GCS 14/15 (E4, V4, M6), PEARL, temperature 38.5°C, CBG 8 mmol/L.
- Exposure: abdomen soft with mild suprapubic tenderness. Normal bowel sounds. Surgical site looks healthy. You notice he is catheterised, and there is cloudy urine in the catheter bag.

INITIAL INVESTIGATIONS

- Haematology: FBC (inflammation or anaemia)
- Biochemistry: U&E (acute kidney injury or dehydration), CRP (inflammation)
- Microbiology: blood, stool and urine cultures (infection)
- Radiology: CXR (chest infection or atelectasis)

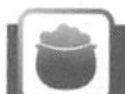

Clinical Tip

Blood lactate should be less than 2 mmol/L. A rising lactate is a bad sign in the context of sepsis.

MAKING A DIAGNOSIS

- Symptoms and signs: a history should be taken when the patient is haemodynamically stable to identify the likely aetiology of the sepsis.
    - Respiratory: productive cough/shortness of breath/pleuritic chest pain
    - Urinary tract: flank pain/dysuria/frequency/cloudy urine
    - Gastrointestinal: abdominal pain/diarrhoea/vomiting
    - Central nervous system: confusion/drowsiness
    - Skin/soft tissue: rashes/abscess/indwelling lines or catheter
    - Surgical site: pain/erythema/swelling

  Also look out for non-specific signs such as confusion, high or low temperature, lethargy, tachycardia, tachypnoea or hypotension.

Clinical Tip

The most serious cases of sepsis have signs of organ failure such as hypotension, confusion, high respiratory rate, reduced urine output and high lactate.

MANAGEMENT

Sepsis accounts for 37,000 deaths a year in the UK and requires prompt diagnosis and treatment. The BUFALO sepsis campaign gives us a guide for our initial management (BUFALO – blood cultures, uring output, fluids, antibiotics, lactate and oxygen).

Give the patient oxygen and obtain a fresh set of observations. An ABG will give you a good idea of his gas exchange, metabolic state and lactate level.

Appropriate fluid resuscitation is crucial in sepsis management: increased respiratory rate and pyrexia can increase fluid loss and sepsis can make blood vessels leaky. Give this elderly man a 250-mL crystalloid fluid bolus and monitor his blood pressure and other measures of perfusion.

Antibiotics have to be started within an hour of suspecting sepsis. Your choice of antibiotic depends on the suspected source and your trust antimicrobial guidelines. In complex cases, with multiple allergies, discussion with the on call microbiologist is highly recommended. Investigating the cause of sepsis should not delay your treatment. The confusion is likely to be sepsis-driven and there is no need for a CT head to be requested immediately.

There are many scoring systems for sepsis. SIRS has the highest sensitivity but low specificity and is no longer recommended for use by most people; NEWS has the second highest sensitivity and a moderate level of specificity. qSOFA has the lowest sensitivity but the second highest specificity.

ESCALATION

You should be comfortable starting the initial management for sepsis, but if there is no response or you feel the patient is deteriorating further, call for the medical registrar early or dial 2222 for the EMRT. Hypotension not responding to fluids or hypoxaemia not responding to simple facemask oxygen requires urgent senior attention and may require escalation to the ICU where inotropes and mechanical ventilation can be offered if deemed appropriate.

FURTHER READING

AAGBI. *Anaphylaxis and allergies*. Available at: https://anaesthetists.org/Home/Resources-publications/Safety-alerts/Anaesthesia-emergencies/Anaphylaxis-and-allergies.

American Heart Association. *About cardiac arrest*. Available at: https://www.heart.org/en/health-topics/cardiac-arrest.

Bishop, S., & Maguire, S. (2012). Anaesthesia and intensive care for major burns. *Continuing Education in Anaesthesia Critical Care and Pain*, *12*(3), 118–122.

Brennan, D. (2021). *What is the rule of nines?* Available at: https://www.webmd.com/skin-problems-and-treatments/what-is-the-rule-of-nines.

Burns Association, British (2002). *Classification of burns*. Available at: www.britishburnassociation.org/european-standards.

Craw, N. (2008). *Gullain–Barré syndrome*. Available at: www.frca.co.uk/article.aspx?articleid=101047. [Accessed 24 July 2022].

Healthwise. *Rule of 9s: First aid and emergencies*. Available at: www.webmd.com/first-aid/rule-of-nines.

Hunt, B. J., Allard, S., & Keeling, D. (2015). A practical guideline for the haematological management of major haemorrhage. *British Journal of Haematology*, *170*, 788–803.

Joint United Kingdom (UK) Blood Transfusion and Tissue Transplantation Services Professional Advisory Committee (2013). *Transfusion guidelines for major haemorrhage*. Available at: www.transfusionguidelines.org.uk/transfusion-handbook/7-effective-transfusion-in-surgery-and-critical-care/7-3-transfusion-management-of-major-haemorrhage [Accessed 24 July 2022].

KSS Acedamic Health Service Network. *Summary of NICE guidelines for sepsis*. Available at: www.kssahsn.net/what-we-do/KSSPatientSafetyCollaborative/sepsis/Pages/resources-and-links.aspx.

Kumar, P. J., & Clark, M. C. (2012). *Kumar & Clark's clinical medicine* (8th ed.). Oxford: Saunders.

McLymont, N., & Glover, G. (2016). Scoring systems for the characterization of sepsis and associated outcomes. *Annals of Translation Medicine*, *4*(24), 527.

NICE. (2019). *Guidelines, burns and scalds*. Available at: https://cks.nice.org.uk/burns-and-scalds#!scenario. [Accessed 24 July 2022].

NICE. (2016). *Mersey Burns for calculating fluid resuscitation volume when managing burns*. Available at: https://www.nice.org.uk/advice/mib58.

NICE. (2016). *Sepsis: recognition, diagnosis and early management*. Available at: https://www.nice.org.uk/guidance/ng51.

Resus, U. K. (2021). *Anaphylaxis guidelines 2021*. Available at: www.resus.org.uk/anaphylaxis. [Accessed 24 July 2022].

Resuscitation Council UK (2021). *Advanced life support 2021 guidelines*. Available at: https://www.resus.org.uk/library/2021-resuscitation-guidelines/adult-advanced-life-support-guidelines.

Singer, M., et al. (2016). The Third International Consensus definitions for sepsis and septic shock (Sepsis-3). *JAMA*, *315*(8), 801–810.

ST Helens, & Knowsley Teaching Hospitals NHS Trust. *Mersey burns*. Available at: https://merseyburns.com.

Sun, W., et al. (2014). Thromboelastography (TEG)-based algorithm reduces blood product utilization in patients undergoing VAD implant. *Journal of Cardiac Surgery*, *29*(2), 238–243.

World Health Organization. *Burns*. Available at: https://www.who.int/news-room/fact-sheets/detail/burns.

Cardiology

6

Content Outline

STATION 6.1: ACUTE CORONARY SYNDROME

The Bleep Scenario

A 64 year old male attended the emergency department (ED) complaining of central chest pain for 40 minutes, radiating to the left side of his jaw with associated nausea. He has a background of hypertension and diet-controlled type 2 diabetes.

His observations are: heart rate (HR) 122 bpm, blood pressure (BP) 136/80 mmHg, respiratory rate (RR) 21 breaths per minute, SpO_2 96% on room air and temperature 36.8°C. You are asked to review him.

DEFINITION

Acute coronary syndrome (ACS) describes a range of conditions associated with a sudden reduction in cardiac perfusion causing ischaemia.

It encompasses ST-segment myocardial infarction (STEMI), non-ST-segment myocardial infarction (NSTEMI) and unstable angina.

INITIAL THOUGHTS

This man has cardiac-sounding chest pain with associated autonomic symptoms, as evidenced by the vomiting and tachycardia.

He has significant cardiovascular risk factors – increased age, male, hypertension and diabetes.

Other risk factors for ischaemic heart disease include personal or family history of coronary artery disease, hyperlipidaemia, obesity, smoking and physical inactivity. This requires urgent investigation and treatment.

DIFFERENTIAL DIAGNOSIS

- Cardiovascular: aortic dissection, aortic stenosis, decompensated arrhythmogenic disease and pericardial pathology
- Gastrointestinal: gastro-oesophageal reflux disease, peptic and duodenal ulceration
- Respiratory: pulmonary embolism and pneumonia
- Locomotor: musculoskeletal chest pain, e.g. Tietze's syndrome

INITIAL INSTRUCTIONS OVER PHONE

Ask the nurse to obtain an electrocardiogram (ECG), intravenous (IV) access and bloods if possible, including troponin.

Early pain relief should be given as sublingual glyceryl trinitrate and IV morphine plus an antiemetic. This can be prescribed after assessment but is important to think of beforehand.

Prescribing Tip

Check with the nurse if one or more of these have already been prescribed as an as-needed medication. If so, the nurse can administer them.

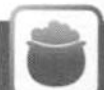

Clinical Tip

Morphine provides symptomatic relief of dyspnoea and decreases preload to the heart, reducing cardiac strain – this could be even more useful if the patient proves to have concomitant pulmonary oedema.

Prescribing Tip

The three most commonly used antiemetics are cyclizine, ondansetron and metoclopramide.

ASSESSMENT AND RESUSCITATION

- End of the bed assessment: patient appears clammy and dyspnoeic
- Airway: patent

- Breathing: RR 21 breaths per minute, SpO_2 95% on room air. On auscultation, there are vesicular breath sounds with good air entry bilaterally
- Circulation: capillary refill time (CRT) < 2 s, HR 122 bpm, regular, BP 136/89 mmHg (both arms), jugular venous pressure (JVP) normal, heart sounds (HS) I + II + 0
  - 12-lead ECG : ST elevation noted on anterolateral leads. Compare with old ECGs as T-wave changes or bundle branch blocks may be old
- Disability: Glasgow Coma Scale (GCS) 15/15, pupils equal and reactive to light (PEARL), temperature 37.2°C, capillary blood glucose (CBG) 8.8 mmol/L
- Exposure: abdomen soft and non-tender, with normal bowel sounds. Calves are unremarkable.

INITIAL INVESTIGATIONS

- Haematology: full blood count (FBC: anaemia or infection)
- Biochemistry: urea and electrolytes (U&Es), liver function tests (LFTs) and troponin upon onset of chest pain and at least 3 hours after (cardiac necrosis)
- Radiology: chest X-ray (CXR: left-heart failure/respiratory pathology), echocardiogram (impaired ventricular function, valvular pathology [most commonly aortic stenosis] and complications of ACS, e.g. ventricular septal defect/aneurysm)

MAKING A DIAGNOSIS

For the diagnosis of unstable angina there must be:

- Cardiac-sounding chest pain (most often retrosternal, radiating to the left arm) that is severe, i.e. at rest, new-onset severe angina, angina increasing in frequency, longer in duration, lower in threshold, or that has occurred after a recent myocardial infarction
- Normal troponin with or without ECG changes

For the definitive diagnosis of a STEMI or NSTEMI, there must be a rise in cardiac troponin with at least one value above the 99th percentile of the upper reference limit and one of the following:

- Cardiac-sounding chest pain
- Evidence of myocardial damage on echocardiography or identification of a coronary artery thrombus on angiography
- Any of the following ECG changes:
  - New ST-segment or T-wave changes; ST depression on an ECG may indicate posterior lead ST elevation (posterior STEMI)
  - Large, peaked T waves occurring in the early phase
  - Pathological Q waves on ECG

For the definitive diagnosis of a STEMI, there must be:

- Chest pain within 12 hours of onset (or ongoing chest pain of > 12 hours duration) plus either ST-segment elevation or new LBBB on ECG. Fig. 6.1 shows ECG changes in STEMI.

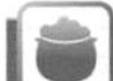

Clinical Tip

CAUSES OF INCREASED TROPONIN

- Cardiac: cardiac failure, myocarditis, cardiomyopathies, traumatic cardiac contusion and postprocedural, e.g cardiac surgery, cardioversion and percutaneous coronary intervention (PCI), aortic dissection, aortic valve disease, cardiotoxic drugs, arrhythmias, Takotsubo cardiomyopathy and rhabdomyolysis
- Renal: renal failure and amyloidosis
- Respiratory: pulmonary embolism and severe pulmonary hypertension
- Systemic: sepsis, severe critical illness and burns
- Neurological: stroke and subarachnoid haemorrhage

MANAGEMENT

It is important to make a diagnosis of STEMI versus NSTEMI within a few minutes as international recommendations aim for a door-to-angioplasty time of less than 90 minutes in STEMI.

The mainstay management of ACS is to give aspirin 300 mg and either clopidogrel 300 mg or ticagrelor 180 mg or prasugrel 60 mg. Fondaparinux 2.5 mg should

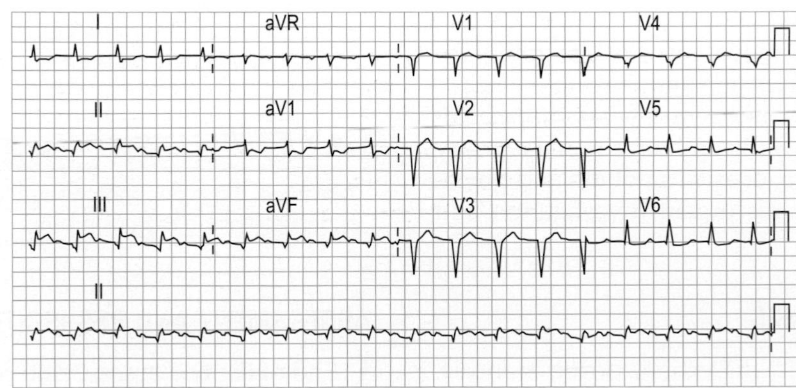

Fig. 6.1 ST-segment myocardial infarction (STEMI) in inferior chest leads. (Source: Mythen, M.M. et al. [2010]. *Anaesthesiology e-book: Churchill's ready reference*. Elsevier.)

also be given subcutaneously, unless the patient is having urgent primary PCI.

These patients will need to be transferred to the coronary care unit (CCU) or cardiology ward for cardiac monitoring depending on the hospital protocol and bed availability. Patients are at high risk of developing arrhythmias. A coronary angiogram should also be arranged.

If the patient has had a STEMI, they should have urgent PCI. If this is contraindicated or unavailable, they should receive thrombolysis.

ESCALATION

The medical registrar should be informed as soon as you suspect acute coronary syndrome. If the patient is likely to need urgent PCI, you should call the cardiac catheter lab as well as the cardiology registrar as soon as possible. Even for NSTEMI you should inform the same people so that arrangements can be made.

STATION 6.2: BRADYCARDIA

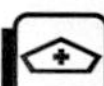

The Bleep Scenario

A 78 year old man on the medical assessment unit is feeling light-headed. He is known to have a background of myocardial infarction, hypertension and diabetes.

His observations are: HR 35 bpm, BP 132/80 mmHg, RR 16 breaths per minute, SpO_2 98% on room air and temperature 37°C. You are asked to review this patient.

DEFINITION

Bradycardia is defined as HR of 50 bpm or less. Bradycardia can be sinus in origin, or can involve the atrioventricular (AV) node, leading to AV block.

AV (heart) block is a delay or failure in the conduction of electrical impulses from the atria to the ventricles.

INITIAL THOUGHTS

This elderly man has a significant cardiovascular history, and is likely to be on multiple medications as a result. Both are well-known risk factors for bradycardia. Other risk factors to consider include surgery, hypothyroidism, electrolyte disorders, acidosis, hypothermia or infections.

Although he is haemodynamically stable, you must monitor for hypotension and syncopal episodes indicative of compromise in cerebral perfusion pressure.

DIFFERENTIAL DIAGNOSES

- Drug-related: beta-blockers, digoxin, non-dihydropyridine calcium channel blockers (e.g. diltiazem and verapamil) or amiodarone
- Cardiac: AV block (primary or secondary to myocardial ischaemia), myocarditis and complications post cardiac intervention
- Non-cardiac: vasovagal syncope and hypothyroidism

INITIAL INSTRUCTIONS OVER PHONE

Ask the nurse to perform a 12-lead ECG. If the patient is unstable, IV access should be obtained immediately. Request the nurse to repeat observations upon arrival and ask the nurse to await review before any regular medications are given, as these may affect the heart rate.

ASSESSMENT AND RESUSCITATION

- End-of-the-bed assessment: patient appears pale and clammy. He is feeling dizzy and lethargic
- Airway: patent
- Breathing: RR 21 breaths per minute, SpO_2 96% on room air. On auscultation, there are vesicular breath sounds with good air entry bilaterally
- Circulation: CRT 5 s, HR 31 bpm, regular. BP 97/69 mmHg. JVP normal, HS I + II + 0. Pale and cool peripheries
- 12-lead ECG: there is complete dissociation of P waves and QRS complexes
- Disability: GCS 15/15, PEARL, temperature 37.0°C, CBG 5.1 mmol/L
- Exposure: abdomen soft and non-tender, with normal bowel sounds. Mild pitting ankle oedema

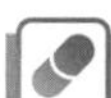

Prescribing Tip

Patients with multiple comorbidities should have regular drug reviews to look for interactions and medications that could be reduced or stopped if no longer indicated.

INITIAL INVESTIGATIONS

- Haematology: FBC (anaemia or infection)
- Biochemistry: U&Es, LFTs, thyroid function tests (TFTs: hypothyroidism), troponin (if ACS is suspected) and digoxin levels (if the patient takes digoxin)

Clinical Tip

Remember to check renal function; there is an increased risk of significant side effects because of reduced renal clearance, for example, in the elderly.

MAKING A DIAGNOSIS

- First-degree AV block: a prolongation of impulse conduction within the AV node (prolonged PR interval >200 ms). In older people, it is mostly secondary to medication. It can be physiological in young people due to high vagal tone.

- Second-degree AV block: categorised as Mobitz type 1, Mobitz type 2 or advanced block. There are multiple causes, including ischaemia, myocarditis, increased vagal tone and medication.
  - Mobitz type 1: PR interval gets progressively longer until one P wave fails to conduct to ventricles. Usually caused by medications (also known as Wenckebach phenomenon).
  - Mobitz type 2: PR interval is unchanged but intermittently fails to conduct to ventricles. Frequently associated with ischaemic heart disease. There is a high risk of asystole.
- Third-degree AV block: complete failure of atrial impulses to conduct to the ventricles, usually a result of structural change secondary to ischaemia.
  - Complete separation of P waves and QRS complexes. QRS complexes are usually broad and infrequent because they originate from an abnormal focus in the ventricle, hence known as an 'escape' rhythm. Fig. 6.2 is an illustration of ECG changes in complete heart block.

MANAGEMENT

The patient's haemodynamic stability should be your priority. Red-flag symptoms and signs that require immediate treatment with IV atropine 500 μg include evidence of shock (systolic BP <90 mmHg), syncope or heart failure and/or signs of insufficient myocardial blood supply (such as ST depression or central chest pain).

The second major concern is the patient's risk of asystole. Risk factors for this include second-degree (Mobitz 2) or third-degree (complete) heart block, having had a recent cardiac arrest or patients who have had a ventricular pause (an absence of QRS complexes on ECG) for >3 s. Symptomatic patients or those at risk of asystole must be monitored closely and further treated with atropine 500 μg IV, up to a maximum of 3 mg.

You may consider administration of IV fluids to support BP. In cardiogenic shock, fluid administration is a difficult decision to make. It is important to put out a periarrest call in order to involve the multidisciplinary team – this will allow discussion with the medical registrar on call and intensive therapy unit (ITU) team. At this point, depending on the significance of symptoms, background cardiac history and performance, a decision will be made either to attempt small-volume fluid resuscitation, e.g. 250 mL over 15 minutes, or to support the patient in a CCU or ITU setting with inotropes.

ESCALATION

If atropine fails to stabilise the patient, the on call medical registrar should be contacted immediately to initiate more advanced therapy, such as an IV adrenaline infusion.

A senior clinician with competence in transvenous pacing may also need to be contacted for patients at risk of asystole or with symptoms refractory to atropine boluses. This will usually be the on call cardiologist.

Transcutaneous pacing can be initiated by a cardiologist as a temporary measure with the consideration of transvenous pacing if required. If the patient is stable and has a low risk of asystole, pacing may not be necessary and observation is sufficient. An implantable pacemaker may then be inserted electively.

STATION 6.3: NARROW-COMPLEX TACHYCARDIA

The Bleep Scenario

A nurse bleeps to inform you that a 45 year old female patient has an HR of 154 bpm. She was previously fit and well, her only history being asthma for which she uses a blue inhaler on occasion. She was admitted for a colonoscopy.

Her observations are: HR 154 bpm, BP 132/98 mmHg, RR 19 breaths per minute, SpO_2 97% on room air and temperature 37.1°C. You are asked to review her.

DEFINITION

A narrow-complex tachycardia is any heart rhythm in which HR is greater than 100 bpm and on ECG the QRS complex is less than 120 ms (three small squares on a normal ECG trace).

INITIAL THOUGHTS

This patient is tachycardic. Your initial assessment should involve consideration of the different causes of tachycardia, which is multifactorial in nature. It is likely that this patient is having a sinus tachycardia. Consider whether the tachycardia could be secondary to a bleed post-colonoscopy or related to salbutamol inhaler use. Other causes of sinus tachycardia include

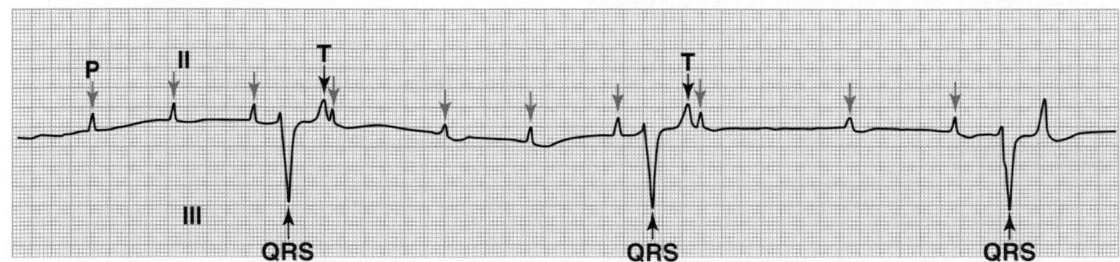

Fig. 6.2 Electrocardiogram (ECG) changes in complete heart block. (Source: Bassert, J.M. [2014]. *McCurnin's clinical textbook for veterinary technicians.* Elsevier.)

sepsis, hypoxia, pulmonary embolism, hyperthyroidism, drugs and certain prescribed medications.

DIFFERENTIAL DIAGNOSIS

- Young patients (<60 years old): sinus tachycardia, AV nodal re-entry tachyarrhythmia (AVNRT), AV re-entry tachyarrhythmia (AVRT)
- Older patients (>60 years old): atrial fibrillation, atrial flutter, atrial tachycardia

INITIAL INSTRUCTIONS OVER PHONE

Request the nursing staff to perform a repeat set of observations, including the patient's GCS, to assess for signs of haemodynamic compromise. A 12-lead ECG and if unstable IV access should also be obtained. Ask the nursing staff to kindly await review before any regular medications are given. Ensure the patient is monitored closely whilst awaiting your arrival, and advise the nursing staff to put out a periarrest call if there is any deterioration in BP, HR or GCS in the meantime.

ASSESSMENT AND RESUSCITATION

- End-of-the-bed assessment: the patient appears anxious but well perfused
- Airway: patent
- Breathing: RR 19 breaths per minute, SpO_2 97% on room air. On auscultation, there are vesicular breath sounds with good air entry bilaterally
- Circulation: CRT < 2 s, HR 154 bpm, regular. BP 132/98 mmHg. JVP normal, HS I + II + 0
    - 12-lead ECG: regular narrow-complex tachycardia with absent P waves
- Disability: GCS 15/15, PEARL, temperature 37.1°C, CBG 4.6 mmol/L
- Exposure: abdomen soft and non-tender, with normal bowel sounds. Calves are unremarkable. Mucous membranes are moist and peripheries appear well perfused

INITIAL INVESTIGATIONS

- Haematology: FBC (anaemia or infection)
- Biochemistry: U&Es (metabolic derangements), TFTs (hyperthyroidism), troponin (if ACS is suspected), toxicology screen (external agents that may cause tachycardia, e.g. stimulants)
- Radiology: CXR (infection)

MAKING A DIAGNOSIS

IN YOUNG PATIENTS (<60 YEARS OLD)

- Sinus tachycardia: rhythm originating from the sinoatrial node, with a rate > 100 bpm. Multiple causes such as sepsis or hyperthyroidism
- AVNRT: a common cause of palpitations in structurally normal hearts, particularly in women. AVNRT is a re-entrant tachycardia involving two pathways within the AV node or perinodal tissue
    - Presents with absent or inverted P waves (due to retrograde conduction of impulse through atria)
- AVRT: occurs due to an accessory pathway from the atria to ventricles and is often associated with preexcitation syndromes, e.g. Wolff–Parkinson–White syndrome
    - P wave will be present but may be abnormal

IN OLDER PATIENTS (>60 YEARS OLD)

- Atrial fibrillation: a supraventricular tachyarrhythmia due to rapid and random conduction of irregular impulses to the ventricle. It is common, especially in patients >65 years. AF may occur due to various causes, such as cardiovascular disease, stress on the body, stimulants, congenital heart disease or metabolic imbalances. Fig. 6.3 gives an illustration of ECG changes in atrial fibrillation

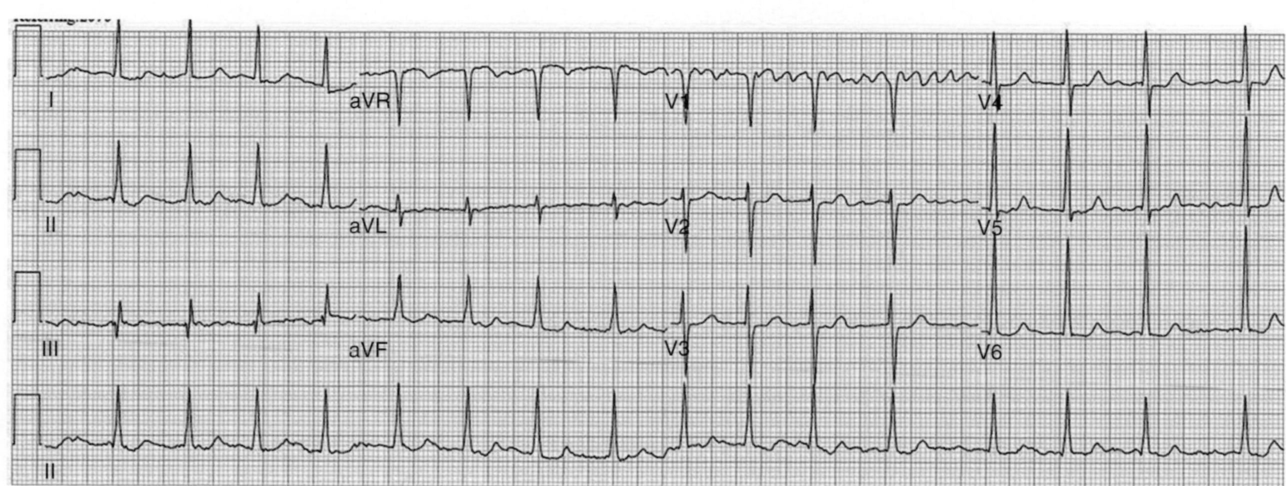

Fig. 6.3 Atrial fibrillation. (Source: Naqvi, T.Z. [2021]. *Point-of-care echocardiography: A clinical case-based visual guide.* Elsevier.)

- Atrial flutter: an organised re-entrant rhythm with atrial rates between 250 and 300 bpm and ventricular rates often at 150 bpm, due to 2:1 block. It may occur due to underlying cardiovascular disease, congenital heart disease, myocarditis or other conditions such as lung disease or hyperthyroidism
  - 'Sawtooth' pattern on baseline ECG
- Atrial tachycardia: a focal or multifocal tachyarrhythmia arising in the atria. Some causes include structural heart disease, catecholamine excess and digoxin toxicity
- Tachycardia with abnormal P-wave morphology

Fig. 6.4 summarises different ECG findings in the context of narrow-complex tachycardia.

MANAGEMENT

Management of a tachyarrhythmia depends on haemodynamic stability and type of arrhythmia.

SHOCK

Regardless of the rhythm, any patient who is haemodynamically unstable will need immediate discussion with the medical registrar, cardiology registrar and intensive care team. They may require the administration of more potent antiarrhythmic agents, such as amiodarone, that will require monitoring, or the initiation of DC cardioversion.

Patients should have continuous telemetry on a monitored bed, or on a specialist CCU bed. It is crucial to assess continually for signs of syncope, myocardial ischaemia, shock (BP < 90 mmHg systolic) or any symptoms or signs indicative of cardiac failure, such as pulmonary or peripheral oedema or the development of ascites.

HAEMODYNAMICALLY STABLE

Management should be based on the nature of the tachyarrhythmia. The most commonly occurring rhythms are sinus tachycardia, atrial fibrillation, atrial flutter and supraventricular tachycardias (AVRT or AVNRT).

- Sinus tachycardia: treat the underlying cause, for example, dehydration or sepsis.
- Atrial fibrillation: an irregular narrow complex tachycardia is very likely to be atrial fibrillation.
  - Rate control: bisoprolol (sometimes IV metoprolol) and diltiazem are the usual first-line drugs. Digoxin can also be used and is especially effective in patients with concurrent heart failure due to reduction in morbidity as well as negative chronotropic effects.
  - Rhythm control: an irregular rhythm can be reverted back to sinus by chemical cardioversion (e.g. with amiodarone or flecainide) or elective DC cardioversion.

ATRIAL FLUTTER

Atrial flutter is managed in the same way as atrial fibrillation. Atrial flutter with a 2:1 block will, on the ECG, appear the same as a supraventricular tachycardia. Carotid massage will make flutter waves more visible.

In most cases, supraventricular tachycardias can be subdivided into two major subtypes (AVRT and AVNRT).

Supraventricular tachycardias are managed with carotid sinus massage initially. This can be used to

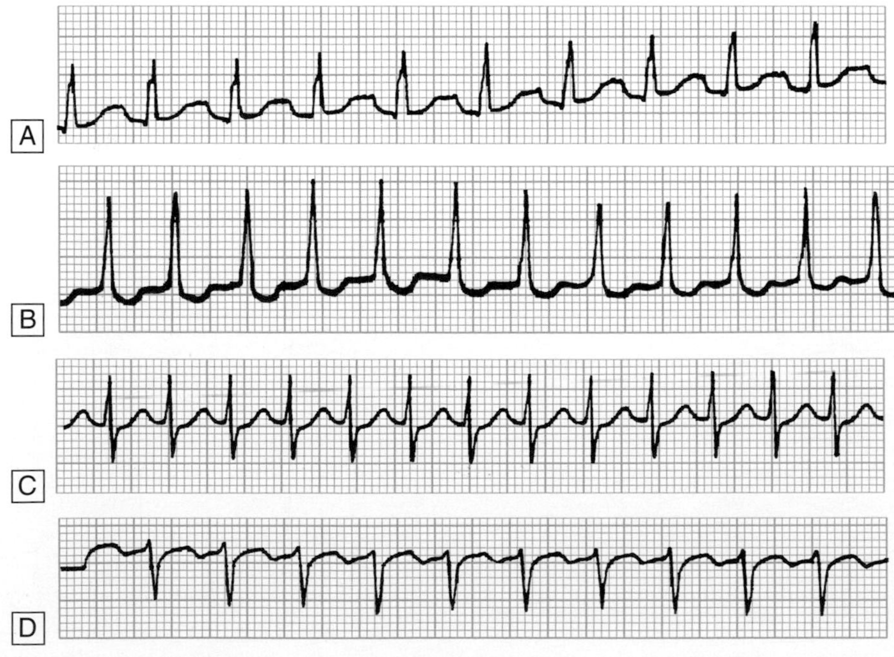

Fig. 6.4 Electrocardiogram (ECG) patterns in narrow-complex tachycardia. (Source: Goldberger, A. [2018]. *Goldberger's clinical electrocardiography*. Philadelphia, PA: Elsevier.)

unmask flutter waves, aiding in clarification of the underlying rhythm if it is unclear, and providing a parasympathetic stimulus to slow down the rate. If vagal manoeuvres fail to work, give a 6-mg bolus of adenosine, followed by 12 mg and then a further 12 mg.

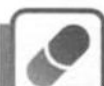
Prescribing Tip

The patient should be warned of sudden-onset chest tightness following an adenosine bolus. Adenosine can be administered in chronic obstructive pulmonary disease (COPD), but if the patient has asthma, discuss with a senior to consider alternative treatments.

ESCALATION

The cardiology registrar should be contacted for further management of any narrow-complex tachycardia that does not respond to adenosine. They may consider IV metoprolol or verapamil (for rate control) and amiodarone or flecainide (for chemical cardioversion).

All patients who are unresponsive to initial lines of medical management or who are haemodynamically unstable should be escalated to CCU/high dependency unit.

STATION 6.4: BROAD-COMPLEX TACHYCARDIA

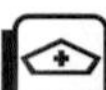
The Bleep Scenario

A 51 year old male patient has recently been stepped down from the CCU after being admitted 4 days ago with a large anterolateral myocardial infarction. He is now complaining of light-headedness and has an HR of 169 bpm. His ECG shows wide QRS complexes.

His observations are: HR 154 bpm, BP 107/78 mmHg, RR 21 breaths per minute, SpO_2 98% on room air and temperature 37.2°C.

DEFINITION

A broad-complex tachycardia is any heart rhythm in which HR is greater than 100 bpm and on ECG the QRS complex is greater than 120 ms (three small squares on a normal ECG trace).

INITIAL THOUGHTS

In this scenario, even if the patient has no ischaemic history, you should assume ventricular tachycardia (VT) until proven otherwise, and anticipate degeneration into pulseless VT or ventricular fibrillation (VF).

DIFFERENTIAL DIAGNOSIS

- Cardiology: structural heart disease (previous myocardial infarctions), coronary artery disease, congenital heart disease (for example, long QT syndrome) and LBBB/right bundle branch block (RBBB)
- Electrolyte imbalances: potassium, magnesium and calcium are of particular importance
- Drug-related: cocaine
- Endocrine: hyperthyroidism and phaeochromocytoma

INITIAL INSTRUCTIONS OVER PHONE

Request a repeat set of observations including GCS and ensure this patient is monitored by a nurse at the bedside until your arrival. Advise the nurse to action a periarrest call if there is any further deterioration in BP, HR or GCS. IV access should be obtained urgently.

ASSESSMENT AND RESUSCITATION

- End-of-the-bed assessment: the patient is clammy and anxious
- Airway: patent
- Breathing: RR 21 breaths per minute, SpO_2 98% on room air. On auscultation, there are vesicular breath sounds with good air entry bilaterally
- Circulation: CRT < 2 s, HR 139 bpm, regular. BP 107/78 mmHg. JVP normal, HS I + II + 0
    - 12-lead ECG: regular broad-complex tachycardia
- Disability: GCS 15/15, PEARL, temperature 37.2°C, CBG 7.7 mmol/L
- Exposure: abdomen soft and non-tender, with normal bowel sounds. Calves unremarkable

INITIAL INVESTIGATIONS

- Haematology: FBC (anaemia or infection)
- Biochemistry: U&Es (metabolic derangements: hypokalaemia and hypomagnesemia), troponin (if ACS is suspected), toxicology screen (external agents that may cause tachycardia, e.g. stimulants)
- Radiology: CXR (infection)

MAKING A DIAGNOSIS

VT can be sustained (lasting longer than 30 s or requiring termination) or non-sustained. Fig. 6.5 shows an example of VT.

- Sustained monomorphic VT: it most commonly arises due to scarring in the ventricle from previous myocardial infarctions or acute coronary ischaemia but may also be associated with cardiomyopathies. It may resemble supraventricular tachyarrhythmia with bundle branch block.
    - All QRS complexes have the same morphology and arise from the same locus in the ventricles.
- Sustained polymorphic VT: the most common cause is torsades de pointes (TdP) VT. Torsades de pointes arises due to long QT syndrome, which may be congenital or acquired. Acquired long QT syndrome is most commonly caused by drugs such as macrolide antibiotics,

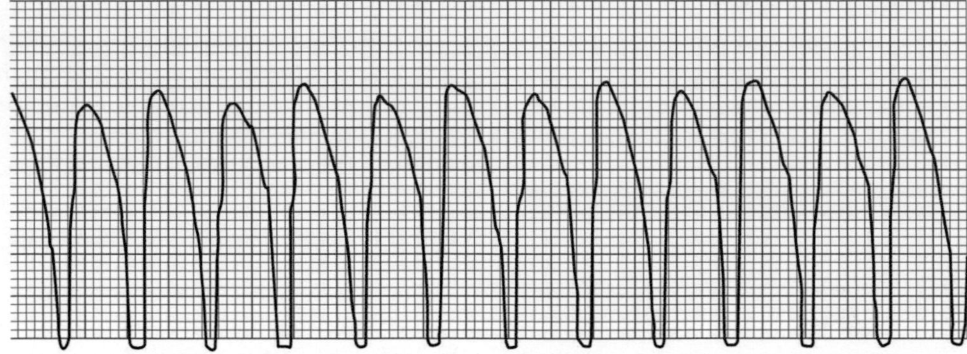

Fig. 6.5 Ventricular tachycardia. (Source: Frownfelter, D. et al. [2022]. *Cardiovascular and pulmonary physical therapy: Evidence to practice*. Elsevier.)

antipsychotics, tricyclic antidepressants and antiarrhythmics, but may also be caused by ischaemic heart disease and electrolyte abnormalities. Sustained polymorphic VT may resolve spontaneously but risks degenerating into ventricular fibrillation.

- QRS complexes show several different or changing morphologies.
- In torsades de pointes, characteristic 'twisting around the isoelectric line' morphology is noted.

An important differential is a supraventricular tachycardias with a bundle branch block. This is more likely if: (1) the rhythm is irregular; (2) there is known bundle branch block already; and (3) there is no AV dissociation (i.e. in VT the QRS complexes are independent of the P waves). However, if there is any doubt, it is always safer to treat as VT.

 **Clinical Tip**

Make the diagnosis – if in doubt, treat as VT. Make sure you consider the patient's haemodynamic stability and call the crash team if cardiac arrest is likely.

MANAGEMENT

Give the patient oxygen and set up continuous ECG monitoring for the duration of their acute management. Assess frequently using the ABCDE approach and be ready to make a cardiac arrest call if the patient starts to lose consciousness.

If the patient shows any signs of syncope, myocardial ischaemia (as assessed by ECG), chest pain, haemodynamic compromise or signs of heart failure, the patient requires emergency DC cardioversion under sedation or general anaesthesia (an anaesthetist should be contacted immediately).

Give IV amiodarone 300 mg over 30–60 minutes, followed by an IV infusion of 900 mg over 24 hours until the patient returns to sinus rhythm, unless there is pre-existing evidence of QT prolongation, in which case, discuss with a senior. Remember to correct potential causes of VT, including electrolyte abnormalities (especially hypokalaemia and hypomagnesaemia) or QT-prolonging medications, as this will help terminate the arrhythmia.

ESCALATION

The medical registrar should be contacted immediately. If the patient is unstable and requires cardioversion, an anaesthetist should also be called for sedation. Once the patient is sedated, cardioversion should be carried out as soon as possible. The patient will warrant level 2 or 3 care for monitoring and may require inotropic support.

STATION 6.5: HYPERTENSIVE EMERGENCIES

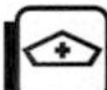 **The Bleep Scenario**

A 39 year old woman has been referred by her general practitioner with a history of severe headache, vomiting and a raised BP of 217/136 mmHg. She is known to have a history of hypertension, which is usually well controlled on antihypertensives.

Her observations in the medical assessment unit are: HR 95 bpm, BP 217/126 mmHg, RR 24 breaths per minute, SpO_2 99% on room air and temperature of 36.8°C. You are asked to review the patient.

DEFINITION

A hypertensive emergency, also known as malignant or accelerated hypertension, is defined as an elevated BP above 220/120 mmHg with signs of end-organ dysfunction.

INITIAL THOUGHTS

The most common cause of a persistently raised BP is undiagnosed or inadequately treated essential hypertension. However, in younger patients, it is important to consider the secondary causes of hypertension. Risk factors of a hypertensive emergency include poorly controlled hypertension, old age, male gender and presence of chronic kidney function.

DIFFERENTIAL DIAGNOSIS

- Renal: renovascular disease (renal artery stenosis or fibromuscular dysplasia) and chronic kidney disease
- Endocrine: Cushing's syndrome, Conn's syndrome, phaeochromocytoma, thyroid disease and acromegaly
- Cardiovascular: uncontrolled essential hypertension, coarctation of the aorta and pre-eclampsia
- Drug-induced: sympathomimetic drugs (including recreational sympathomimetics), steroids, vasopressin and monoamine oxidase inhibitor drug reactions

INITIAL INSTRUCTIONS OVER PHONE

Ask the nurse to obtain a 12-lead ECG, IV access and initial bloods if possible.

ASSESSMENT AND RESUSCITATION

- End-of-the-bed assessment: the patient is extremely agitated, sweaty and flushed
- Airway: patent
- Breathing: RR 26 breaths per minute, SpO_2 100% on room air. On auscultation, there are vesicular breath sounds with good air entry bilaterally
- Circulation: CRT <2 s, HR 98 bpm, regular, BP 217/136 mmHg, JVP normal, HS I + II + 0
  - 12-lead ECG: T-wave inversion in leads V5–V6 with large associated QRS complexes
- Disability: GCS 15/15, PEARL, temperature 36.8°C. CBG 5.1 mmol/L
- Exposure: abdomen soft and non-tender. On fundoscopy, she has evidence of AV nipping, retinal exudates and flame haemorrhages. No optic disc swelling or neurological deficit noted.

Clinical Tip

Assessment should identify signs of end-organ dysfunction, which will require a full neurological examination and fundoscopy. Signs of hypertensive retinopathy on fundoscopy include cotton-wool spots, retinal haemorrhages, retinal arteriolar narrowing, compression of venules (AV nipping) and optic disc swelling.

INITIAL INVESTIGATIONS

- Haematology: FBC (polycythaemia)
- Biochemistry: U&Es (end-organ damage), lactate dehydrogenase, TFTs (secondary cause: thyroid disease), toxicology screen (secondary causes: drug-related), plasma renin and aldosterone levels (secondary causes: Conn's syndrome), 24-hour urine free cortisol (secondary causes: Cushing's syndrome, phaeochromocytoma), urinalysis (end-organ damage)
- Radiology: CXR (secondary cardiac/vascular causes, as well as signs of fluid overload), renal ultrasound (secondary renal causes)
- Others: 12-lead ECG (signs of myocardial damage) and echocardiography (heart failure/ischaemia)

Clinical Tip

If there are signs to suggest an aortic dissection, an urgent CT aortogram should be requested. If the patient has focal neurological signs that suggest intracranial haemorrhage or ischaemic stroke, you should request an urgent CT head scan.

MAKING A DIAGNOSIS

Diagnosis of a hypertensive emergency requires an elevated BP above 220/120 mmHg and signs of end-organ dysfunction.

SYMPTOMS OF END-ORGAN DYSFUNCTION:

- Neurological: blurred vision, dizziness, headaches, seizures, altered mental status, weakness or sensory disturbance
- Cardiac: chest pain, shortness of breath, palpitations or oedema
- Renal: reduced urine output
- Opthalmological: Fig. 6.6 is an example of ocular changes in patients with hypertensive retinopathy, found in chronic disease.

MANAGEMENT

In most cases, a slow and controlled reduction in systolic BP is recommended to avoid cardiac, cerebral or renal ischaemia. IV labetolol may be considered in a HDU setting.

In malignant hypertension associated with stroke, treatment is complex and should be initiated with direction from the senior medical team and a neurologist or stroke specialist.

After initial management, a target BP of 160/110 mmHg should be achieved over the next 6 hours. Following this, oral antihypertensive medication can be prescribed.

Prescribing Tip

As a junior doctor, you will often be bleeped to the ward to manage stage 1 and 2 hypertension. If no end-organ damage is present, there is no need to treat unless there is a recurring pattern. If so, you can either increase existing therapy or prescribe an additional agent regularly; if it is safe to do so, it is often better to do this following discharge from hospital.

ESCALATION

In general, patients with hypertensive crises are monitored in the CCU. In the event that there is renal failure requiring haemofiltration or a GCS < 8 which may require ventilation, intensive care should be contacted.

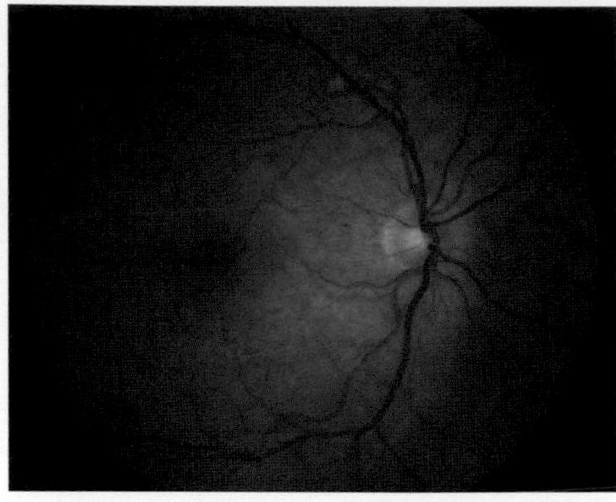

Fig. 6.6 Hypertension – grade III retinopathy (arteriovenous nipping, cotton-wool exudates, flame haemorrhages). (Source: Sainani, G. S. [2010]. *Manual of clinical & practical medicine*. Elsevier India.)

STATION 6.6: ACUTE EXACERBATION OF CONGESTIVE HEART FAILURE

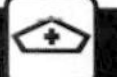 **The Bleep Scenario**

A 76 year old woman has been admitted after becoming short of breath in the early hours of the morning. She reports a new-onset cough, productive of frothy sputum. She is known to have a history of hypertension, diabetes, CHF and rheumatoid arthritis. No history of respiratory illness is reported.

Her observations are: HR 120 bpm, BP 106/75 mmHg, RR 31 breaths per minute, SpO_2 87% on room air and a temperature of 37.2°C.

DEFINITION

Acute exacerbation of congestive heart failure (CHF) refers to the clinical deterioration in a patient with heart failure, abnormal heart structure and/or function. This can be left-sided, right-sided or biventricular.

INITIAL THOUGHTS

Acute heart failure should be the main differential in the case of this patient with a history of acute shortness of breath, on a background of CHF. Additionally, she reports well-known risk factors: old age, history of hypertension and diabetes.

 **Clinical Tip**

In any clinical picture suspicious of acute pulmonary oedema, you should be thinking of the potential cause: cardiogenic (acute or decompensated chronic heart failure) or non-cardiogenic (such as renal failure or acute respiratory distress syndrome).

DIFFERENTIAL DIAGNOSIS

- Cardiology: acute exacerbation of CHF, ACS, bradycardia or pericardial tamponade
- Respiratory: acute exacerbation of asthma or COPD, pulmonary embolism, pneumonia, pneumothorax, pleural effusions or upper-airway obstruction
- Vascular: aortic dissection
- Drug-related: anaphylaxis

INITIAL INSTRUCTIONS OVER PHONE

Request the nurse to commence the patient on a 15 L/minute oxygen via a non-rebreather (NRB) mask. A 12-lead ECG and IV access with bloods should be obtained. Observations should be repeated. Await review before any regular medications are given.

ASSESSMENT AND RESUSCITATION

- End-of-the-bed assessment: the patient is sat forward and holding the sides of the bed tightly (tripod posturing)
- Airway: patent
- Breathing: RR 31 breaths per minute, SpO_2 94% on 15 L/minute oxygen via NRB mask. On auscultation, bibasal crackles can be heard. Dullness noted on percussion of bases
- Arterial blood gas on room air: PaO_2 7.0 kPa, $PaCO_2$ 4.8 kPa, pH 7.36, HCO_3^- 18 mmol/L (type 1 respiratory failure)
- Circulation: CRT 3 s, HR 127 bpm, regular, BP 106/75 mmHg. JVP is visible above the level of the mandibular angle. HS are present with a S3 gallop rhythm audible
  - 12-lead ECG: left ventricular strain pattern
- Disability: GCS 15/15, PEARL, temperature 37.2°C, CBG 7.5 mmol/L
- Exposure: abdomen soft and non-tender, normal bowel sounds. Pitting oedema present up to the level of the knee

INITIAL INVESTIGATIONS

- Haematology: FBC (anaemia)
- Biochemistry: U&Es, LFTs, TFTs (derangement can cause acute CHF), troponin (ACS) and nt-pro BNP (if diagnosis of CHF is unclear)
- Radiology: CXR (pulmonary oedema -see Fig. 6.7)

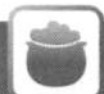 **Clinical Tip**

Radiological signs of acute pulmonary oedema include upper-lobe venous diversion, increased alveolar markings, Kerley B lines, fluid in the horizontal fissure and blunting of the costophrenic angles.

MAKING A DIAGNOSIS

CLASSIFICATION

- Left-sided heart failure is the most common type and occurs when there is reduced left ventricular output, resulting in pulmonary congestion. Common presenting symptoms include dyspnoea, tachypnoea and hypoxia (typically type 1 respiratory failure). Common physical signs include bibasal coarse crackles, and signs of respiratory distress.
- Right-sided heart failure occurs when there is reduced right ventricular output, resulting in systemic venous congestion. It is commonly associated with

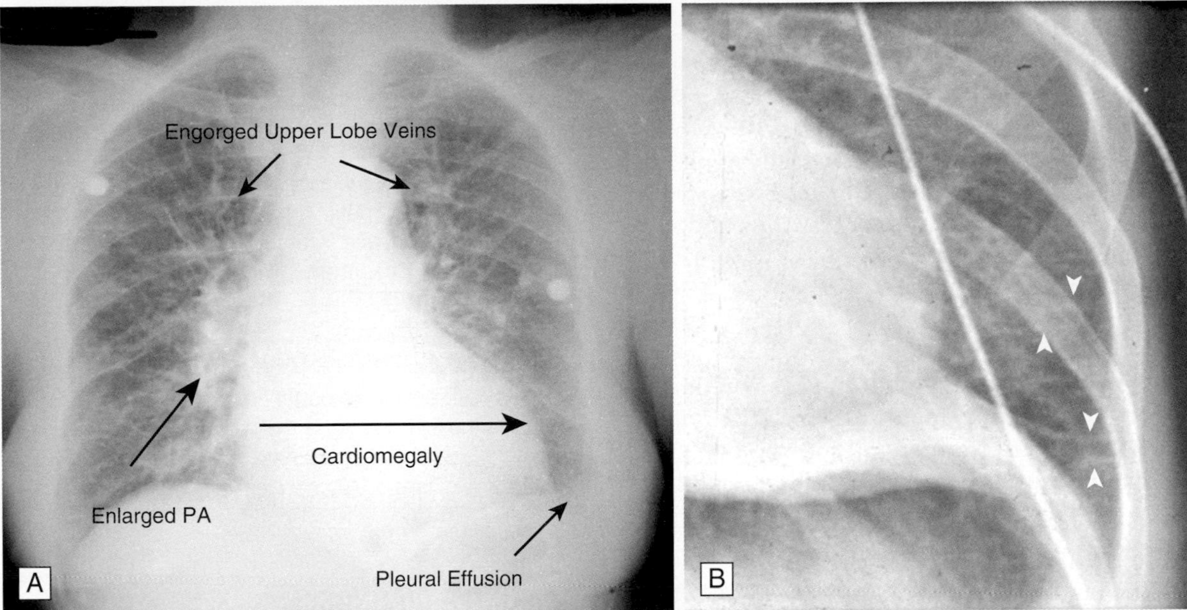

Fig. 6.7 Chest X-ray in a heart failure patient. (A) Cardiac and vascular features of heart failure are depicted. (B) Kerley B lines (arrows) are apparent as horizontal linear densities that extend to the pleural surface of the lung. PA, pulmonary artery. (Source: Felker, G.M. and Mann, D.L. [2020]. *Heart failure: A companion to Braunwald's heart disease*. Elsevier.)

chronic lung disease (cor pulmonale). Symptoms are generally varied but can include peripheral oedema, ascites, right upper abdominal discomfort or pain and any sequelae of existing primary pulmonary disease.
- Biventricular failure occurs when both sides of the heart are affected.

MANAGEMENT

Initial treatment of diuresis aims to reduce fluid overload and decrease preload to the heart and thereby cardiac strain.

In general, treatment is commenced with a loading dose of IV furosemide 80 mg followed by 40 mg once or twice daily, according to BP readings. In severe cases, 240 mg by slow infusion over 24 hours can be considered. The initiation of furosemide requires close monitoring of urine output, weight and renal function. A urinary catheter and fluid balance chart are usually required.

This patient is in acute decompensated cardiac failure with type 1 respiratory failure. Do not administer fluids and await review from the medical registrar and intensive care team, who may consider continuous positive airway pressure (CPAP). It is important to review her previous functional status, as this will determine her suitability for escalation.

 **Prescribing Tip**

Nitrate infusions such as glyceryl trinitrate are no longer recommended as first-line treatment but may still have a useful role, especially in severe renal disease after discussion with a senior clinician. If recommended, you should facilitate stepping the patient up to level 2 care to ensure appropriate monitoring.

 **Prescribing Tip**

Many patients presenting with acute heart failure will be suffering from decompensated chronic heart failure and will already be taking long-term diuretics; in these patients a higher furosemide dose may be warranted.

ESCALATION

Severe refractory pulmonary oedema or any deterioration of the patient's condition warrants immediate escalation to the medical registrar and ITU/critical care outreach team for the consideration of CPAP, which will be performed in a high dependency area.

STATION 6.7: ENDOCARDITIS

 **The Bleep Scenario**

A 37 year old woman has presented to the ED complaining of a gradually worsening history of rigors, fever and malaise over the last 4 weeks. She has a past history of heroin dependence. On initial assessment, she was noted to have a temperature of 39.8°C and has an audible heart murmur.

Her observations are: HR 110 bpm, BP 105/72 mmHg, RR 20 breaths per minute, SpO_2 96% on room air and temperature 39.8°C. You are asked to review the patient.

DEFINITION

Infective endocarditis is an infection of the lining of the heart, often involving the heart valves.

INITIAL THOUGHTS

This woman has clinical features of sepsis. The patient's history and demographics are important to consider when determining the aetiology: patients with prosthetic cardiac valves and IV drug users, for example, are at particularly high risk of infective endocarditis. Other risk factors for endocarditis include previous endocarditis and congenital heart defects.

DIFFERENTIAL DIAGNOSES

- Infective causes: infective endocarditis, rheumatic fever, chest infection, urinary tract infection, hepatitis and sexually transmitted infections
- Inflammatory causes: myocarditis and pericarditis

INITIAL INSTRUCTIONS OVER PHONE

Ask the nurse to obtain a 12-lead ECG and IV access. Request a sepsis screen including bloods, urine sample and a CXR.

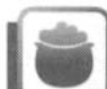 **Clinical Tip**

Your assessment should identify heart failure and embolic complications such as pulmonary or systemic arterial embolism which may be evidenced clinically by the development of focal neurological deficits.

ASSESSMENT AND RESUSCITATION

- End-of-bed assessment: patient is pale, clammy and shivering
- Airway: patent
- Breathing: RR 22 breaths per minute, SpO_2 96% on room air. On auscultation, there are vesicular breath sounds with good air entry bilaterally
- Circulation: CRT 4 s, HR 108 bpm, regular, BP 103/70 mmHg, JVP normal. A systolic murmur can be heard at the left sternal border, loudest during inspiration
  - 12-lead ECG: normal
- Disability: GCS 15/15, PEARL, temperature 39.8°C, CBG 8.9 mmol/L
- Exposure: abdomen soft and non-tender, normal bowel sounds. Finger clubbing is noted. Fundoscopic examination is unremarkable. No neurological deficit noted. Calves unremarkable

INITIAL INVESTIGATIONS

- Haematology: FBC (anaemia or infection)
- Biochemistry: U&Es, LFTs, inflammatory markers (infection)
- Microbiology: blood cultures and urine microscopy, culture and sensitivity (infection screen)
- Radiology: CXR (infection screen), transthoracic echocardiogram (to confirm diagnosis of infective endocarditis)

 **Clinical Tip**

If the transthoracic echocardiogram does not reveal any vegetations, but the patient has a high probability of infective endocarditis by Duke's criteria, you should refer to a cardiologist for a transoesophageal echocardiogram.

 **Prescribing Tip**

Blood cultures should be taken before initiating antibiotic therapy, as the first dose of antibiotics may mask bacteraemia. At least two positive cultures are required for a definitive microbiological diagnosis, so sequential cultures should be taken.

MAKING A DIAGNOSIS

Infective endocarditis should be assessed using the modified Duke's criteria. The patient must have two major criteria or one major and three minor criteria or five minor criteria.

MAJOR CRITERIA

Positive Blood Culture for Infective Endocarditis

- A typical organism in two separate blood cultures (look for *Streptococcus viridans*, *Streptococcus bovis*, *Staphylococcus aureus* or a HACEK organism – *Haemophilus*, *Actinobacillus*, *Cardiobacterium*, *Eikenella*, *Kingella*)
  or
- Consistently positive blood cultures: two over 12 hours apart, or three positive blood cultures with the first and last at least 1 hour apart, or a majority of four blood cultures positive

Features of Endocardial Involvement

- Oscillating intracardiac mass with no anatomical explanation, abscess or prosthetic valve dehiscence detected by echocardiogram
  or
- New valve regurgitation

MINOR CRITERIA

- Predisposing condition: pre-existing heart condition or IV drug use
- Fever >38°C
- Vascular signs such as arterial emboli or Janeway lesions; or immunological signs such as glomerulonephritis, Roth spots, Osler's nodes
- Positive blood culture that fails to meet major criteria
- Positive echocardiogram finding that fails to meet major criteria

Fig. 6.8 shows an example of right atrial vegetations on a transoesophageal echocardiogram.

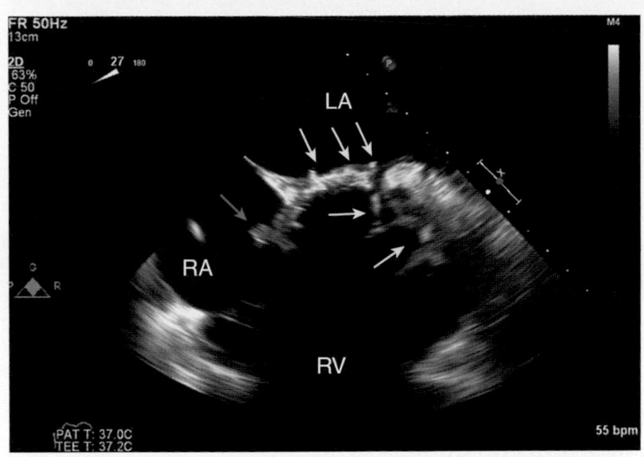

Fig. 6.8 Aortic root abscess with extension into right atrium. Transoesophageal echocardiogram. Midoesophageal aortic valve short-axis view demonstrating an aortic bioprosthesis enveloped by a large aortic root abscess (yellow arrows). Abscess extension into the right atrium (RA) is demonstrated by the presence of a vegetative mass on the RA surface of the aortic abscess (green arrow). LA, left atrium; RV, right ventricle. (Source: Solomon, S.D., Wu, J. and Gillam, L.D. [2019]. *Essential echocardiography*. Elsevier.)

MANAGEMENT

Patients may present with septic shock or acute heart failure, which must be managed before definitive treatment.

This patient may require support with IV fluids to assist perfusion, e.g. 1 L over 1 hour, but as she demonstrates evidence of cardiac decompensation with a new-onset murmur, this should first be discussed with cardiology. Importance must be given to controlling the septic source.

Empirical antibiotic therapy can be initiated even when a definitive causative organism has not yet been confirmed, in communication with the local microbiology team. The choice of antibiotic is dependent on local guidelines and the affected valve.

The most common organisms that cause infective endocarditis include *Staphylococcus aureus, Streptococcus viridans* and culture-negative organisms, including *Coxiella burnetii* and the HACEK organisms.

ESCALATION

Early input from the cardiology and microbiology team is vital. Patients with features of complicated endocarditis such as systemic emboli, heart failure and periannular complications such as abscesses may require surgical intervention. Thus, involvement of the cardiothoracic team may be appropriate.

FURTHER READING

BMJ Best Practice. (2021). *Assessment of tachycardia*. Available at: https://bestpractice.bmj.com/topics/en-gb/830. [Accessed 16 January 2022].

BMJ Best Practice. (2021). *Atrioventricular block*. Available at: https://bestpractice.bmj.com/topics/en-gb/728. [Accessed 16 January 2022].

BMJ Best Practice. (2021). *Bradycardia*. Available at: https://bestpractice.bmj.com/topics/en-gb/832. [Accessed 16 January 2022].

Clinical Audit and Research Unit. (2019). *London Ambulance Service NHS Trust*. Available at: www.londonambulance.nhs.uk/wp-content/uploads/2020/01/Cardiac-Arrest-Annual-Report-2018-2019.pdf. [Accessed 16 January 2022].

Habib, G., et al. (2015). ESC guidelines for the management of infective endocarditis. The task force for the management of infective endocarditis of the European Society of Cardiology (ESC). Endorsed by: European Association for Cardio-Thoracic Surgery (EACTS), the European Association of Nuclear Medicine (EANM). *European Heart Journal, 36*(44), 3075–3128.

ICNARC. (2022). *NCAA key statistics for 2020–21*. Available at: www.icnarc.org/Our-Audit/Audits/Ncaa/Reports/Key-Statistics. [Accessed 16 January 2022].

Kumar, P., & Clark, L. M. (2012). *Kumar & Clark's clinical medicine* (8th ed.). London: Elsevier Health Sciences.

Longmore, M., et al. (2010). *Oxford handbook of clinical medicine* (8th ed.). Oxford: Oxford University Press.

Mahajan, V. S., & Jarolim, P. (2011). Clinician update: how to interpret elevated cardiac troponin levels. *Circulation, 124*, 2350–2354.

Mancia, G., et al. (2013). ESH/ESC guidelines for the management of arterial hypertension: The task force for the management of arterial hypertension of the European Society of Hypertension (ESH) and of the European Society of Cardiology (ESC). *Journal of Hypertension, 31*(7), 1281–1357.

NICE. (2005). *Dual-chamber pacemakers for symptomatic bradycardia due to sick sinus syndrome and/or atrioventricular block*. Available at: www.nice.org.uk/guidance/ta88/chapter/2-Clinical-need-and-practice. [Accessed 16 January 2022].

NICE. (2014). *Acute heart failure: Diagnosis and management. CG187*. Available at: www.nice.org.uk/guidance/cg187. [Accessed 16 January 2022].

NICE. (2017). *Breathlessness*. Available at: https://cks.nice.org.uk/topics/breathlessness. [Accessed 16 January 2022].

Peters, R. J., Mehta, S., & Yusuf, S. (2007). Acute coronary syndromes without ST segment elevation. *BMJ, 334*(7606), 1265–1269.

Resuscitation Council UK. (2017). *Peri-arrest arrhythmias*. Available at: https://lms.resus.org.uk/modules/m10-v2-cardiac-arrest/10346/resources/chapter_11.pdf.

Resuscitation Council UK. (2021). *Adult-advanced life support guidelines*. Available at: www.resus.org.uk/library/2021-resuscitation-guidelines/adult-advanced-life-support-guidelines. [Accessed 16 January 2022].

Resuscitation Council UK. (2021). *Advanced life support book* (8th ed.). London: Resuscitation Council UK.

Resuscitation Council UK. (2021). *Adult bradycardia algorithm*. Available at: www.resus.org.uk/sites/default/files/2021-04/Bradycardia%20Algorithm%202021.pdf. [Accessed 16 January 2022].

Resuscitation Council UK. (2022). *The ABCDE approach*. Available at: www.resus.org.uk/resuscitation-guidelines/abcde-approach. [Accessed 16 January 2022].

Roffi, M., et al. (2015). ESC guidelines for the management of acute coronary syndromes in patients presenting without persistent ST-segment elevation: Task force for the management of acute coronary syndromes in patients presenting without persistent ST-segment elevation of the European Society of Cardiology (ESC). *European Heart Journal, 37*, 267–315.

Simon, C., et al. (2014). *Oxford handbook of general practice* (4th ed.). Oxford: Oxford University Press.

Williams, B., et al. (2018). ESC/ESH guidelines for the management of arterial hypertension: The task force for the management of arterial hypertension of the European Society of Cardiology (ESC) and the European Society of Hypertension (ESH). *European Heart Journal, 39*(33), 3021–3104.

7 Respiratory

Content Outline

STATION 7.1: ACUTE EXACERBATION OF ASTHMA

The Bleep Scenario

A 24 year old female has attended the emergency department (ED) with increasing shortness of breath and wheeze. She has a background of asthma, atopic dermatitis and allergic rhinitis.

Her observations are: heart rate (HR) 100 bpm, blood pressure (BP) 120/90 mmHg, respiratory rate (RR) 24 breaths per minute, SpO_2 92% on room air and temperature 37.2°C. You are asked to review her.

DEFINITION

An acute exacerbation of asthma is an episode of progressive worsening of symptoms of asthma, including breathlessness, wheeze, cough and chest tightness.

Exacerbations are marked by decreases from baseline in measures of pulmonary function, such as peak expiratory flow rate (PEFR) and forced expiratory volume in 1 second (FEV_1).

INITIAL THOUGHTS

This young woman with known asthma is experiencing worsening respiratory symptoms. Your initial diagnosis is likely an acute exacerbation of asthma; however, it is important to consider other causes of acute breathlessness when planning further investigations and not just assume it must be the asthma.

DIFFERENTIAL DIAGNOSIS

- Respiratory: acute asthma exacerbation, acute exacerbation of chronic obstructive pulmonary disease (COPD), pneumonia, pneumothorax, pulmonary embolism (PE), hyperventilation, acute respiratory distress syndrome and foreign-body inhalation. More chronic causes may include severe/poorly controlled asthma/COPD, chronic PE, pleural effusions, bronchial carcinoma and interstitial lung disease
- Cardiac: acute coronary syndrome, acute pulmonary oedema, congestive cardiac failure
- Other: symptomatic anaemia, metabolic acidosis

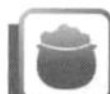

Clinical Tip

Aspiration pneumonia is particularly common in those with a poor swallow, e.g. the elderly, those with neurological conditions (Parkinson's disease, multiple sclerosis) and those with additional needs (learning disabilities, Down's syndrome). Aspiration pneumonia more commonly presents as consolidation in the right lower lobe due to bronchial anatomy.

INITIAL INSTRUCTIONS OVER PHONE

Ask the nurse to put the patient in an upright position, give supplemental oxygen and obtain intravenous (IV) access and bloods as soon as possible. Observations should be repeated, and PEFR measured. You can also ask the nurse to administer salbutamol nebulisers immediately (after checking for allergies) to provide the patient with short-term relief whilst you are on your way.

ASSESSMENT AND RESUSCITATION

- End of the bed assessment: patient appears dyspnoeic and is tiring
- Airway: patent
- Breathing: RR 30 breaths per minute, SpO_2 92% on room air. Symmetrical chest expansion. On auscultation, there is widespread expiratory wheeze. Resonant to percussion throughout. Patient unable to complete sentences
  - Arterial blood gas: pH 7.35, PaO_2 6.3 kPa, $PaCO_2$ 3.5 kPa, HCO_3^- 24 mmol/L (type 1 respiratory failure)
  - Administer oxygen at 2 L/minute and titrate. Aim for saturations of 94–98%

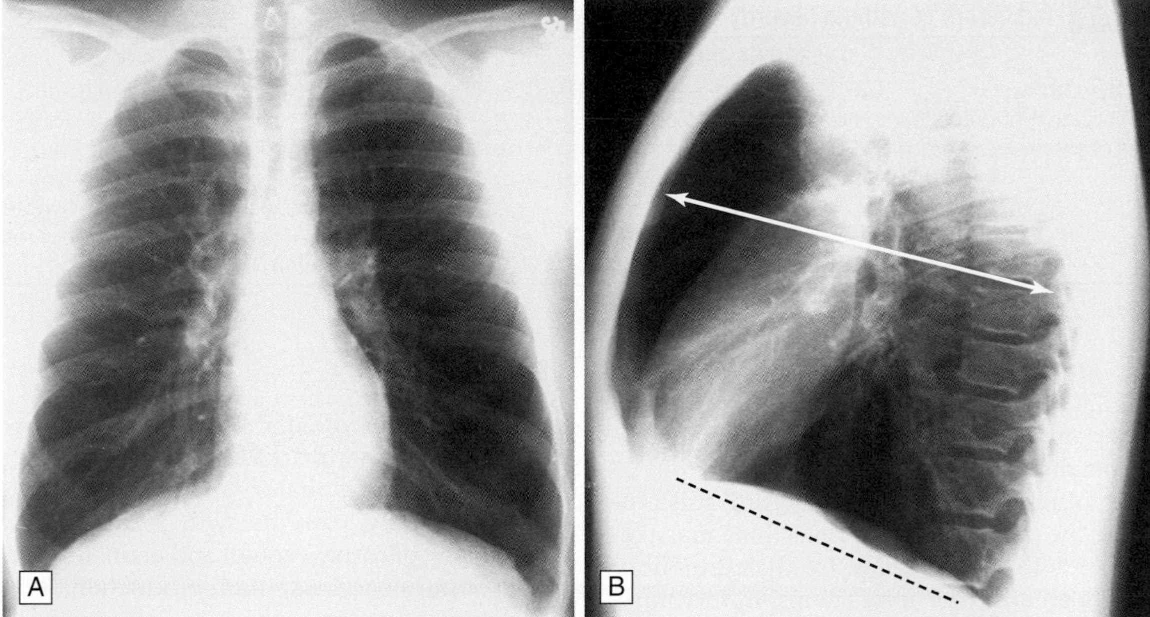

Fig. 7.1 Asthma. During a severe asthma attack, hyperinflation, similar to that seen in chronic obstructive pulmonary disease (COPD), can be seen. In this case, hyperinflation is seen, with the superior aspect of the hemidiaphragms located at the level of the posterior 11th ribs (A); a slight increase in the anteroposterior diameter and some flattening of the hemidiaphragm appear (B). The patient does not have the barrel-shaped chest seen in COPD. Most patients with asthma have normal chest X-rays. (Source: Mettler, F.A. [2014]. *Essentials of radiology*. Elsevier.)

- Circulation: capillary refill time (CRT) 3s, HR 110 bpm, regular, BP 126/74 mmHg, jugular venous pressure (JVP) not raised, heart sounds (HS) I + II + 0
  - 12-lead electrocardiogram (ECG): regular sinus tachycardia
- Disability: Glasgow Coma Scale (GCS) 15/15, pupils equal and reactive to light (PEARL), temperature 36.4°C, capillary blood glucose (CBG) 5.7 mmol/L
- Exposure: abdomen soft and non-tender, with normal bowel sounds. Calves are unremarkable

 **Prescribing Tip**

Remember that salbutamol nebulisers can cause hypokalaemia and increase lactate levels. It is important to take this into account when interpreting blood gas results.

INITIAL INVESTIGATIONS

- Haematology: full blood count (FBC: anaemia or infection)
- Biochemistry: urea and electrolytes (U&Es: risk of hypokalaemia with salbutamol) and troponin if experiencing chest pain (cardiac necrosis)
- Radiology: chest X-ray (CXR: hyperinflation (Fig. 7.1), consolidation, pleural effusion, pneumothorax)

MAKING A DIAGNOSIS

Determine the severity of the exacerbation using objective criteria and note the patient's degree of agitation and consciousness. Look for signs of exhaustion, cyanosis and use of accessory muscles (Table 7.1).

MANAGEMENT

The aim of asthma treatment is to relieve airflow obstruction and maintain arterial oxygen saturations. Treatment begins with the administration of supplemental oxygen, short-acting beta-2 agonists and systemic corticosteroids.

Sit the patient as upright as possible and give supplemental oxygen. Give oxygen-driven nebulised salbutamol (5 mg every 30–60 minutes titrated according to response). Aim for oxygen saturations of 94–98%.

If there is no improvement or the exacerbation is severe/life-threatening, an inhaled anticholinergic should be added: nebulised ipratropium bromide (500 µg every 4 hours) in addition to the salbutamol nebulisers. Give the first dose of prednisolone 40 mg (if unable to tolerate orally, consider IV hydrocortisone 100 mg) and start IV fluids as required. Consider a single dose of magnesium sulphate 1.2–2 g IV over 20 minutes; however, this must be discussed with a senior clinician.

Further medical management includes the consideration of IV aminophylline and IV salbutamol which are given in an intensive care setting. It is crucial to ask about any previous intensive therapy unit admissions; patients who have required organ support in the past will likely require timely escalation to critical care.

Remember that infections are a common cause of an exacerbation of asthma. However, do not prescribe

Table 7.1 Indicators of asthma severity

MODERATE	SEVERE, ANY ONE OF:	LIFE-THREATENING, ANY ONE OF:
Increasing symptoms PEF >50–75% best or predicted No features of acute severe asthma	PEFR 33–50% best or predicted Heart rate ≥110 bpm Respiratory rate ≥25 breaths per minute Inability to complete sentences in one breath	PEFR <33% best or predicted SpO_2 <92%, or PaO_2 <8 kPa Normal $PaCO_2$ (3.6–6.0 kPa) Clinical signs: altered conscious level, exhaustion, arrhythmia, hypotension, cyanosis, silent chest, poor respiratory effort

PEFR, peak expiratory flow rate.

antibiotics routinely, unless symptoms and signs suggest a bacterial infection.

It is important to determine compliance with medication and details of previous exacerbations.

After the initial exacerbation is resolved, it is crucial to ensure the patient's long-term asthma management is revised through review by the respiratory team. Many hospitals have access to respiratory nurses who will be able to give initial advice. Some patients can benefit from chest physiotherapy which can potentially help alleviate wheezing and frequency of exacerbations.

Prescribing Tip

Prescribe salbutamol and ipratropium nebulisers regularly and as needed. Oral prednisolone is prescribed as a 5-day course.

ESCALATION

Evidence of poor response to initial treatment includes: reducing PEFR, persistent/worsening hypoxia, hypercapnia, acidosis, exhaustion, reduction in GCS, respiratory arrest.

At this point, it is likely that the patient will require continuous monitoring and additional respiratory support in the intensive care unit. Examples of treatment given in this setting include the administration of IV aminophylline and IV salbutamol, both of which require intensive monitoring of respiratory and cardiovascular function, and in some instances, intubation and ventilatory support.

STATION 7.2: ACUTE EXACERBATION OF COPD

The Bleep Scenario

A 60 year old man has been admitted to the acute medical unit complaining of increasing shortness of breath and productive cough. He has a background of COPD, hypertension and gout.

His observations are: HR 75 bpm, BP 140/85 mmHg, RR 19 breaths per minute, SpO_2 85% on room air and temperature 36.7°C. You are asked to review him.

DEFINITION

An acute exacerbation of COPD is an acute worsening of symptoms that marks a deterioration from the patient's baseline respiratory function.

It classically presents with increasing dyspnoea, worsening of chronic cough and an increase in the volume or purulence of sputum production.

INITIAL THOUGHTS

This man with known COPD is experiencing an acute deterioration of respiratory function associated with hypoxia. Your top differential is likely an acute exacerbation of COPD; given his symptoms of shortness of breath and productive cough, however, you should be mindful of other causes when assessing the patient.

DIFFERENTIAL DIAGNOSIS

- Respiratory: acute exacerbation of COPD, acute exacerbation of asthma, pneumonia, pleural effusion, pneumothorax, PE, airway obstruction, lung/lobar collapse, interstitial lung disease and malignancy
- Cardiovascular: acute pulmonary oedema, congestive cardiac failure and acute coronary syndrome
- Gastrointestinal: gastro-oesophageal reflux disease
- Other: drugs such as angiotensin-converting enzyme inhibitors, non-steroidal anti-inflammatory drugs, beta-blockers and adenosine or sarcoidosis

INITIAL INSTRUCTIONS OVER PHONE

Ask the nurse to commence the patient on supplemental oxygen, aiming for saturations 94–98%. Ask the nurse to repeat observations and to obtain IV access, bloods and an ECG as soon as possible. You should also ask the nurse to administer salbutamol and ipratropium nebulisers to provide immediate relief for the patient whilst you are on your way.

ASSESSMENT AND RESUSCITATION

- End of the bed assessment: patient appears cachectic and flushed
- Airway: patent

- Breathing: RR 30 breaths per minute, SpO_2 85% on room air. On auscultation, there are right mid-zone crepitations with a widespread expiratory wheeze. There is dullness to percussion in the right mid and lower zones
- Arterial blood gas: pH 7.29, PaO_2 7.1 kPa, $PaCO_2$ 7.4 kPa, HCO_3^- 33 mmol/L (type 2 respiratory failure and respiratory acidosis)
  - Make sure the patient receives high-flow oxygen
- Circulation: CRT 3 s, HR 80 bpm, regular, BP 135/80 mmHg, JVP not visible, HS I + II + 0
  - 12-lead ECG: may show right heart enlargement, arrhythmia or evidence of ischaemia
- Disability: GCS 15/15, PEARL, temperature 37.5°C, CBG 5.7 mmol/L
- Exposure: Evidence of finger clubbing and tar staining in the fingers. Barrel-shaped chest. Abdomen soft and non-tender with normal bowel sounds. Calves unremarkable

INITIAL INVESTIGATIONS

- Haematology: FBC (infection, anaemia)
- Biochemistry: U&Es and LFTs (check for any renal or liver injury secondary to chest sepsis), C-reactive protein (CRP): infection and serum theophylline (if the patient is on theophylline/aminophylline)
- Microbiology: sputum microscopy, culture and sensitivity (common isolates include *Haemophilus influenzae, Streptococcus pneumoniae and Moraxella catarrhalis*)
- Radiology: CXR (hyperinflation, flattened diaphragm, focus of infection), computed tomography (CT) chest (only if suspicion of malignancy, PE, bronchiectasis or considering surgery)

MAKING A DIAGNOSIS

An acute exacerbation of COPD is a clinical diagnosis, dependent on the clinical presentation and past medical history.

- Symptoms: dyspnoea, cough, increased sputum volume/purulence
- Signs: hyperinflated chest, wheeze, crackles if concurrent infection

A CXR is used to identify any potential focus of infection and to exclude other diagnoses. Spirometry is used to confirm the diagnosis of COPD; however, this is not appropriate during an acute exacerbation.

MANAGEMENT

Encourage the patient to sit upright for comfort and prescribe air-driven salbutamol (5 mg every 4 hours) and ipratropium (500 μg every 6 hours) nebulisers.

Using a Venturi mask, provide the patient with controlled oxygen and target saturations of 88–92% (however some COPD patients may have target saturations of 94% to 98%). Ensure that serial arterial blood gases are taken to monitor for respiratory failure and acidosis; for example, on admission, 30–60 minutes after commencing oxygen therapy and if the patient deteriorates.

Commence oral prednisolone 30 mg for 7–14 days, or IV hydrocortisone 100 mg if the oral route is unavailable. If there is evidence of infection, for example, the CXR shows consolidation or clinical findings are suggestive of infection, then antibiotics should be prescribed according to local guidelines and any previous culture results for the patient. If you suspect sepsis, then initiate the sepsis protocol.

The patient should be closely monitored until clinically stable through clinical assessment, repeat observations including pulse oximetry and arterial blood gas measurements.

All patients should also receive appropriate fluid management and venous thromboembolism prophylaxis. You can also consider nicotine replacement therapy and nutritional supplements.

ESCALATION

If the patient fails to respond to initial management or deteriorates, then you should escalate immediately to the medical registrar and to the intensive care unit. Signs that the patient needs urgent escalation include respiratory acidosis, severe dyspnoea and persistent hypoxaemia.

Further interventions might include IV aminophylline, non-invasive ventilation and invasive mechanical ventilation. The patient's ceiling of care should also be considered.

STATION 7.3: COMMUNITY-ACQUIRED PNEUMONIA

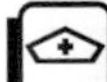

The Bleep Scenario

A 63 year old woman is admitted to the acute medical unit with confusion, shortness of breath and productive cough. She has a background of osteoarthritis.

Her observations are: HR 90 bpm, BP 110/90 mmHg, RR 28 breaths per minute, SpO_2 92% on room air and temperature 38.4°C. The nurse calls you to review her.

DEFINITION

Community-acquired pneumonia (CAP) is pneumonia acquired outside of hospital or healthcare facilities.

Pneumonia develops when pathogens invade the lung parenchyma and commonly presents with fever, cough, mucopurulent sputum and focal signs on clinical examination of the chest.

INITIAL THOUGHTS

CAP is a common cause of hospital admissions in the UK and is likely your initial diagnosis in this patient, based on her symptoms.

 Clinical Tip

The patient's past medical history will provide you with vital clues to determine the most likely diagnosis and appropriate management.

DIFFERENTIAL DIAGNOSIS

- Respiratory: acute bronchitis, COPD exacerbation, asthma exacerbation, bronchiectasis exacerbation, pneumothorax, PE and empyema. More chronic respiratory causes include hypersensitivity pneumonitis, interstitial lung disease, tuberculosis, lung cancer or metastatic disease
- Cardiovascular: congestive cardiac failure

 Clinical Tip

The distinction between CAP and hospital-acquired pneumonia (develops >48 hours after hospital admission) is important due to the differing pathogens which are responsible and which antimicrobial medications are most likely to be effective.

INITIAL INSTRUCTIONS OVER PHONE

Ask the nurse to sit the patient upright and give her supplemental oxygen, as well as obtain IV access and bloods, if possible before you arrive. Remind the nurse to monitor the patient continuously for any changes in her observations until you arrive, and request the nurse to await your review before any further medications are given.

ASSESSMENT AND RESUSCITATION

- End of the bed assessment: the patient is dyspnoeic and using accessory muscles of respiration
- Airway: patent
- Breathing: RR 30 breaths per minute, SpO_2 90% on room air. On auscultation, there is reduced air entry with bronchial breathing at the right lower zone. There is dullness to percussion at the right lower zone associated with reduced chest expansion on the right side
- Arterial blood gas: pH 7.33, PaO_2 10.0 kPa, $PaCO_2$ 3.2 kPa, HCO_3^- 20 mmol/L, lactate 3.0 mmol/L (raised lactate, metabolic acidosis, hypoxaemia)
  - Give nasal cannulae oxygen 2 L/minute. Aim for oxygen saturations of 94–98%
- Circulation: CRT 3 s, HR 94 bpm, regular, BP 100/82 mmHg, JVP not visible, HS I + II + 0
  - 12-lead ECG: sinus tachycardia
- Disability: GCS 14/15, PEARL, temperature 38.4°C, CBG 5.7 mmol/L, Abbreviated Mental Test Score (AMTS) 7/10
- Exposure: rigors noted. Abdomen soft and non-tender, with normal bowel sounds. Calves unremarkable

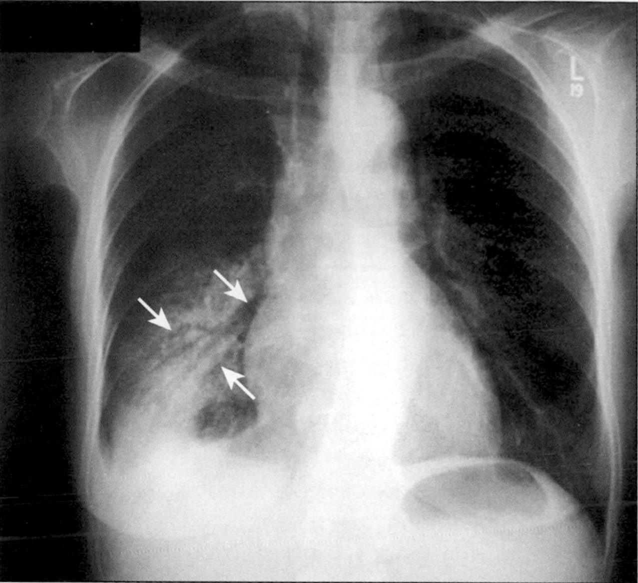

Fig. 7.2 Right lower-lobe consolidation. The abnormal whiteness in the right lower and mid zones is poorly defined and 'fluffy'. There is a trident-shaped lucency, which is an air bronchogram (arrows). The right heart border remains visible. (Source: Cross, J. et al. [2008]. *Respiratory physiotherapy: an on call survival guide*. Elsevier.)

INITIAL INVESTIGATIONS

- Haematology: FBC (leukocytosis)
- Biochemistry: U&Es (urea part of CURB-65 score), CRP (inflammation), LFTs
- Microbiology: sputum for MCS, blood cultures, urinary antigens (*Legionella*, pneumococcal antigens)
- Radiology: CXR (lobar or multilobar infiltrates) (Fig. 7.2)

 Clinical Tip

Note that any patient with a known cognitive impairment automatically receives 1 point for confusion on the CURB-65 score.

MAKING A DIAGNOSIS

You should suspect CAP in any patient with symptoms and signs consistent with an acute lower respiratory tract infection and with new radiographic changes (consolidation). You must also be mindful of sepsis when managing patients with any type of infection, even if their temperature is normal. Use your local sepsis protocol within 1 hour for any patient with suspected sepsis.

- Symptoms: cough, dyspnoea, pleuritic chest pain, mucopurulent sputum, myalgia and/or confusion
- Signs: pyrexia, tachypnoea, crackles, decreased breath sounds, dullness to percussion and/or wheeze

You should determine the clinical severity of CAP using the CURB-65 score (Table 7.2).

Table 7.2 CURB-65 scoring

Confusion (AMTS ≤8)	1 point
Urea >7 mmol/L	1 point
Respiratory rate >30 breaths per minute	1 point
Blood pressure: diastolic <60 mmHg or systolic <90 mmHg	1 point
Age ≥65 years	1 point

AMTS, Abbreviated Mental Test Score.

Clinical Tip

The most common causative pathogen is *Streptococcus pneumoniae*. Other pathogens include *Haemophilus influenzae*, *Staphylococcus aureus* and *Moraxella catarrhalis*. Remember to consider atypical pathogens and their respective presentations (*Mycoplasma pneumoniae, Chlamydophila pneumoniae, Legionella pneumophila).*

MANAGEMENT

In terms of oxygenation, you should target saturations of 94–98% in acutely ill patients not at risk of hypercapnia, and target saturations of 88–92% in patients at risk of hypercapnia once you have access to their past history and know if they are likely to develop type 2 respiratory failure. Use arterial blood gas measurements to monitor for respiratory failure.

Treat hypotension with IV fluid resuscitation and seek senior support if the patient has a history of cardiac failure or chronic kidney disease. Consider catheterisation for fluid balance monitoring.

Remember to prescribe adequate analgesia if the patient is experiencing pleuritic chest pain.

Commence antibiotics as per the patient's CURB-65 score and your local antibiotic guidelines and your patient's allergies (Table 7.3).

Of note, you should also arrange a follow-up clinical review and chest x-ray 6 weeks after the initial presentation to rule out any underlying malignancy.

ESCALATION

The medical registrar should be notified with a view to initiating further escalation measures, including CPAP or non-invasive ventilation, or invasive mechanical ventilation in an intensive care setting if any of the following apply: refractory or progressive hypoxia, hypercapnia, acidosis, respiratory failure or evidence of sepsis.

STATION 7.4: PLEURAL EFFUSION

The Bleep Scenario

A 60 year old woman is admitted with shortness of breath. She does not normally have any difficulties in breathing. She is normally fit and well with no significant past medical history.

Her observations are: HR 88 bpm, BP 135/80 mmHg, RR 30 breaths per minute, SpO_2 92% on room air and temperature 39.0°C. You are asked to review her.

Table 7.3 Treatment according to CURB-65 scores

CURB SCORE	SEVERITY	TREATMENT
0–1	Low	Home-based care Oral antibiotics according to local guidelines
2	Moderate	Hospital-based care Oral/IV antibiotics according to local guidelines
≥3	High	Hospital-based care IV antibiotics according to local guidelines Urgent discussion with senior colleague and ICU

ICU, intensive care unit; IV, intravenous.

DEFINITION

A pleural effusion is a collection of fluid between the parietal and visceral pleural surfaces of the thorax. Effusions can be classified according to their protein content as transudates (<25 g/L) or exudates (>35 g/L), using Light's criteria.

INITIAL THOUGHTS

You should consider causes of acute dyspnoea in patients ≥60 years with no pre-existing respiratory disease. These include pleural effusion, PE, pneumonia, pneumothorax, COPD and pulmonary oedema. You should also attempt to rule out other causes such as malignancy, bronchiectasis and lung/lobar collapse. One of the first investigations to request (if not completed already) is a CXR.

DIFFERENTIAL DIAGNOSIS

TRANSUDATIVE PLEURAL EFFUSION

A transudative pleural effusion is caused by an imbalance of oncotic and hydrostatic pressures, resulting in pleural fluid with low protein and lactate dehydrogenase (LDH) levels.

Reasons include cardiac failure, cirrhosis, hypoalbuminaemia, nephrotic syndrome, hypothyroidism, constrictive pericarditis and Meigs' syndrome.

EXUDATIVE PLEURAL EFFUSION

An exudative pleural effusion is caused by accumulation of fluid from leaky pleural capillaries, resulting in pleural fluid with high protein and LDH levels.

Reasons include infection (tuberculosis, bacterial pneumonia), inflammation (systemic lupus erythematosus, sarcoidosis), malignancy (bronchial carcinoma, mesothelioma), pulmonary infarction, post-myocardial infarction and acute pancreatitis.

INITIAL INSTRUCTIONS OVER PHONE

Ask the nurse to make sure the patient is sat upright and to give supplemental oxygen, aiming for saturations of

94–98%. You can also ask the nurse to obtain IV access and bloods and to repeat her observations. You can also ask for the patient to have paracetamol (if not contraindicated) prior to your arrival to make her feel more comfortable.

ASSESSMENT AND RESUSCITATION

- End of the bed assessment: the patient is short of breath and sweating
- Airway: patient appears flushed, breathing pattern is shallow and fast
- Breathing: RR 30 breaths per minute, SpO_2 91% on room air. On auscultation, there are reduced breath sounds at the right lower zone. Percussion note is stony dull in the right lower zone.
    - Arterial blood gas: pH 7.32, PaO_2 9.1 kPa, $PaCO_2$ 2.9 kPa, lactate 3.4 mmol/L, HCO_3^- 18.0 mmol/L (metabolic acidosis, hypoxaemia, hypocapnia)
    - Give high-flow oxygen 15 L/minute. Aim for saturations of 94–98%
- Circulation: CRT 3 s, HR 90 bpm, regular, BP 135/80 mmHg, JVP not visible, HS I + II + 0
    - 12-lead ECG: may show arrhythmias or cardiac pathologies
- Disability: GCS 15/15, PEARL, temperature 39.0°C, CBG 5.7 mmol/L
- Exposure: abdomen soft and non-tender, with normal bowel sounds. No shifting dullness. No peripheral or sacral oedema

INITIAL INVESTIGATIONS

- Haematology: FBC (infection)
- Biochemistry: serum LDH and protein levels (to determine nature of effusion), CRP (inflammation), NT-Pro BNP (cardiac failure) and troponin (myocardial ischaemia)
- Microbiology: blood cultures, sputum for MCS
- Pleural fluid analysis: biochemistry (protein, LDH, glucose, pH, amylase), bacteriology (microscopy and culture, tuberculosis culture, auramine stain), cytology, immunology (rheumatoid factors, antinuclear antibody and complement levels)
- Radiology: CXR (blunting of costophrenic angle(s)), pleural ultrasound (fluid in pleural space), CT chest (suspicion of malignancy)

MAKING A DIAGNOSIS

A diagnosis of pleural effusion is made clinically, and radiologically confirmed with a CXR (Fig. 7.3), but can also be diagnosed and more clearly anatomically defined, by a chest ultrasound.

Light's criteria are then used to differentiate a transudative from an exudative effusion if there is diagnostic uncertainty. Light's criteria suggest an exudative effusion if any of the following are present:

- Pleural protein-to-serum ratio >0.5
- Pleural LDH-to-serum LDH ratio >0.6
- Pleural LDH greater than two-thirds of upper limit of normal for serum

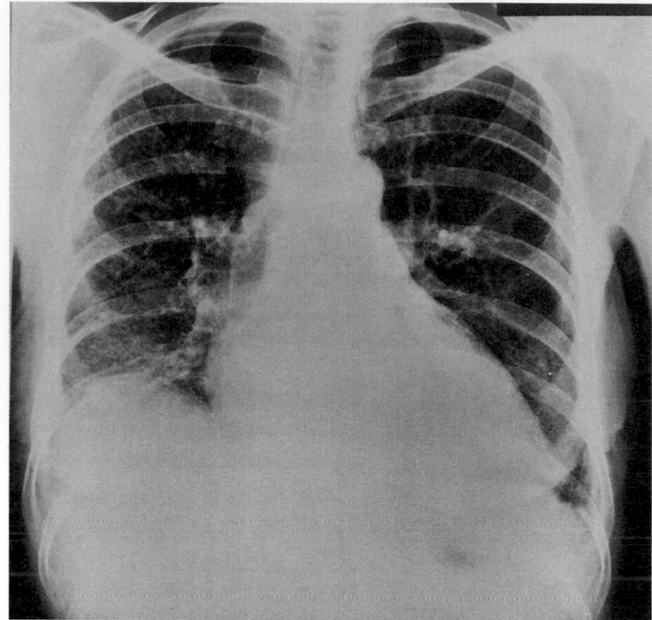

Fig. 7.3 An example of a chest X-ray showing a pleural effusion. (Source: Heuer, A. [2021]. *Wilkins' clinical assessment in respiratory care*. Elsevier.)

Given this patient's pyrexia and unilateral findings, the most likely diagnosis is an exudative effusion secondary to an infective process.

- Symptoms: dyspnoea, pleurisy
- Signs: decreased chest expansion, stony dullness to percussion, diminished breath sounds, decreased vocal resonance/tactile fremitus and tracheal deviation away from the side of effusion if large

Once you have confirmed the presence of a pleural effusion, you should try to identify the cause using the patient's history and the investigations above. Pleural ultrasound is often used for diagnostic or therapeutic aspiration, though this will most likely be performed by a respiratory physician.

MANAGEMENT

This patient should be sat upright and given high-flow oxygen via a non-rebreather mask to target saturations of 94–98%. An arterial blood gas is essential to determine the presence of respiratory failure. This patient should also be initiated on antibiotics, given the high suspicion of infection.

Ongoing management will be determined by the cause of the effusion and by senior team members. Interventions may include diuretics in the case of cardiac effusions, antibiotics in the case of parapneumonic effusions, therapeutic aspiration if the effusion is large and significantly symptomatic, chest drain insertion or the consideration of pleurodesis or surgical intervention (lysis of adhesions, decortication) if unresponsive to medical management.

ESCALATION

You should involve the medical registrar and respiratory physician as soon as possible as the patient will need an ultrasound-guided pleural aspiration for diagnostic and/or therapeutic purposes. If this patient's observations of hypoxia, tachypnoea or pyrexia do not improve with the measures described above, then aspiration may need to occur more urgently.

STATION 7.5: PNEUMOTHORAX

 **The Bleep Scenario**

A 21 year old male is admitted to the ED with sudden-onset shortness of breath and unilateral chest pain. He has no known past medical history.

His observations are: HR 80 bpm, BP 130/80 mmHg, RR 28 breaths per minute, SpO_2 80% on room air and temperature 36.4°C. You are asked to review him.

DEFINITION

Pneumothorax is air in the pleural space that can be classified as primary or secondary. Primary pneumothorax arises in people without pre-existing lung disease whereas secondary pneumothorax arises in people with pre-existing lung disease.

INITIAL THOUGHTS

This patient is experiencing acute dyspnoea with tachypnoea and borderline hypoxia. Your initial assessment should involve consideration of the life-threatening causes of shortness of breath in this age group. Immediate causes to consider include pneumothorax, pneumonia, PE, pleural effusion and exacerbation of asthma. Remember, if the patient has a tension pneumothorax, this requires immediate decompression. You should not await CXR confirmation if a tension pneumothorax is clinically suspected as any delay may be fatal.

DIFFERENTIAL DIAGNOSIS

- Respiratory: acute asthma exacerbation, pneumonia acute COPD exacerbation, PE, pleural effusion, bronchopleural fistula and interstitial lung disease
- Cardiovascular: myocardial ischaemia and pericarditis
- Gastrointestinal: oesophageal perforation and gastro-oesophageal reflux

INITIAL INSTRUCTIONS OVER PHONE

Ask the nurse to monitor the patient continuously, importantly, being vigilant of hypoxia and hypotension, which are both potential indicators of a tension pneumothorax with systemic decompensation.

ASSESSMENT AND RESUSCITATION

- End of the bed assessment: patient's breathing is shallow and fast
- Airway: patent
- Breathing: RR 30 breaths per minute, SpO_2 80% on room air. Trachea is central. Equal chest expansion bilaterally. On auscultation, there are reduced breath sounds on the right side. Percussion note is hyperresonant on the right side
  - Arterial blood gas: pH 7.2, $PaCO_2$ 5.5 kPa, PaO_2 8.2 kPa, HCO_3^- 18 mmol/L
  - Give high-flow oxygen 15 L/minute. Aim for saturations of 94–98%
- Circulation: CRT 2 s, HR 84 bpm, regular, BP 130/80 mmHg, JVP not visible, HS I + II + 0
  - 12-lead ECG: normal sinus rhythm
- Disability: GCS 15/15, PEARL, temperature 36.4°C, CBG 5.7 mmol/L
- Exposure: Patient is tall and slender. No obvious signs of chest trauma. Abdomen soft and non-tender, with normal bowel sounds. Calves unremarkable

INITIAL INVESTIGATIONS

- Haematology: FBC (signs of superimposed infection)
- Biochemistry: CRP (inflammation/infection), U&Es (electrolytes/renal function)
- Radiology: CXR (pneumothorax, evidence of pre-existing lung disease), CT scan (occult pneumothorax, traumatic pneumothorax and evidence of pre-existing lung disease)

MAKING A DIAGNOSIS

Primary pneumothorax is common in tall, slender young males. Risk factors include smoking history, Marfan's syndrome or a positive family history. Predisposing respiratory conditions for secondary pneumothorax include COPD, asthma, *Pneumocystis jirovecii*, cystic fibrosis and tuberculosis. Also, be sure to ask the patient about any recent trauma or invasive medical procedure.

- Symptoms: sudden-onset breathlessness, pleuritic chest pain and sudden respiratory deterioration in patients with asthma/COPD; ventilated patients experience sudden hypoxia or increased ventilatory pressures
- Signs: reduced chest expansion on the affected side, hyperresonance to percussion and/or decreased breath sounds

In the context of a tension pneumothorax, it is particularly important to be vigilant of tracheal deviation away from the affected side, haemodynamic instability and distended neck veins.

 **Clinical Tip**

Remember that if there is clinical suspicion of a tension pneumothorax, do not await CXR confirmation. The patient requires emergency decompression.

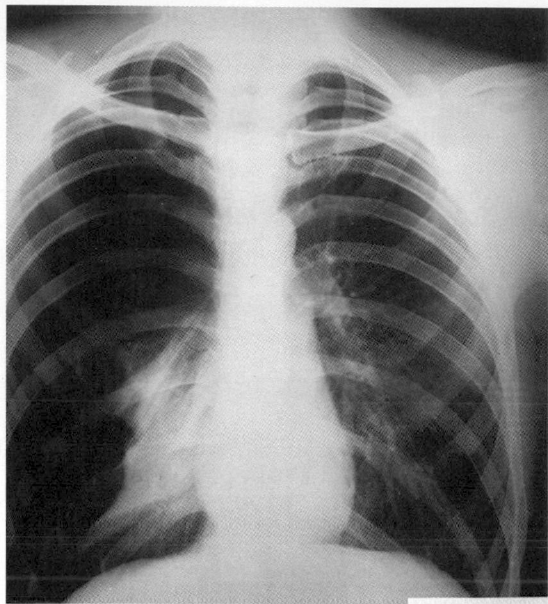

Fig. 7.4 Chest X-ray showing pneumothorax. (Source: Kowalczyk, N. [2021]. *Radiographic pathology for technologists*. Elsevier.)

MANAGEMENT

Encourage the patient to sit upright for comfort and arrange CXR as soon as possible (as long as tension pneumothorax is not suspected; Fig. 7.4). Given that this patient has no pre-existing lung disease, this is most likely to be a primary spontaneous pneumothorax.

- Primary pneumothorax <2 cm: consider discharge with outpatient review in 2–4 weeks.
- Primary pneumothorax >2 cm: simple aspiration using 16–18G cannula. Insert cannula at the intersection between the midclavicular line and the second or third intercostal space and aspirate less than 2.5 L. If unsuccessful, proceed to chest drain insertion.
- Secondary pneumothorax <1 cm, no acute dyspnoea: admit for 24 hours observation and oxygen therapy.
- Secondary pneumothorax 1–2 cm, or acute dyspnoea: simple aspiration using 16–18G cannula. If successful, admit for 24 hours observation and oxygen therapy. If unsuccessful, proceed to chest drain insertion.
- Secondary pneumothorax >2 cm: insert a chest drain.

All patients having aspiration or chest drain insertion should have a repeat CXR to ensure the intervention was successful. The patient should also be advised against air travel for 1 week and diving permanently (unless there is a bilateral pleurectomy and normal lung function is satisfactory on CT thorax).

ESCALATION

If simple aspiration of a primary pneumothorax is unsuccessful, you should contact the medical registrar to consider insertion of a chest drain (8–14 Fr). The patient should then be transferred to the respiratory ward for further observation and management.

STATION 7.6: PULMONARY EMBOLISM

The Bleep Scenario

A 55 year old male has presented to the ED complaining of shortness of breath and chest pain worsened by deep inspiration. Of note, he returned from Thailand 24 hours before presentation. He has a background of prostate cancer.

His observations are: HR 95 bpm, BP 145/100 mmHg, RR 23 breaths per minute, SpO_2 88% on room air and temperature 37.5°C. You are asked to review him.

DEFINITION

PE is a consequence of venous thrombus formation, most commonly in the pelvis or lower limb, that embolises to the pulmonary vasculature.

Thrombus formation results from a triad of risk factors, known collectively as Virchow's triad: venous stasis, trauma and hypercoagulability.

INITIAL THOUGHTS

This man has pleuritic-sounding chest pain associated with dyspnoea, tachypnoea, hypoxia and low-grade pyrexia – highly suggestive of PE.

He has at least two significant risk factors for venous thromboembolic disease: malignancy and recent immobilisation (long-haul flight).

Other risk factors suggestive of venous thromboembolism include current/previous venous thromboembolism, malignancy, recent surgery or immobilisation, recent travel, medication history, family history and smoking history.

DIFFERENTIAL DIAGNOSIS

- Respiratory: pneumothorax, CAP, exacerbation of asthma, exacerbation of COPD
- Cardiovascular: acute coronary syndrome, angina, congestive cardiac failure, pericarditis, cardiac tamponade, aortic dissection
- Locomotor: costochondritis, chest wall injury, herpes zoster

INITIAL INSTRUCTIONS OVER PHONE

Ask the nurse to sit the patient upright and administer high-flow oxygen. An ECG, IV access and bloods should be obtained as soon as possible.

Clinical Tip

Morphine can be used as effective analgesia and to relieve symptomatic dyspnoea.

ASSESSMENT AND RESUSCITATION

- End of the bed assessment: patient appears dyspnoeic and distressed
- Airway: patent
- Breathing: RR 30 breaths per minute, SpO_2 88% on room air. Equal and bilateral chest expansion. On auscultation, there are vesicular breath sounds with good air entry bilaterally
    - Arterial blood gas: pH 7.47, PaO_2 7.5 kPa, $PaCO_2$ 2.5 kPa, HCO_3^- 25 mmol/L (hypoxaemia, hypocapnia, mild respiratory alkalosis)
- Circulation: CRT 3 s, HR 100 bpm, regular, BP 94/60 mmHg, JVP normal, HS I + II + 0
    - 12-lead ECG: sinus tachycardia
- Disability: GCS 15/15, PEARL, temperature 37.5°C, CBG 5.7 mmol/L
- Exposure: abdomen soft and non-tender, with normal bowel sounds. Right calf unremarkable. Left calf mildly swollen and tender on palpation.

INITIAL INVESTIGATIONS

- Haematology: FBC (thrombocytopenia, anaemia, polycythaemia), coagulation studies (prothrombin time, activated partial thromboplastin time, international normalized ratio and fibrinogen) and D-dimer (according to Wells' score).
- Biochemistry: U&Es, LFTs and troponin (myocardial ischaemia)
- Radiology: CXR (usually normal), CT pulmonary angiogram (CT PA: intraluminal filling defect of the pulmonary artery or one of its branches), echocardiogram (R ventricular strain or R ventricular hypokinesis) and V/Q scan (area of ventilation that is not perfused)

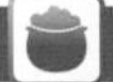 **Clinical Tip**

V/Q scan may be performed in patients with contraindications to CT PA (renal impairment, contrast allergy, young patients, pregnant patients) but is of limited use in patients with underlying lung disease or cardiac failure.

MAKING A DIAGNOSIS

You should determine the clinical probability of PE using the modified Wells' two-level PE score and manage accordingly (Table 7.4).

It is important to suspect PE in any patient who develops acute dyspnoea, pleuritic chest pain or haemoptysis. Similarly, patients who become acutely tachypnoeic or experience a sudden drop in their oxygen saturations should be treated with a high index of suspicion.

You must be cautious in patients who present with 'syncope' or 'collapse'. The presence of a thrombus in the pulmonary vasculature increases pulmonary vascular resistance, which leads to overdistension of the right ventricle and decreases left ventricular preload. This decreases cardiac output, causing significant haemodynamic compromise, and is often fatal.

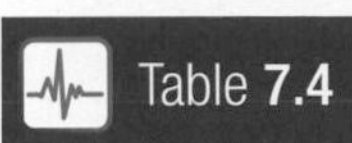

Table 7.4 Wells' pulmonary embolism (PE) scoring system

CLINICAL FEATURE	POINT
Clinically suspected DVT	3.0
Alternative diagnosis less likely than PE	3.0
Tachycardia (HR >100 bpm)	1.5
Recent surgery or immobilisation	1.5
History of DVT or PE	1.5
Haemoptysis	1.0
Malignancy	1.0

DVT, deep-vein thrombosis; HR, heart rate.

MANAGEMENT

If there is PE with evidence of haemodynamic compromise, you should alert the medical registrar and critical care for consideration of thrombolysis.

The modified two-level Wells' score is useful to guide the investigation and management of these patients.

- If the Wells' score is >4 then request an immediate CT PA (or V/Q scan); if this is unavailable then give therapeutic dose low-molecular-weight heparin.
- If the Wells' score is ≤4 then request a D-dimer. If the D-dimer is positive, then proceed as for Wells' score >4. If the D-dimer is negative, then no further immediate action is required to exclude or treat PE unless there is significant clinical suspicion (you should discuss with a senior if this is the case).

Any patient with an unprovoked venous thromboembolism (no preceding risk factors) should have a full history and examination (including breast or prostate exam) and consideration of further investigations. This may include a chest x-ray, myeloma screen, serum calcium, tumour markers, CT of the thorax, abdomen and pelvis and thrombophilia screen.

When considering anticoagulation you should keep in mind comorbidities and contraindications (including age, weight and renal function) as well as local guidelines. Anticoagulation should be started as soon as possible if there are no contraindications. A direct oral anticoagulant is usually first-line for ongoing treatment; however, low-molecular-weight heparin, fondaparinux, warfarin can also be used depending on local guidance.

 **Prescribing Tip**

Direct oral anticoagulants should never be co-prescribed with parenteral anticoagulation.

ESCALATION

In the context of haemodynamic compromise, the patient should be assessed for suitability for thrombolysis by a medical registrar. Indications for potential escalation to intensive care include refractory hypoxia or hypotension requiring support from continuous positive airway pressure, non-invasive ventilation, intubation and mechanical ventilation or vasopressors.

FURTHER READING

Almirall, J., et al. (2007). Differences in the etiology of community-acquired pneumonia according to site of care: a population-based study. *Respiratory Medicine, 101*(10), 2168–2175.

Bennett, J. (2021). *BMJ best practice. Community-acquired pneumonia (non covid-19)*. Available at https://bestpractice.bmj.com/topics/en-gb/3000108. [Accessed 10 January 2022].

Bennett, J., & Russell, R. (2016). *BMJ best practice. Acute exacerbation of asthma in adults*. Available at https://bestpractice.bmj.com/topics/en-gb/3000085. [Accessed 10 January 2022].

BTS/SIGN. (2019). *Guideline for the management of asthma*. Available at www.brit-thoracic.org.uk/quality-improvement/guidelines/asthma. [Accessed 10 January 2022].

Cilloniz, C., et al. (2014). Community-acquired lung respiratory infections in HIV-infected patients: microbial aetiology and outcome. *European Respiratory Journal, 43*(6), 1698–1708.

Davies, H. E., et al. (2010). Management of pleural infection in adults: British Thoracic Society pleural disease guideline 2010. *Thorax, 65*(Suppl 2), ii41–ii53.

Global Initiative for Chronic Obstructive Lung Disease. (2018). *Global strategy for diagnosis, management, and prevention of COPD*. Available at: https://goldcopd.org/wp-content/uploads/2017/11/GOLD-2018-v6.0-FINAL-revised-20-Nov_WMS.pdf. [Accessed 10 January 2022].

Hooper, C., et al. (2010). Investigation of a unilateral pleural effusion in adults: British Thoracic Society pleural disease guideline 2010. *Thorax, 65*(Suppl 2), ii4–ii17.

Huisman, M. V., et al. (1989). Unexpected high prevalence of silent pulmonary embolism in patients with deep venous thrombosis. *Chest, 95*(3), 498–502.

Jantz, M. A., & Pierson, D. J. (1994). Pneumothorax and barotrauma. *Clinical Chest Medicine, 15*(1), 75–91.

Lieberman, D., et al. (2001). Infectious etiologies in acute exacerbation of COPD. *Diagnosis of Microbiological Infectious Disease, 40*(3), 95–102.

Light, R. W. (1995). *Pleural diseases* (3rd ed.). Baltimore, MD: Williams & Wilkins.

McIntyre, K. M., & Sasahara, A. A. (1971). The hemodynamic response to pulmonary embolism in patients without prior cardiopulmonary disease. *American Journal of Cardiology, 28*(3), 288–294.

NICE. (2018). *Chronic obstructive pulmonary disease in over 16s: Diagnosis and management*. Available at www.nice.org.uk/guidance/ng115/chapter/recommendations#managing-exacerbations-of-copd. [Accessed 10 January 2022].

NICE. (2019). *Pneumonia (community-acquired): Antimicrobial prescribing*. Guideline NG 138. Available at www.nice.org.uk/guidance/NG138. [Accessed 10 January 2022].

NICE. (2020). *Venous thromboembolic diseases: Diagnosis, management and thrombophilia testing*. Guideline NG 158. Available at www.nice.org.uk/guidance/ng158. [Accessed 10 January 2022].

NICE. (2021). *Asthma: Acute exacerbation of asthma*. Available at https://cks.nice.org.uk/topics/asthma/management/acute-exacerbation-of-asthma/. [Accessed 10 January 2022].

Rice, L. B. (2006). Antimicrobial resistance in Gram-positive bacteria. *American Journal of Medicine, 119*(6 Suppl 1), S11–S19 discussion, pp. S62–S70.

Ridsdale, H. A., & Hurst, J. R. (2016). Dyspnoea perception and susceptibility to exacerbation in COPD. *Thorax, 72*(2), 107–108.

Sapey, E., & Stockley, R. A. (2006). COPD exacerbations. 2: Aetiology. *Thorax, 61*(3), 250–258.

Sevitt, S. (1974). The structure and growth of valve-pocket thrombi in femoral veins. *Journal of Clinical Pathology, 27*(7), 517–528.

Singh, A. M., & Busse, W. W. (2006). Asthma exacerbations 2: Aetiology. *Thorax, 61*, 809–816.

Gastroenterology

8

Content Outline

STATION 8.1: ABDOMINAL SEPSIS

The Bleep Scenario

A nurse bleeps to inform you that a 68 year old male patient on the oncology ward, with a recent diagnosis of colon cancer, has been complaining of severe abdominal pain for the last 30 minutes. His early-warning system (EWS) score has increased to 11 from 3 earlier in the day. His observations are: heart rate (HR) 138 bpm, blood pressure (BP) 110/85 mmHg, respiratory rate (RR) 32 breaths per minute, SpO_2 97% on room air and temperature 38°C. You are asked to review him.

DEFINITION

Abdominal sepsis is life-threatening organ dysfunction caused by a dysregulated response to an intra-abdominal infection. It encompasses both primary or secondary and localised or generalised peritonitis.

INITIAL THOUGHTS

These observations should alert you to the high possibility of abdominal sepsis from a suspected perforated colon, given the patient's background of colon cancer, which is a risk factor. It would be helpful to obtain more history, including the extent of cancer that the patient has and treatments he has undergone or that are planned.

DIFFERENTIAL DIAGNOSIS

- Upper gastrointestinal tract: peptic ulcer perforation, oesophageal rupture, malignancy
- Lower gastrointestinal tract: obstruction, appendicitis, diverticulitis, ischaemic bowel, incarcerated hernia, a flare of inflammatory bowel disease (IBD) malignancy (all of which can cause perforation/abscess)
- Hepatobiliary tract: cholangitis, cholecystitis, pancreatitis, malignancy, gallstone ileus
- Genitourinary tract: pelvic inflammatory disease, malignancy

INITIAL INSTRUCTIONS OVER PHONE

Ask the nurse to commence intravenous (IV) fluid resuscitation, with 500 mL crystalloid, which you will prescribe on arrival. Ask for initial bloods and an electrocardiogram (ECG) to be taken before your arrival. The patient should be moved to a monitored area as he is very unwell.

ASSESSMENT AND RESUSCITATION

- End of the bed assessment: patient is lying rigid in bed as any movement causes him severe pain
- Airway: patent
- Breathing: RR 34 breaths per minute, SpO_2 96% on room air. On auscultation, there are vesicular breath sounds with good air entry bilaterally
  - Arterial blood gas (pH 7.35, PaO_2 10.2 kPa, $PaCO_2$ 5.2 kPa, HCO_3^- 18 mmol/L, lactate 5.0 mmol/L)
- Circulation: capillary refill time (CRT) 3 s, HR 136 bpm, low-volume regular pulse, BP 86/51 mmHg, jugular venous pressure (JVP) normal, heart sounds (HS) I + II + 0
  - 12-lead ECG: sinus tachycardia
- Disability: Glasgow Coma Scale (GCS) 15/15, pupils equal and reactive to light (PEARL), temperature 38.2°C, capillary blood glucose (CBG) 9.0 mmol/L
- Exposure: on abdominal palpation, there is guarding with poorly localised rebound tenderness suggestive of peritonism. Bowel sounds are absent. Per rectum (PR) exam is not possible due to pain. There is no overt bleeding

INITIAL INVESTIGATIONS

- Haematology: full blood count (FBC: leukocytosis), coagulation screen, cross-match / group and save

- Biochemistry: urea and electrolytes (U&Es: dehydration), liver function tests (LFTs: suspicion of biliary tract pathology), amylase/lipase (suspicion of pancreatitis), C-reactive protein (CRP: acute inflammatory marker)
- Microbiology: blood cultures (exclude bacteraemia), urine microscopy, culture and sensitivity (MCS: exclude urinary sepsis), stool MCS
- Radiology: erect chest X-ray (CXR: pneumoperitoneum), urgent computed tomography abdomen and pelvis (CT AP: to investigate aetiology of symptoms), abdominal X-ray (AXR: suspect flare of IBD, to exclude toxic megacolon)

MAKING A DIAGNOSIS

You should risk stratify the patient for sepsis; this reveals that he meets several high-risk criteria.

- Symptoms: one of the principal symptomatic features of abdominal sepsis is pain. Depending on the site of the infection and the underlying pathology, it may be dull and poorly localised, becoming progressively worse and more localised as the infection irritates the local parietal peritoneum. More generalised pain may develop if the inflammation spreads to involve more of the peritoneum.
- Signs: tachypnoea, tachycardia, hypotension and pyrexia (although normothermia and hypothermia are also reported). On abdominal examination, there is tenderness to palpation, guarding and rebound tenderness. PR examination may intensify the abdominal pain. Severely ill patients will lie rigid with their knees flexed to minimise irritation of the abdominal wall and underlying parietal peritoneum. Bowel sounds may be absent.

MANAGEMENT

You can then implement the 'sepsis six':

1. Oxygen
2. Cultures: blood, urine, stool, sputum, wound swabs as indicated
3. Antibiotics: broad-spectrum IV antibiotics within an hour of diagnosis
4. Fluids: IV resuscitation (250–500 mL crystalloid over 10–15 minutes depending on cardiovascular and renal function), repeated according to the BP. Then prescribed maintenance fluids as required
5. Lactate: a reading >2 mmol/L indicates tissue hypoperfusion and ischaemia
6. Urine output: catheterise the patient and target a urine output of >0.5 mL/kg/hour

If the patient's BP stabilises, you can then take a more comprehensive history. You can also review notes to obtain sufficient history to enable you to understand the context and provide appropriate information with regard to escalation of the patient.

Communication with the patient and next of kin is an essential component of care, and they can provide further information about performance status to guide decisions about the escalation of care.

Observations and alert, verbal, pain, unresponsive (AVPU) level should be taken every 30 minutes, and the patient should be kept nil by mouth in anticipation of emergency surgery.

ESCALATION

You should be comfortable with starting the initial management. If the patient's BP fails to improve after a fluid bolus, you must seek urgent advice from senior team members. In this case, peritonitis due to a surgical cause is high on your differential diagnosis, and the patient is at risk of further deterioration, so you will need to ring for help early.

Contact the on call medical registrar and request an urgent review by the surgical team to consider definitive surgical treatment.

Discussion with intensive care or the critical care outreach team is indicated in high-risk patients and those with refractory hypotension and hypoxia. These patients require urgent review and may receive inotropic support and/or mechanical ventilation if appropriate.

STATION 8.2: ACUTE DIARRHOEA AND VOMITING

The Bleep Scenario

You are called by the acute medical unit (AMU) ward sister about a 36 year old woman who has a 48-hour history of watery diarrhoea associated with vomiting and abdominal cramps. She returned the previous day from a business trip to West Africa. Her observations are: HR 100 bpm, BP 100/60 mmHg, RR 22 breaths per minute, SpO_2 97% on room air and temperature 37.6°C.

DEFINITION

- Diarrhoea: passage of three or more abnormally loose stools per day
- Vomiting: a centrally mediated forceful expulsion of gastric contents through the mouth (not regurgitation or reflux)

INITIAL THOUGHTS

Acute diarrhoea associated with vomiting in travellers is highly likely to be caused by infective gastroenteritis. The most likely diagnosis here is travellers' diarrhoea caused by enterotoxigenic *Eschericia coli* (ETEC), norovirus or rotavirus. Risk factors include travel, food, unwell close contacts and drugs, especially proton pump inhibitors (PPIs) and antibiotics.

Clinical Tip

Remember that *Clostridium difficile* can present atypically with pain, diarrhoea and vomiting. Risk factors include antibiotics, recent hospital stay, immunosuppression and PPI use.

DIFFERENTIAL DIAGNOSIS

- Infective (viral): rotavirus, norovirus, COVID-19
- Infective (bacterial): *E. coli* (ETEC, also called travellers' diarrhoea, enteroinvasive or enterohaemorrhagic *E. coli*), *Campylobacter*, *Shigella*, cholera, *Salmonella*, *Clostridium difficile* and typhoid
- Infective (parasitic): malaria, *Cryptosporidium*, *Giardia*, *Entamoeba* and *Cyclospora*

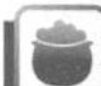

Clinical Tip

With any recent travel from high-risk areas you will also need to consider viral haemorrhagic fever.

INITIAL INSTRUCTIONS OVER PHONE

The patient is likely to be hypovolaemic with deranged electrolytes from persistent diarrhoea and vomiting. Ask the nurse to commence initial fluid resuscitation which you will prescribe on arrival. Ask for initial bloods to be taken before your arrival. The patient should be moved to a side room for isolation purposes, given that she is likely highly infective.

ASSESSMENT AND RESUSCITATION

- End of the bed assessment: the patient has sunken eyes and appears fatigued
- Airway: patent
- Breathing: RR 22 breaths per minute, SpO_2 97% on room air. On auscultation, there are vesicular breath sounds with good air entry bilaterally
- Circulation: CRT 4 s, HR 115 bpm with a low-volume regular pulse, BP 92/57 mmHg with a postural drop of 20 mmHg, JVP not visible, HS I + II + 0, dry mucous membranes, cold/pale peripheries, 1 L Hartmann's solution running at a rate of 1000 mL/h
  - Arterial blood gas: pH 7.46, PaO_2 10.2 kPa, $PaCO_2$ 5.0 kPa, HCO_3^- 30 mmol/L
  - 12-lead ECG: sinus tachycardia
- Disability: GCS 15/15, PEARL, temperature 37.6°C, CBG 5.6 mmol/L
- Exposure: abdomen soft and non-tender with hyperactive bowel sounds. PR examination is normal. Calves unremarkable

INITIAL INVESTIGATIONS

- Haematology: FBC (leukocytosis/leukopenia, eosinophilia, haemoglobin, haematocrit, platelet count), coagulation screen, group and save
- Biochemistry: U&Es (dehydration, electrolyte derangements), LFTs, CRP (inflammatory marker), urinalysis (to exclude haemoproteinuria and pregnancy)
- Microbiology: blood cultures, stool for MCS (including hot stool for ova, cysts and parasites – call lab first; freshly passed stool needs to be kept warm and taken to the lab fast), stool for viral polymerase chain reaction (PCR)
  - Urgent (same-day result) thick and thin films for malaria on 3 consecutive days (lab will also measure parasitaemia level if malaria is found) / rapid diagnostic testing
  - Nasopharyngeal swab for COVID-19 (stool testing not routinely available)
- Radiology: AXR (if persistent diarrhoea, to rule out toxic megacolon), CT abdomen-pelvis with IV contrast (to rule out obstruction or perforation)
- Other: urine dip (to exclude haemoproteinuria), pregnancy test

MAKING A DIAGNOSIS

The patient may be very unwell with features of dehydration and hypovolaemic shock: dry mucous membranes, reduced skin turgor, prolonged CRT, tachycardia and hypotension (including significant postural drop).

Once the patient is stable, you should take a full history, including:

- Frequency, appearance and volume of diarrhoea and vomiting
- Presence of any blood, mucus and pus visible in the stools
- Associated symptoms, including fever, abdominal pain, weight loss
- Ability to tolerate oral intake
- Ingestion of potentially contaminated food, untreated water or known gastrointestinal irritant
- Recent travel – where to, how long, which particular areas?
- Contact with certain animals or similarly ill people
- Recent use of medications, especially antibiotics and PPIs

MANAGEMENT

Goals of initial management include:

- Rehydration as needed. If the patient does not already have a catheter, this should be inserted.

- Correct any electrolyte abnormalities.
- Treat symptoms, e.g. fever (paracetamol), pain (buscopan).
- Fill in a stool chart to record frequency, stool consistency, presence of blood.
- Identify cause where possible – send suitable investigations to identify cause.
- Ensure the patient is isolated for infection control.
- Treat certain cases with specific or empirical antibiotic therapy (liaise with microbiology).
- Notify Public Health England as needed.
- Explain diagnosis and plan to patient / next of kin.

After the initial ABCDE approach with appropriate fluid resuscitation and electrolyte replacement, for any volume-depleted patient you should prescribe a fluid challenge and monitor the response (caution in elderly patients, those with chronic kidney disease or congestive heart failure). Further fluid boluses may be required. Once the patient has been fluid-resuscitated, you will need to prescribe maintenance fluids. Once the vomiting has settled, the patient should be encouraged to drink clear fluids, such as diluted fruit juice. Oral rehydration solution is probably unnecessary in otherwise fit and healthy patients. You should also initiate a fluid balance chart, aiming for a urine output of >0.5 mL/kg/hour.

Loperamide can help to reduce the frequency of bowel motions but should be avoided in bloody diarrhoea (dysentery), severe abdominal pain or high-grade fever. Public Health England will need to be informed of notifiable diseases. In terms of further treatment, antibiotics are usually unnecessary in self-limiting gastroenteritis. However, you should discuss severe cases with microbiology as antimicrobials may confer benefit. You should also stop PPIs and any precipitating antibiotics. Table 8.1 lists notifiable organisms causing diarrhoea and vomiting.

ESCALATION

Cases of acute diarrhoea and vomiting with severe abdominal tenderness, high-grade fever with dysentery or signs of sepsis indicate potential bacteraemia and should be escalated to the medical registrar.

STATION 8.3: ACUTE LIVER FAILURE

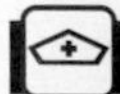 **The Bleep Scenario**

A nurse on AMU bleeps you to request an urgent review of a 34 year old woman who is becoming increasingly drowsy and confused. She has deranged LFTs and was admitted 12 hours earlier having taken a staggered overdose of paracetamol. She is currently on *N*-acetylcysteine treatment. She is normally fit and well. Her observations are: HR 90 bpm, BP 110/70 mmHg, RR 16 breaths per minute, SpO_2 92% on room air and temperature 36.5°C.

DEFINITION

Acute liver failure is a severe reduction in synthetic liver function in a person with previously normal liver function. It is characterised by jaundice, coagulopathy and hepatic encephalopathy. It is also known as fulminant hepatic failure.

INITIAL THOUGHTS

Paracetamol overdose is the most common cause of acute liver failure in the UK. Paracetamol overdose causes depletion of hepatic glutathione stores and results in accumulation of *N*-acetyl-*p*-benzoquinone imine and direct hepatocyte injury.

This patient is exhibiting signs of hepatic failure, including deranged LFTs and altered mental state. She requires urgent review due to the risk of rapid deterioration and further complications, including infection, renal failure, hypoglycaemia, acidosis and shock. Though alcohol, obesity and hepatitis infection are the most common chronic causes of liver disease in the UK, they are important to remember in the context of suspected paracetamol overdose as they may be concurrent and may be included in the differentials of acute-on-chronic decompensated chronic liver disease which may overlap in their presentation.

Table 8.1 Notifiable diseases/organisms causing diarrhoea and/or vomiting

Enteric fever (typhoid or paratyphoid fever)	Food poisoning
Haemolytic uraemic syndrome (HUS)	Infectious bloody diarrhoea
Bacillus cereus (only if associated with food poisoning)	*Campylobacter* species
Cholera	*Clostridium botulinum*
Clostridium perfringens (only if associated with food poisoning)	COVID-19
Cryptosporidium species	*Entamoeba histolytica*
Giardia lamblia	*Salmonella* species
Shigella species	Verocytotoxigenic *Escherichia coli* (including *E. coli* O157)
Vibrio cholerae	*Yersinia pestis*

DIFFERENTIAL DIAGNOSIS

- Drugs: prescription medications (paracetamol, antituberculosis medications, statins, non-steroidal anti-inflammatory drugs (NSAIDs), phenytoin, carbamazepine, flucloxacillin, illicit drugs (e.g. ecstasy) and herbal supplements
- Hepatitis and other viruses (e.g. acute hepatitis B, A, E; less often, cytomegalovirus, herpes simplex virus (HSV), varicella-zoster virus, dengue)
- Toxins: *Amanita phalloides*, phosphorus, alcohol
- Autoimmune hepatitis
- Metabolic liver disease: Wilson's, non-alcoholic fatty liver disease
- Pregnancy: haemolysis, elevated liver enzymes and low platelets (HELLP), acute fatty liver of pregnancy
- Vascular: shock, sepsis, hypotension causing ischaemic, hypoxic hepatitis; diseases of veins in the liver, e.g. Budd–Chiari syndrome
- Malignancy, lymphoma, haemophagocytic lymphohistiocytosis

Many cases have no identifiable cause. As mentioned above, it is important to check for evidence of chronic liver disease in patients who present with an acute liver injury.

INITIAL INSTRUCTIONS OVER PHONE

Ask the nurse to repeat the patient's observations, including a formal GCS. The patient should be given supplemental oxygen to target oxygen saturations of 94–98% and needs to have regular observations every 30 minutes. She should be moved to a monitored area as soon as possible.

ASSESSMENT AND RESUSCITATION

- End of the bed assessment: the patient is drowsy and confused. She is clinically jaundiced.
- Airway: you are concerned about the patient's ability to protect her airway from aspiration of vomit.
  - Ensure the airway is clear of any obstruction.
  - Perform a head tilt, chin lift manoeuvre and insert an airway adjunct (oropharyngeal or nasopharyngeal airway) if the patient tolerates it.
  - If a patient needs airway management due to reduced GCS, then call an Emergency Medical Response Team. Don't wait until she arrests.
- Breathing: RR 16 breaths per minute, SpO_2 92% on room air. On auscultation, there are vesicular breath sounds with good air entry bilaterally.
  - Arterial blood gas: pH 7.45, PaO_2 8.5 kPa, $PaCO_2$ 5.5 kPa, HCO_3^- 28 mmol/L.
- Circulation: CRT 2 s, HR 95 bpm, regular, BP 101/68 mmHg, JVP normal, HS I + II + 0.
  - 12-lead ECG: sinus rhythm.
- Disability: GCS 9/15 (E2V3M4), PEARL, temperature 36.5°C, CBG 4.1 mmol/L.
- Exposure: abdomen generally tender but soft, with normal bowel sounds. Two-fingerbreadth hepatomegaly. Positive asterixis; no signs of chronic liver disease. No evidence of bleeding.

INITIAL INVESTIGATIONS

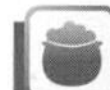

Clinical Tip

In cases of staggered overdose, treatment is started irrespective of level as there is no defined time of overdose against which to measure a level.

Review any bloods that have already been sent. You should send a repeat screen now to track progress, as whilst encephalopathy has worsened, international normalised ratio (INR) and kidney function are likely to have altered too.

- Haematology: FBC (leukocytosis, anaemia, thrombocytopenia), clotting screen (INR >1.5), cross-match (in case a transfusion is required)
- Biochemistry: U&Es (50% of acute liver failure patients will have significant renal dysfunction; it is more common in acute liver failure due to paracetamol overdose), LFTs (hyperbilirubinaemia, elevated liver enzymes), ammonia (sign of encephalopathy), CRP (acute inflammatory marker), blood glucose (risk of hypoglycaemia)
- Liver screen: paracetamol levels, salicylate levels, viral hepatitis serology (anti-hepatitis A immunoglobulin M (IgM), hepatitis B surface antigen, anti-HBc IgM, anti-HSV IgM), viral PCR for cytomegalovirus, HSV, Epstein–Barr virus, parvovirus, and vesicular stomatitis virus G PCR, autoimmune hepatitis serology (antinuclear antibody, antimitochondrial antibody, anti-smooth-muscle antibody, liver kidney microsomal antibody), human immunodeficiency virus (HIV) serology, serum caeruloplasmin
- Microbiology: cultures – blood, urine, ascitic fluid if present (patients susceptible to infection)
- Radiology: CXR, ultrasound scan of the abdomen with Doppler (assess the patency of hepatic vessels), cross-sectional imaging, e.g. CT may be needed (can help distinguish which patients have underlying chronic liver disease)

MAKING A DIAGNOSIS

A diagnosis of acute liver failure is made if there is evidence of jaundice (hyperbilirubinaemia and deranged LFTs), coagulopathy (INR >1.5) and encephalopathy (drowsiness, confusion, changes in mental status) in a patient without underlying chronic liver disease. In a patient with acute-on-chronic liver disease, it is crucial to look for stigmata such as ascites and telangiectasia.

If the cause is not known, the patient history and clinical findings should be used with appropriate clinical testing to determine the underlying cause. The collateral history is key to confirming a reliable alcohol

Table 8.2 **Modified West Haven criteria**

GRADE OF ENCEPHALOPATHY	GCS	CONSCIOUSNESS LEVEL AND COGNITIVE FUNCTION	CLINICAL AND NEUROPSYCHIATRIC FINDINGS
1	14–15	• Impaired computation • Mild confusion	• Shortened attention span • Minor lack of awareness
2	12–15	• Inattentive • Disoriented to time • Moderate confusion	• Irritability • Disinhibition • Asterixis • Slurred speech
3	7–12	• Somnolent but rousable • Marked confusion	• Inappropriate/bizarre behaviour • Paranoia • Aggression • Asterixis plus ataxia • Slurred speech • Hypo- or hyperreflexia
4	<7	• Unrousable	• Unresponsive to pain • Pupillary abnormalities • Flexor/extensor posturing

GCS, Glasgow Coma Scale.

history, medication history as well as herbal, alternative and illicit drug use. It may be helpful to understand the patient's mental health during and before this episode, including past involvement with psychiatry and general practitioner (GP), as the transplant centre will require this information.

- Symptoms: abdominal pain, confusion, malaise, anorexia
- Signs: jaundice, hepatomegaly, right upper quadrant tenderness, reduced GCS, motor dysfunction, fetor hepaticus, haemodynamic instability, evidence of bleeding
- Signs of cerebral oedema: obtundation, coma, bradycardia, hypertension

MANAGEMENT

Given this patient's reducing GCS, your first concern must be to maintain her airway and breathing. Follow the ABCDE approach to stabilise the patient and seek urgent senior review.

You should give fluid resuscitation and monitor the CBG. If the patient develops hypoglycaemia, a 10–20% dextrose infusion is required, but this would be a sign of significant liver dysfunction requiring level 2/3 care monitoring in the intensive therapy unit (ITU).

Early restoration of intravascular volume and systemic perfusion may prevent or mitigate the severity of organ failure – catheterisation will be helpful to monitor urine output.

- *N*-acetyl cysteine is used (even in non-paracetamol acute liver failure).
- Give stress ulcer prophylaxis.
- Nutrition: enteral feeding may be indicated, although you should discuss with a senior first.
- Avoid sedatives, nephrotoxic and hepatotoxic drugs.

An urgent ultrasound Doppler will show portal or hepatic venous thrombosis if present. If ascites is present, an ascitic tap should be sent to investigate spontaneous bacterial peritonitis (SBP).

The patient is showing signs of hepatic encephalopathy. You can determine the grade of encephalopathy using the modified West Haven criteria, detailed in Table 8.2.

This patient has grade 3 hepatic encephalopathy. This indicates that medical and ITU senior support is required and she may need a liver transplant. The transplant centre will usually ask for broad-spectrum prophylactic antimicrobial therapy as well as antifungal cover (e.g. fluconazole).

Regular neurological observations will be needed to monitor the patient's consciousness level. You should stop all hepatotoxic and anticoagulant medications; you may consider giving a stat dose of 10 mg IV vitamin K if the INR or bilirubin is significantly raised, but if there is no active bleeding, it is worth checking with the gastroenterology team/tertiary liver team first. Do not give fresh frozen plasma (FFP) and clotting products unless there is evidence of bleeding – measures of blood clotting (INR, prothrombin time) are used by the transplant centre as prognostic markers. Please refer to Haematology chapter for further information.

ESCALATION

Call for the periarrest team if there are any concerns regarding the airway.

If a patient has impaired or worsening mental status, an urgent senior review is needed as the development of reduced conscious level or confusion (encephalopathy or raised intracranial pressure) is a serious sign, and patients can rapidly develop coma. ITU will need to consider invasive ventilation, close monitoring

Table 8.3 King's College criteria

PARACETAMOL-INDUCED ACUTE LIVER FAILURE	NON-PARACETAMOL-INDUCED ACUTE LIVER FAILURE
pH <7.30 after resuscitation and >24 hours after ingestion Lactate >3 mmol/L or The three following criteria: • HE >grade 3 • Serum creatinine >300 µmol/L • - INR >6.5	INR >6.5 (PT >100 s) or Any three of the five following criteria: • Age <10 or >40 years • Aetiology: indeterminate aetiology, hepatitis, drug-induced hepatitis • Interval jaundice – encephalopathy >7 days • INR >3.5 (PT >50 s) • Serum bilirubin >300 µmol/L

HE, hepatic encephalopathy; INR, international normalised ratio; PT, prothrombin time.

and management in close liaison with the transplant centre. Whilst a CT head should be performed to rule out intracranial causes and/or cerebral oedema, this will need to be done with senior support.

Acute liver failure can rapidly lead to multiorgan failure, so early involvement of senior medics, intensive care and a specialist liver centre is vital. This patient would be admitted to ITU and needs to be urgently discussed with your local specialist tertiary liver transplant centre so that the best possible specialist care can be provided, and the patient can be considered for transfer to the specialist centre ± liver transplant if appropriate. Signs that the patient needs urgent liver transplantation are included in the King's College criteria detailed in Table 8.3.

Intensive care treatment includes:

- Controlled ventilation
- Blood glucose monitoring ± 10–20% dextrose infusions
- IV mannitol and hypertonic saline for encephalopathy and intracranial hypertension
- Vasopressors, inotropes and invasive monitoring for hypotension
- Renal replacement therapy for renal failure

STATION 8.4: ACUTE UPPER GASTROINTESTINAL BLEED

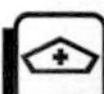 **The Bleep Scenario**

You are bleeped by a nurse on the elderly care ward about a 79 year old woman who has just vomited a large amount of fresh red blood. The patient has a background of ischaemic heart disease and osteoarthritis and is on aspirin. Her observations are: HR 126 bpm, BP 81/59 mmHg, RR 22 breaths per minute, SpO_2 96% on room air and temperature 36.9°C. You are asked to review her urgently.

DEFINITION

An acute upper gastrointestinal bleed is bleeding from the upper gastrointestinal tract, i.e. proximal to the ligament of Treitz at the duodenojejunal junction.

INITIAL THOUGHTS

The most important diagnosis is acute upper gastrointestinal bleeding. In this case, one of your initial thoughts may be peptic ulceration ± perforation secondary to aspirin use for her ischaemic heart disease. The patient is shocked from acute blood loss (haematemesis) and needs urgent resuscitation.

DIFFERENTIAL DIAGNOSIS

- Common: peptic ulcer disease, oesophageal varices, oesophagitis, gastritis, Mallory–Weiss tear
- Uncommon: Boerhaave syndrome, gastric varices, arteriovenous malformations, upper gastrointestinal tumours, aortoenteric fistulae

INITIAL INSTRUCTIONS OVER PHONE

Ask the nurse to keep the BP cuff and pulse oximeter attached to the patient and repeat the observations every 10 minutes, including lying and standing BP, if possible. The patient should be moved to a monitored area as soon as possible, given the evidence of hypovolaemia and haemodynamic instability.

ASSESSMENT AND RESUSCITATION

- End of the bed assessment: patient is alert. Vomit bowel at bedside contains 500 mL bright-red blood.
- Airway: patent.
- Breathing: RR 24 breaths per minute, SpO_2 96% on room air. On auscultation, there are vesicular breath sounds and good entry bilaterally.
    - Venous blood gas: pH 7.35, PaO_2 10.2 kPa, $PaCO_2$ 4.9 kPa, HCO_3^- 22 mmol/L.
- Circulation: CRT 3 s, HR 134 bpm, regular, BP 79/53 mmHg, JVP normal, HS I + II + 0, peripheries are cold to touch.
    - Insert a wide-bore IV cannula into each antecubital fossa and simultaneously take blood for haematological and biochemical investigations.
    - Prescribe and administer a fluid challenge of 250 mL crystalloid over 10 minutes.

- 12-lead ECG: sinus tachycardia (to rule out acute coronary syndrome given the patient's cardiac history).
- Disability: GCS 15/15, PEARL, temperature 36.9°C, CBG 9.6 mmol/L.
- Exposure: no blood on the bedsheets. Abdomen tender to palpation in the epigastric region, with normal bowel sounds. No signs of chronic liver disease. PR examination confirms melaena.

Clinical Tip

Note that the initial haemoglobin on the venous blood gas can be normal as haemodilution takes time to manifest.

INITIAL INVESTIGATIONS

- Haematology: FBC (haemoglobin trend, platelets), coagulation screen (clotting abnormalities), samples for group and save and cross-matching (so the appropriate blood can be issued)
- Biochemistry: U&Es (raised urea), LFTs (underlying liver disease), troponin (myocardial ischaemia)
- Radiology: erect CXR (exclude perforated viscus), AXR (exclude ileus), CT imaging may also be indicated

MAKING A DIAGNOSIS

Acute upper gastrointestinal bleeding is a gastroenterological emergency. Bleeding from the upper gastrointestinal tract is four times more common than bleeding from the lower gastrointestinal tract.

- Symptoms: haematemesis, coffee-ground vomiting, haematochezia, melaena, features of the underlying cause (weight loss, dyspepsia, jaundice), syncope or dizziness due to hypotension (may have postural drop)
- Signs: abdominal tenderness, haemodynamic instability, pallor, features of the underlying cause (abdominal mass, palpable supraclavicular lymph nodes), subcutaneous emphysema (Boerhaave's syndrome)

You can calculate the Glasgow-Blatchford score (Table 8.4) to predict the need for intervention; scores of 5 or more are associated with a greater than 50% chance of requiring intervention as an inpatient (i.e. blood transfusion and endoscopic, surgical or radiological intervention).

MANAGEMENT

Most hospital trusts will have a specific care bundle for gastrointestinal bleeding, which you should familiarise yourself with.

Given that the patient is shocked due to blood loss, and showing signs of hypovolaemia, your priority is to stabilise her using the ABCDE approach and call for help.

Table 8.4 Glasgow-Blatchford score

PARAMETER	PARAMETER VALUE (AND SCORE)
Systolic blood pressure (mmHg)	100–109 (1) 90–99 (2) <90 (3)
Serum urea (mmol/L)	6.5–7.9 (2) 8.0–9.9 (3) 10.0–24.9 (4) ≥25.0 (6)
Haemoglobin for men (mg/dL)	120–129 (1) 100–119 (3) <100 (6)
Haemoglobin for women (mg/dL)	100–11.9 (1) <100 (6)
Pulse (bpm)	≥100 (1)
Melaena	Present (1)
Syncope	Present (2)
Liver disease	Present (2)
Cardiac failure	Present (2)

You should determine the need for an urgent transfusion. Use your clinical judgement to determine the number of red cell units to be transfused as there are risks with overtransfusing (e.g. fluid overload or coagulopathy) as well as undertransfusing (e.g. coronary ischaemia or anaemia). Recent evidence suggests a transfusion threshold of 80 g/dL in patients with known ischaemic heart disease such as this patient (haemoglobin target 80–100 g/L) compared to a threshold of 70 g/L in a patient without vascular comorbidities (target range 70–90 g/L).

If the patient continues to show signs despite fluid resuscitation, there is ongoing bleeding or severe anaemia on the venous blood gas, group O Rhesus-negative blood is available for immediate transfusion.

Group-specific blood takes around 15 minutes to arrange via blood bank. A full cross-match takes around 45 minutes to complete.

You should keep the patient nil by mouth. IV or intramuscular analgesia would be appropriate if needed and use antiemetics if vomiting is ongoing.

Prescribing Tip

Metoclopramide can help as a prokinetic to empty the stomach, facilitating endoscopy.

Clinical Tip

In variceal bleeding, terlipressin IV can help vasoconstrict the splanchnic circulation, leading to a decrease in propensity to bleed. This has limited efficacy in the context of non-variceal bleeding. Terlipressin is also used in hepatorenal syndrome, where it increases renal blood flow.

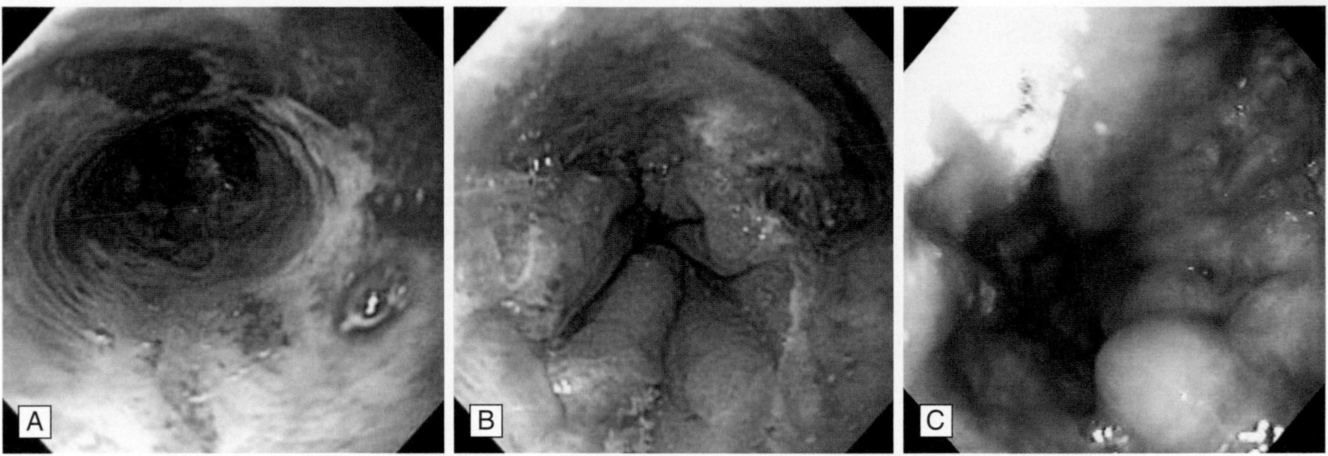

Fig. 8.1 Endoscopic changes in upper gastrointestinal bleeding. (A) Erosive oesophagitis. (B) Deep oesophageal ulcer. (C) Oesophageal varices. (Source: Zitelli, B.J. et al. (Eds.) [2022]. *Zitelli and Davis' atlas of pediatric physical diagnosis*. Elsevier.)

You should review the patient's drug chart and suspend any antiplatelets, anticoagulants or NSAIDs. If on warfarin, reversal may be required depending on the INR. For patients at high risk of cardiovascular events, seek advice from the cardiology, haematology or stroke team regarding the management of antiplatelet drugs, warfarin and direct oral anticoagulants (DOACs). The indication for the anticoagulation will dictate the management before and after the endoscopy (e.g. appropriate to suspend in atrial fibrillation). Discuss with haematology to determine the use of FFP, Beriplex and vitamin K.

For patients with suspected variceal bleeding, immediately give terlipressin 2 mg IV (caution in ischaemic heart disease) as well as prophylactic antibiotics according to local antimicrobial guidelines.

 **Prescribing Tip**

PPIs should not be given before endoscopy unless you are advised otherwise by a senior member of the medical or gastroenterological team.

ESCALATION

Call for help early. If the patient doesn't respond to initial management or is periarrest, you should call the medical emergency team. You may need to activate the major haemorrhage protocol to request urgent blood products – this provides O-negative packed red cells, FFP, platelets and cryoprecipitate. For ongoing blood product use, ensure you have the patient's most recent blood results and clinical status to discuss with the haematology team.

The patient should be discussed with the on call gastroenterologist as soon as possible. Given that this patient with ischaemic heart disease is in shock due to blood loss, early endoscopy would need to be considered even if she responds to fluid. If the patient remains haemodynamically unstable following resuscitation, or you suspect bleeding varices, this would be an indication for emergency endoscopy, likely in theatre with anaesthetic support (to protect airway given the likelihood of a stomach full of blood). Otherwise, endoscopy should happen within 24 hours. Fig. 8.1 illustrates endoscopic changes found in the most common causes of upper gastrointestinal bleeding.

STATION 8.5: EXACERBATION OF INFLAMMATORY BOWEL DISEASE

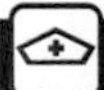 **The Bleep Scenario**

You are bleeped by the AMU nurse to review a new admission. A 28 year old man has presented via his GP with a 4 day history of frequent bloody diarrhoea, fever and abdominal pain. He has a background of ulcerative colitis (UC).

His observations are: HR 110 bpm, BP 110/70 mmHg, RR 20 breaths per minute, SpO_2 98% on room air and temperature 37.9°C.

DEFINITION

An acute flare of ulcerative colitis (UC) or Crohn's disease is usually managed as an outpatient but can require admission to hospital when severe.

INITIAL THOUGHTS

The most likely diagnosis, given the patient's past medical history, is an acute exacerbation of UC. However, infective gastroenteritis, particularly from a bacterial pathogen, is a sensible differential diagnosis at this early stage. You should recognise that the patient is showing signs of hypovolaemia and will require fluid resuscitation.

DIFFERENTIAL DIAGNOSIS

- Diarrhoea: UC, Crohn's disease, coeliac disease, diverticulitis, infective colitis, ischaemic colitis, radiation colitis, irritable bowel syndrome, acquired immunodeficiency syndrome (AIDS), colorectal malignancy, vasculitis, laxative use
- Abdominal pain and gastrointestinal bleeding: UC, Crohn's disease, ischaemic colitis, radiation colitis, arteriovenous malformations, NSAID enteropathy, intestinal tuberculosis, colorectal malignancy, vasculitis

INITIAL INSTRUCTIONS OVER PHONE

You can ask the nurse to commence a fluid challenge, for example 500 mL crystalloid over 10–15 minutes, which you will prescribe on arrival. Ask for initial bloods and, if possible, venous blood gas.

ASSESSMENT AND RESUSCITATION

- End of the bed assessment: patient is alert and complaining of abdominal pain.
- Airway: patent.
- Breathing: RR 20 breaths per minute, SpO_2 98% on room air. On auscultation, there are vesicular breath sounds with good air entry bilaterally.
- Circulation: CRT 2 s, HR 115 bpm, regular, BP 100/64 mmHg, JVP normal, HS I + II + 0, warm and well-perfused peripheries.
  - Venous blood gas: pH 7.47, K 3.0 mmol/L, Hb 105 g/L (hypokalaemic metabolic alkalosis).
  - 12-lead ECG: sinus tachycardia.
- Disability: GCS 15/15, PEARL, temperature 37.9°C, CBG 7.8 mmol/L.
- Exposure: abdomen is soft and non-tender, with normal bowel sounds. PR examination shows loose stool mixed with fresh blood; no irregular masses felt.

INITIAL INVESTIGATIONS

- Haematology: FBC (anaemia, leukocytosis, thrombocytosis), coagulation screen, group and save
- Biochemistry: U&Es (dehydration, deranged electrolytes), LFTs (cholestatic picture possible in primary sclerosing cholangitis), bone profile, glucose, CRP and erythrocyte sedimentation rate (inflammatory markers), haematinics (deficiencies). CRP can be normal even in extensive disease
- Microbiology: stool MCS, including *Clostridium difficile* testing (to exclude infective cause), blood cultures (if suspicion of bacteraemia), faecal calprotectin.
- Radiology: erect CXR (colonic perforation), AXR (toxic megacolon, dilatation >5.5 cm), CT abdomen and pelvis may be indicated (look for evidence of perforation, abscess or toxic megacolon)

MAKING A DIAGNOSIS

- Symptoms: an acute exacerbation of IBD often begins insidiously, with increased urgency to defecate, lower abdominal cramps, blood and mucus in the stools. Patients may also experience fatigue and weight loss, as well as feeling generally unwell. You need to know the type and extent of IBD the patient has.
- Signs: abdominal tenderness, erythema nodosum, pyoderma gangrenosum, uveitis, iritis or episcleritis, joint pain, ankylosing spondylitis, clubbing and pallor.

Patients with Crohn's may also have mouth ulcers, anal/perianal skin tags, abdominal masses and anal fissures/fistulae.

MANAGEMENT

Once the patient is stable, you can take a more detailed history, including travel and medication history. Stratify the patient with markers of exacerbation (Table 8.5) to confirm an acute, severe UC exacerbation. Some patients flare up whilst on a course of steroids or immunosuppression and may not meet these criteria but will still be having a severe flare. A patient presenting with an acute flare on no therapy or occasional use of 5-aminosalicylic acid is a different management challenge to a patient already on second-line biologic medication and a recently started on an oral course of steroids.

Follow the trust's acute severe colitis protocol, prior to review of the patient by the gastroenterology team.

You should initiate IV hydrocortisone 100 mg four times daily to induce a remission of the acute flare, pending the results of the stool MCS and *C. difficile*. As the patient has a known diagnosis of UC, this is the most likely cause of symptoms, and the initiation of hydrocortisone treatment should not be delayed.

IBD exacerbation is a procoagulant state (incidence of venous thromboembolism (VTE) 2–3 times higher than inpatients without IBD), so you should prescribe VTE prophylaxis with low-molecular-weight heparin and thromboembolic deterrent stockings. You should also review the patient's drug chart and stop any opiates, antidiarrhoeal and antispasmodic agents to prevent colonic dilatation.

The Bristol stool chart is essential to monitor the frequency, consistency and presence of blood in the patient's bowel movements as falling frequency and thickening up of the stools to semiformed or formed will show response to therapy. See Table 8.5 for the grading of IBD severity.

Crohn's disease management requires an early specialist opinion and will depend on what areas of the bowel are affected by Crohn's disease and which bits are flaring up.

- Perianal disease causes fever, perianal pain, discharge, fluctuant perianal mass (e.g. perianal abscess).
- Colonic Crohn's (colitis) can cause diarrhoea, pain, bleeding.

Table 8.5 Severity measures of inflammatory bowel disease

MEASURE OF SEVERITY	MILD	MODERATE	SEVERE
Bowel movements/day	<4	4–6	>6 plus one of: • Temperature >37.8°C • Pulse >90 bpm • Hb <100 g/L • ESR >30
Blood in stools	Small amounts	Between mild and severe	Visible blood
Fever (temperature > 37.8°C)	No	No	Yes
Pulse >90 bpm	No	No	Yes
Anaemia (Hb <10^5 g/L)	No	No	Yes
ESR (mm/h)	≤30	≤30	>30

ESR, erythrocyte sedimentation rate; Hb, haemoglobin.

Small-bowel disease can cause symptoms from areas of active inflammation, stricturing, perforation, abscess or fistulation – symptoms can include incomplete obstruction, vomiting, weight loss, diarrhoea. A right iliac fossa mass may be palpable.

The decision on whether to start steroids and the choice of steroids will depend on the scenario and should be discussed with the specialist team. They may also advise flexible sigmoidoscopy, but this is often used to confirm active disease-prior to considering second-line medical therapy. It may not be needed if the patient settles on IV then PO steroids. Table 8.6 gives a comparison of ulcerative colitis and Crohn's disease.

ESCALATION

You should inform the gastroenterology registrar and IBD clinical nurse specialist of the new admission. A dietician and pharmacist review may also be indicated. If you suspect an infection from perforation, fistulation or abscess formation, then antibiotics and CT or magnetic resonance imaging plus urgent surgical review are indicated. Similarly, patients should be referred urgently if there is any evidence of toxic megacolon.

An early review by gastroenterology and colorectal surgery helps ensure that the patient is on the correct management plan, but also helps the patient understand the situation they are in through explanations of their management options; this will allow for time to come to terms with a difficult situation if they need an operation or stoma.

In line with British Society of Gastroenterology guidance, if on day 3 of IV hydrocortisone the patient is till passing >8 bowel movements per day or has 3–8 bowel motions per day with CRP >45 mg/L, then a surgical review is indicated to consider a colectomy. If there has been no or insufficient improvement within 72 hours on IV steroids, the gastroenterology and colorectal teams will need to consider second-line medical therapy or surgery. Whilst many patients would prefer to avoid surgery, it may still be needed if they don't respond to the second-line therapy within the next 3–5 days, and many will subsequently need surgery even if they respond to medical therapy on this admission.

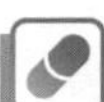

Prescribing Tip

Second-line therapy is usually infliximab, which is simpler to use and of equal efficacy to ciclosporin (which National Institute for Health and Care Excellence (NICE) guidance recommends in favour of infliximab), and most centres have more experience with infliximab.

STATION 8.6: SPONTANEOUS BACTERIAL PERITONITIS

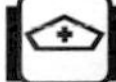

The Bleep Scenario

You are bleeped by the nurse asking you to review a patient newly admitted to AMU. He is a 54 year old man presenting with shortness of breath caused by large volume ascites from decompensated liver cirrhosis. He is now complaining of chills and abdominal pain. His observations are: HR 115 bpm, BP 105/60 mmHg, RR 24 breaths per minute, SpO_2 94% on room air and temperature 38.4°C.

DEFINITION

Spontaneous bacterial peritonitis (SBP) is an infection of ascitic fluid with ≥ 250 neutrophils/mm^3, and a single organism may or may not be cultured from the ascitic fluid. SBP usually occurs in patients with advanced chronic liver disease and is associated with high mortality. Translocation of bacteria through a leaky gut mucosa is a possible mechanism.

INITIAL THOUGHTS

This patient has an EWS of 7 for pyrexia, tachypnoea, tachycardia and hypotension, which should alert you to an acutely unwell patient with the potential for rapid deterioration. SBP should always be ruled out in any patient presenting with ascites.

Table 8.6 Comparing ulcerative colitis and Crohn's disease

DISEASE FEATURE	ULCERATIVE COLITIS	CROHN'S DISEASE
GI tract involvement	Always involves rectum. May affect the entire colon with confluent lesions	Can affect the whole GI tract from mouth to anus. Skip lesions
Histology	Acute and chronic inflammatory cells; crypt abscesses	Giant cell granuloma
Bowel wall involvement	Mucosal ulceration; thumbprinting on abdominal X-ray	Full-thickness ulceration; cobblestone appearance on endoscopy
Increased risk of GI tract cancer?	Yes (colon)	Yes (colon, small-bowel adenocarcinoma)
Fistulae/abscesses?	No	Yes

GI, gastrointestinal.

DIFFERENTIAL DIAGNOSIS

- Hepatic causes of ascites: liver cirrhosis (viral hepatitis, alcohol excess), malignancy (primary hepatocellular carcinoma, metastatic deposit)
- Non-hepatic causes of ascites: pancreatitis, congestive cardiac failure, hypoalbuminaemia (nephrotic syndrome, malnutrition, malabsorption)

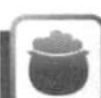

Clinical Tip

SBP versus secondary bacterial peritonitis: secondary bacterial peritonitis is due to a perforated abdominal viscus or potentially due to infection being introduced at the patient's last paracentesis or ascitic tap. This often leads to more than one – sometimes multiple – bacteria being isolated on blood culture (bacteraemia). This is a surgical emergency needing urgent review and cross-sectional imaging.

Clinical Tip

Bacterascites is when ascitic fluid contains culture-positive bacteria with a neutrophil count > 250 cells/mm^3. This is treated with antibiotics.

INITIAL INSTRUCTIONS OVER PHONE

Ask the nurse to commence initial measures, including supplementary oxygen and IV fluid resuscitation, which you will prescribe on arrival. Ask for bloods, including venous blood gas, and an ECG to be taken before your arrival. The patient should be moved to a monitored area and be clear that this patient may deteriorate rapidly.

ASSESSMENT AND RESUSCITATION

- End of the bed assessment: patient appears clammy, and his breathing is shallow.
- Airway: patent.
- Breathing: RR 26 breaths per minute, SpO_2 92% on room air. On auscultation, there is globally reduced air entry, although vesicular breath sounds are heard.
- Arterial blood gas: pH 7.36, PaO_2 7.5 kPa, $PaCO_2$ 3.4 kPa, lactate 3.0 mmol/L (raised lactate, type 1 respiratory failure).
  - Give high-flow oxygen 15 L/minute. Aim for saturations of 94–98%.
- Circulation: CRT 2 s, HR 115 bpm, regular, BP 104/59 mmHg, JVP normal, HS I + II + 0.
  - 12-lead ECG: sinus tachycardia.
- Disability: GCS 15/15, PEARL, temperature 38.4°C, CBG 4.6 mmol/L.
- Exposure: abdomen is distended and diffusely tender, bowel sounds are just audible. Positive for shifting dullness. Features of cirrhosis; evidence of protein calorie malnutrition, portal hypertension.

INITIAL INVESTIGATIONS

- Haematology: FBC (leukocytosis, anaemia), coagulation screen (coagulopathy)
- Biochemistry: U&Es (hepatorenal syndrome), LFTs (hypoalbuminaemia, deranged LFTs), calcium, phosphate, magnesium, CRP
- Microbiology: blood cultures, urine MCS
- Radiology: abdominal ultrasound scan and portal or hepatic vein Doppler (bedside ultrasound can be used to guide diagnostic paracentesis), CT abdomen (confirms ascites, excludes pneumoperitoneum), CXR (part of septic screen)

MAKING A DIAGNOSIS

Patients with end-stage liver disease are at high risk for SBP. You can make a clinical diagnosis by eliciting the presence of ascites and of peritoneal inflammation, but patients can be non-specifically unwell or have a fever and/or tachycardia without localising signs. Other patients with cirrhosis can develop encephalopathy or have an upper gastrointestinal bleed as the presenting issue. See Table 8.7 for additional information on ascitic fluid analysis.

- Symptoms: fever, abdominal pain, nausea, vomiting, diarrhoea, confusion
- Signs: pyrexia/hypothermia, hypotension, tachycardia, altered mental status, abdominal distension

Table 8.7 Ascitic fluid sampling

ASCITIC FLUID TEST	SAMPLE CONTAINER	DEPARTMENT TO SEND SAMPLE TO	RESULTS TO CHASE WHILE ON CALL
White cell count (WCC) and differential	Full blood count (purple) tube	Microbiology	≥ 250 neutrophils/mm^3
Microscopy, culture and sensitivity (MC&S)	Universal (white-top) container and blood culture bottles	Microbiology	Initial microscopy/culture after 24 hours
Cytology	Universal (white-top) container	Pathology	Not going to be available immediately
Total protein, albumin, glucose, LDH, pH, ALP and serum albumin allow calculation of serum ascites albumin gradient (to help determine causes of the ascites)	Universal (white-top) container	Biochemistry	In secondary bacterial peritonitis: • High total protein (>1 g/dL) • Glucose <50 mg/dL • LDH >225 mU/mL • ALP >240 U/L

ALP, alkaline phosphatase; LDH, lactate dehydrogenase.

and tenderness, presence of ascites (flank dullness, shifting dullness)
- Diagnostic paracentesis: ascites white cell count / neutrophil count (≥ 250 neutrophils/mm^3 is diagnostic)

MANAGEMENT

You should follow guidance from the British Society of Gastroenterology or the British Association for the Study of the Liver (or your own trust's guidance) to ensure you complete all the management steps required. This should be completed in the first 6 hours of admission and aims to ensure that patients receive the correct care ahead of a gastroenterology review within the first 24 hours.

The patient's chances of survival are highest with early diagnosis and treatment. You should seek senior help for diagnostic paracentesis (ultrasound-guided at the bedside may be available), contact the microbiology technician to forewarn of the imminent samples and request urgent results for the cell count (same-day results required). The ascitic fluid is sent in blood culture bottles and universal (white-top) containers to increase diagnostic yield.

It is important to get a detailed history about alcohol intake, either from the patient and/or collateral, to manage the patient correctly in terms of preventing irreversible cognitive impairment (Korsakoff). If the patient has a history of current excess alcohol consumption (>8 units/day males or >6 units/day females), then:

- Start Clinical Institute Withdrawal Assessment (CIWA) score, and prescribe as per trust guideline (e.g. diazepam via CIWA symptom-triggered alcohol withdrawal regime)
- Refer to the alcohol team

INFECTIONS

You should confirm the suspected source, then treat with antibiotics (Table 8.8). If the patient is showing signs of sepsis or ascitic fluid neutrophil count is ≥ 250 cells/mm^3, you should immediately start empirical broad-spectrum antibiotics. You do not need to wait for full ascitic fluid/blood culture results. Check the local microbiology guidelines and the patient's previous microbiology results and you may need to discuss the choice of antimicrobial therapy with microbiology as local antibiotic resistance profiles vary.

IF THERE IS ACUTE KIDNEY INJURY AND/OR HYPONATRAEMIA (SODIUM <125 MMOL/L)

1. Suspend all diuretics and nephrotoxic drugs.
2. Fluid-resuscitate with 5% human albumin solution or 0.9% sodium chloride (250-mL boluses with regular reassessment).
3. Initiate fluid balance chart or daily weights.
4. Aim for mean arterial pressure (MAP) > 80 mmHg to achieve urine output > 0.5 mL/kg/h based on the dry weight.

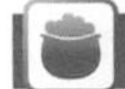 Clinical Tip

Acute Kidney Injury defined by Modified RIFLE Criteria

1. Increase in serum creatinine ≥ 26 μmol/L within 48 hours or
2. ≥50% rise in serum creatinine over the last 7 days or
3. Urine output <0.5 mL/kg/h for more than 6 hours based on dry weight or
4. Clinically dehydrated

GASTROINTESTINAL BLEEDING – IF VARICES ARE SUSPECTED

- Fluid-resuscitate according to BP, pulse and venous pressure (aim for MAP >65 mmHg)

Table 8.8 Common causes of spontaneous bacterial peritonitis (SBP)

BACTERIAL CAUSES OF SBP		IN WHAT SETTING IS THE PATHOGEN MOST COMMONLY FOUND?
Gram-negative bacteria	*Escherichia coli* *Klebsiella*	Community
Gram-positive bacteria	*Streptococcus* *Enterococcus* *Staphylococcus*	Hospital (nosocomial)

- Prescribe IV terlipressin 2 mg four times daily (caution if known ischaemic heart disease or peripheral vascular disease; perform ECG in >65 years).
- Prescribe prophylactic antibiotics.
- If indicated, give IV vitamin K, FFP and/or IV platelets, based on clotting test results and platelet count.
- Transfuse blood if Hb <7.0 g/L or massive bleeding (aim for Hb >8 g/L).
- Early endoscopy after resuscitation (ideally within 12 hours).

ENCEPHALOPATHY

You should look for the precipitant (gastrointestinal bleed, constipation, dehydration, sepsis Lactulose 20–30 mL four times daily or phosphate enema (aiming for two soft stools per day) should be prescribed. If there is clinical doubt in a confused patient, request CT head to rule out subdural haematoma.

OTHER

Prescribe prophylactic low-molecular-weight heparin for VTE prophylaxis. Patients with cirrhosis are at high risk of thromboembolism, even with a prolonged prothrombin time or raised INR. Withhold only if actively bleeding or platelet count <50 × $10^{(9)}$/L.

ESCALATION

Involve the on call gastroenterologist or medical registrar as soon as SBP is suspected. Additionally, any signs of secondary bacterial peritonitis should be escalated to the surgeons and urgently investigated with cross-sectional imaging, e.g. CT scan.

IV 20% human albumin 1.5 g/kg day 1 (and 1 g/kg on day 3) is indicated in patients with SBP and may require discussion with the on call gastroenterologist or medical registrar. This will benefit patients who are at high risk of developing hepatorenal syndrome as a complication of SBP.

If the patient does not become stable with ward level treatment, escalation to high dependency unit/ITU may be required.

FURTHER READING

Arroyo, V., Moreau, R., & Jalan, R. (2020). Acute-on-chronic liver failure. *New England Journal of Medicine*, *28*(22), 2137–2145 382.

Barrett, J., & Brown, M. (2016). Travellers' diarrhoea. *BMJ*, *353*, i1937.

Bernal, W., & Wendon, J. (2013). Acute liver failure. *New England Journal of Medicine*, *369*(26), 2525–2534.

Bernstein, C. N., et al. (2001). The incidence of deep venous thrombosis and pulmonary embolism among patients with inflammatory bowel disease: a population-based cohort study. *Thrombosis and Haemostasis*, *85*(3), 430–434.

Bert, F., et al. (2003). Nosocomial and community-acquired spontaneous bacterial peritonitis: comparative microbiology and therapeutic implications. *European Journal of Clinical Microbiology and Infectious Disease*, *22*(1), 10–15.

Blatchford, O., Murray, W. R., & Blatchford, M. (2000). A risk score to predict need for treatment for upper-gastrointestinal haemorrhage. *Lancet*, *356*(9238), 1318–1321.

BNF. (2021). *Poisoning, emergency treatment*. Available at: https://bnf.nice.org.uk/treatment-summary/poisoning-emergency-treatment. [Accessed 16 January 2022].

Bone, R. C., et al. (1992). Definitions for sepsis and organ failure and guidelines for the use of innovative therapies in sepsis. The ACCP/SCCM Consensus Conference Committee. American College of Chest Physicians/Society of Critical Care Medicine. *Chest*, *101*(6), 1644–1655.

Chiva, M., et al. (2003). Intestinal mucosal oxidative damage and bacterial translocation in cirrhotic rats. *European Journal of Gastroenterology and Hepatology*, *15*(2), 145–150.

DuPont, H. L. (2014). Acute infectious diarrhea in immunocompetent adults. *New England Journal of Medicine*, *370*(16), 1532–1540.

European Association for the Study of the Liver. (2010). EASL clinical practice guidelines on the management of ascites, spontaneous bacterial peritonitis, and hepatorenal syndrome in cirrhosis. *Journal of Hepatology*, *53*(3), 397–417.

European Association for the Study of the Liver. (2017). EASL clinical practice guidelines on the management of acute (fulminant) liver failure. *Journal of Hepatology*, *66*, 1047–1081.

Glare, P. A., et al. (2008). Treatment of nausea and vomiting in terminally ill cancer patients. *Drugs*, *68*(18), 2575–2590.

Hearnshaw, S. A., et al. (2011). Acute upper gastrointestinal bleeding in the UK: Patient characteristics, diagnoses and outcomes in the 2007 UK audit. *Gut*, *60*(10), 1327–1335.

Hunt, B. J., et al. (2015). A practical guideline for the haematological management of major haemorrhage. *British Journal of Haematology*, *170*(6), 788–803.

Johnston, V., et al. (2009). Fever in returned travellers presenting in the United Kingdom: recommendations for investigation and initial management. *Journal of Infection*, *59*(1), 1–18.

Lamb, C. A., et al. (2019). British Society of Gastroenterology consensus guidelines on the management of inflammatory bowel disease in adults. *Gut*, *68*, s1–s106.

McPherson, S., et al. (2014). Available at: www.bsg.org.uk/clinical-resource/bsg-basl-decompensated-cirrhosis-care-bundle-first-24-hours/. [Accessed 16 January 2022].

Mowat, C., et al. (2011). Guidelines for the management of inflammatory bowel disease in adults. *Gut*, *60*(5), 571–607.

NICE. (2012). *Acute upper gastrointestinal bleeding in over 16s: Management*. Clinical guideline CG141. Available at: www.nice.org.uk/guidance/cg141. [Accessed 16 January 2022].

NICE. (2013). *Intravenous fluid therapy in adults in hospital*. Clinical guideline CG174. Available at: www.nice.org.uk/Guidance/CG174. [Accessed 16 January 2022].

NICE. (2016). *Sepsis: recognition, diagnosis and early management*. Clinical guideline 51. Available at www.nice.org.uk/guidance/ng51. [Accessed 16 January 2022].

NICE. (2019). *Crohn's disease: Management*. Clinical guideline NG 129. Available at www.nice.org.uk/guidance/ng129. [Accessed 16 January 2022].

NICE. (2019). *Ulcerative colitis: Management*. Clinical guideline CG166. Available at: www.nice.org.uk/guidance/ng130. [Accessed 16 January 2022].

Norfolk, D. (Ed.). (2013). *Handbook of transfusion medicine* Available at www.transfusionguidelines.org/transfusion-handbook/7-effective-transfusion-in-surgery-and-critical-care/7-3-transfusion-management-of-major-haemorrhage. [Accessed 16 January 2022].

Ortiz, J., et al. (1997). Early microbiologic diagnosis of spontaneous bacterial peritonitis with BacT/ALERT. *Journal of Hepatology*, *26*(4), 839–844.

Public Health England. (2010). *Notifiable diseases and causative organisms:howtoreport*.Availableat:www.gov.uk/guidance/notifiable-diseases-and-causative-organisms-how-to-report. [Accessed 16 January 2022].

Resuscitation Council UK (n.d.) ABCDE approach. Available at: www.resus.org.uk/library/abcde-approach. [Accessed 16 January 2022].

Rhodes, A., et al. (2017). Surviving sepsis campaign: International guidelines for management of sepsis and septic shock: 2016. *Intensive Care Medicine*, *43*(3), 304–377.

Shah, N., DuPont, H. L., & Ramsey, D. J. (2009). Global etiology of travelers' diarrhea: systematic review from 1973 to the present. *American Journal of Tropical Medicine Hygiene*, *80*(4), 609–614.

Singer, M., et al. (2016). The Third International Consensus definitions for sepsis and septic shock (sepsis-3). *JAMA*, *315*(8), 801–810.

Stanley, A. J., et al. (2017). Comparison of risk scoring systems for patients presenting with upper gastrointestinal bleeding: international multicentre prospective study. *BMJ*, *356*, i6432.

Travis, S., Satsangi, J., & Lémann, M. (2011). Predicting the need for colectomy in severe ulcerative colitis: A critical appraisal of clinical parameters and currently available biomarkers. *Gut*, *60*(1), 3–9.

Truelove, S. C., & Witts, L. J. (1955). Cortisone in ulcerative colitis; final report on a therapeutic trial. *British Medical Journal*, *2*(4947), 1041–1048.

Turner, D., et al. (2007). Response to corticosteroids in severe ulcerative colitis: A systematic review of the literature and a meta-regression. *Clinics in Gastroenterology and Hepatology*, *5*(1), 103–110.

Veitch, A. M., et al. (2016). Endoscopy in patients on antiplatelet or anticoagulant therapy, including direct oral anticoagulants: British Society of Gastroenterology (BSG) and European Society of Gastrointestinal Endoscopy (ESGE) guidelines. *Gut*, *65*(3), 374–389.

Villanueva, C., et al. (2013). Transfusion strategies for acute upper gastrointestinal bleeding. *New England Journal of Medicine*, *368*(1), 11–21.

Wiest, R., & Garcia-Tsao, G. (2005). Bacterial translocation (BT) in cirrhosis. *Hepatology*, *41*(3), 422–433.

Wiest, R., Krag, A. and Gerbes, A. (2012) Spontaneous bacterial peritonitis: recent guidelines and beyond. *Gut*, *61*(2), pp. 297–310.

World Gastroenterology Organisation. (2012). *Global guidelines. Acute diarrhea in adults and children: a global perspective*. Available at: www.worldgastroenterology.org/guidelines/global-guidelines/acute-diarrhea/acute-diarrhea-english. [Accessed 16 January 2022].

Zollner-Schwetz, I., & Krause, R. (2015). Therapy of acute gastroenteritis: role of antibiotics. *Clinics in Microbiology and Infection*, *21*(8), 744–749.

9 Endocrinology

Content Outline

STATION 9.1: DIABETIC KETOACIDOSIS

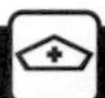

The Bleep Scenario

The nurse in the emergency department (ED) calls regarding a 27 year old male with abdominal pain. He is known to have type 1 diabetes. His current capillary blood glucose (CBG) is 22.0 mmol/L. His observations are: heart rate (HR) 100 bpm, blood pressure (BP) 120/80 mmHg, respiratory rate (RR) 25 breaths per minute, SpO_2 95% on room air and temperature 36.5°C. You have been asked to review him.

DEFINITION

Diabetic ketoacidosis (DKA) is an acute metabolic complication of diabetes. It is characterised by a biochemical triad of hyperglycaemia, ketonaemia (or significant ketonuria) and acidosis.

INITIAL THOUGHTS

DKA is the prime diagnosis to consider with history. DKA may be the first presentation of diabetes, or it may be a complication of an acute illness such as myocardial infarction, stroke, infection, non-compliance with insulin therapy, alcohol misuse or drugs that affect carbohydrate metabolism.

The most crucial initial thought for the treatment of DKA is that of fluid resuscitation. DKA protocols vary by hospital, but detailed treatment is discussed in the management section below.

Clinical Tip

When you are asked to see a patient with diabetes make sure you ascertain:

- the type of diabetes the patient ha
- previous and current medications
- compliance with medication use and monitoring such as HbA1c/blood sugar monitoring

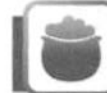

Clinical Tip—cont'd

Be aware of euglycaemic DKA, where patients have normal blood glucose levels. This can occur in children and young people on insulin in pregnancy, or in patients taking sodium-glucose cotransporter-2 (SGLT-2) inhibitors. These patients will still be acidotic and ketotic, and this is an important differential to consider.

DIFFERENTIAL DIAGNOSIS

- Metabolic: hyperosmolar hyperglycaemic state (HHS), lactic acidosis, starvation ketosis, alcoholic ketoacidosis, salicylate poisoning

INITIAL INSTRUCTIONS OVER PHONE

Ask the nurse to consider supplementary oxygen, obtain intravenous (IV) access, take initial bloods and start IV fluids for resuscitation as required. Advise to check urinary or blood ketones.

ASSESSMENT AND RESUSCITATION

- End of the bed assessment: the patient is sweaty and holding a vomit bowl
- Airway: patent
- Breathing: RR 25 breaths per minute, SpO_2 95% on room air. The patient is visibly short of breath with laboured breathing. On auscultation, there are vesicular breaths sounds with good air entry bilaterally
- Circulation: capillary refill time (CRT) <2 s, HR 100 bpm, regular, BP 120/80 mmHg, jugular venous pressure (JVP) normal, heart sounds (HS) I + II + 0. Mucous membranes are moist and normal skin turgor noted
- Disability: Glasgow Coma Scale (GCS) 15/15, pupils equal and reactive to light (PEARL), temperature 36.5°C, CBG 22.0 mmol/L

- Exposure: mild, generalised abdominal pain on palpation. Normal bowel sounds

Prescribing Tip

Review the patient's drug chart. Look for drugs that may precipitate DKA, e.g. corticosteroids, thiazide diuretics, sympathomimetic agents (e.g. dobutamine), terbutaline, second-generation antipsychotic agents and SGLT-2 inhibitors.

INITIAL INVESTIGATIONS

- Bedside: 12-lead electrocardiogram (ECG): to rule out cardiac pathology
- Haematology: full blood count (FBC): leukocytosis or anaemia
- Biochemistry: urea and electrolytes (U&Es): acute kidney injury, electrolyte imbalance, blood/urine ketone and random glucose (diagnose DKA). Venous blood gas (VBG): pH, bicarbonate – diagnose DKA. Consider further electrolyte testing, C-reactive protein (CRP), liver function tests (LFTs), amylase or myocardial enzymes (if indicated to look for precipitating causes, particularly sepsis)
- Microbiology: blood cultures and urine midstream specimen of urine (MSU: septic screen)
- Radiology: chest X-ray (CXR: septic screen)

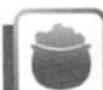

Clinical Tip

The blood gas measurement can be venous or arterial. Venous is more commonly performed as it is often easier and less painful to obtain. Literature suggests equivalence in accuracy.

MAKING A DIAGNOSIS

DKA is characterised by a biochemical triad of hyperglycaemia (>11 mmol/L or known diabetes mellitus), ketonaemia ≥ 3.0 mmol/L or significant ketonuria (more than 2+ on urinary dipstick) and acidaemia (venous pH <7.3 and/or bicarbonate <15 mmol/L). The anion gap, though not strictly part of the protocol for a diagnosis of DKA, tends to be greater than 10 mmol/L in moderate DKA and greater than 12 mmol/L in severe DKA.

Severe DKA is diagnosed in cases where blood pH <7.3, bicarbonate < 18 mmol/L, ketones > 3 mmol/L, haemodynamic instability, hypoxia or reduced GCS is present.

SYMPTOMS

- symptoms of hyperglycaemia (polyuria and polydipsia), as well as non specific symptoms, including abdominal pain, nausea, reduced level of consciousness or confusion. Symptoms of the precipitating cause

SIGNS

- ketotic breath with a characteristic peardrop smell and Kussmaul hyperventilation (deep, laboured breathing to normalise the acidosis)

MANAGEMENT

Fluid replacement is the first essential therapeutic intervention in DKA management. To determine the most appropriate treatment regime, you must first determine the patient's hydration status, potassium levels, age and comorbidities.

FLUID THERAPY

Fluid therapy of 1–1.5 litres (15–20 mL/kg body weight) of 0.9% NaCl, given over 1 hour, should be started immediately, unless the patient is hypotensive (systolic BP <90 mmHg), in which case give a fluid challenge. If the patient's BP is stable, use the following fluid regimen: 1 L of 0.9% NaCl over 1 hour, then another 1 L over 2 hours, 2 hours, 4 hours, 4 hours and 6 hours. Administration may need to be slower in elderly, pregnant, heart or renal failure patients depending on their cardiac index and performance. If the patient's CBG is <14 mmol/L, an IV infusion of 10% dextrose at 125 mL/hour can be given alongside the 0.9% NaCl infusion to prevent hypoglycaemia.

INSULIN THERAPY

A fixed-rate IV insulin (FRII) infusion (50 units Actrapid made up to 50 mL with 0.9% NaCl) at a rate of 0.1 unit/kg/hour should be initiated as soon as possible. If the patient is usually on long-acting insulin, e.g. Levemir, Lantus or Tresiba, this should be continued alongside the FRII.

ELECTROLYTE IMBALANCE

Careful monitoring of potassium is required, as insulin will shift potassium into cells. After the first bag of fluids, if the patient's potassium is 3.5–5.5 mmol/L, 0.9% NaCl + 40 mmol KCl is given. Some trusts may require cardiac monitoring or a higher level of care if potassium is given at a rate >20 mmol/hour. Potassium replacement will depend on levels at each measurement (see Table 9.1).

Table 9.1 Potassium replacement in a patient with diabetic ketoacidosis

SERUM POTASSIUM (MEQ//L)	AMOUNT OF POTASSIUM TO BE ADDED TO EACH LITRE OF REPLACEMENT FLUID (MEQ)
>5	No supplementation
4-5	20 mEq
3-4	40 mEq
<3	Hold insulin, infuse potassium at 10-20 mEq/hour til serum K^+ >3.3 mEq/L, then at 40 mEq/L fluid infusion

MONITORING

Electrolytes should be checked at least hourly, to guide potassium replacement. Urea, venous pH, creatinine and blood glucose should be checked 2-hourly initially, and then 2–4-hourly once numbers begin trending down, until resolution of DKA.

ONGOING MANAGEMENT

Resolution of DKA is achieved when pH >7.3, HCO_3^- >18 mmol/L and blood ketones <0.6 mmol/L. Once this has been achieved the FRII can be stopped. If the patient is not yet eating and drinking they should be started on a variable-rate insulin infusion (VRII). If the patient is eating and drinking they can resume their normal subcutaneous insulin regime (the first dose of which should be given ~30–60 minutes before cessation of the FRII).

SUPPORTIVE AND ADJUNCTIVE THERAPY

The patient will require a nasogastric tube if there is a fluctuating level of consciousness or they are vomiting, to reduce the risk of aspiration. Venous thromboembolism prophylaxis is also essential due to the prothrombotic state.

ESCALATION

Common complications of DKA that may require support from the high dependency unit (HDU) or intensive care unit (ICU) include cerebral oedema, resulting in a significant compromise of GCS, severe hypokalemia, renal failure due to dehydration that may require renovascular support or pulmonary oedema requiring cardiorespiratory support. Remember to seek immediate care from anaesthetics if there is any sign of airway compromise.

STATION 9.2: HYPEROSMOLAR HYPERGLYCAEMIC STATE

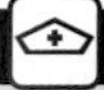

The Bleep Scenario

An ED nurse calls regarding a 56 year old male with type 2 diabetes who has been admitted with a leftleg cellulitis. He has been commenced on IV antibiotics. The nurse has just checked his blood sugars and the reading says 'HI'. His observations are: HR 105 bpm, BP 86/66 mmHg, RR 24 breaths per minute, SpO_2 95% on room air and temperature 37.5°C. You aro asked to review the patient.

DEFINITION

HHS is a serious complication, most often of type 2 diabetes mellitus, which consists of hypovolaemia, profound hyperglycaemia resulting in increased serum osmolality and absence of significant ketonaemia or acidosis.

INITIAL THOUGHTS

If a patient's CBG is very high the glucometer will simply read 'HI' instead of giving a number. When reviewing a patient with an elevated CBG you need to ensure his regular diabetic medications have not been missed. In addition, you must consider whether the patient has a more serious complication such as DKA or HHS.

Remember, HHS may be the first presentation of type 2 diabetes.

Risk factors for HHS include acute illness in a patient with known diabetes, infection, trauma, postoperative state, non compliance with diabetic medications, dehydration and pharmacological precipitants.

Clinical Tip

Patients with HHS present similarly to DKA. However they tend to be older and have multiple comorbidities. HHS also confers a higher mortality than DKA. HHS has a mortality rate of 10-20%.

DIFFERENTIAL DIAGNOSIS

- Metabolic: DKA, lactic acidosis, starvation ketosis, alcoholic ketoacidosis and salicylate poisoning

INITIAL INSTRUCTIONS OVER PHONE

Ask the attending nurse to consider supplementary oxygen aiming for saturations above 94% (in the majority of instances), obtain IV access, take bloods and start IV fluids for resuscitation as required. Advise to check urinary or blood ketones.

ASSESSMENT AND RESUSCITATION

- End of the bed assessment: the patient is sweaty.
- Airway: patent.
- Breathing: RR 24 breaths per minute, SpO_2 95% on room air. On auscultation, there are vesicular breath sounds with good air entry bilaterally.
- Circulation: CRT 3 s, HR 105 bpm, regular but low-volume pulse. BP 86/66 mmHg, JVP normal, HS I + II + 0. Mucous membranes are dry and reduced skin turgor is noted.
  - Administer IV fluids as appropriate, e.g. 500 mL 0.9% saline stat.
- Disability: GCS 15/15, PEARL, temperature 37.5°C, CBG 36.0 mmol/L.
- Exposure: the abdomen is soft and non-tender. Normal bowel sounds.

Clinical Tip

Abdominal pain is an uncommon presentation in HHS. The presence of abdominal pain should raise the possibility of an alternative diagnosis, such as DKA.

Prescribing Tip

Review the patient's drug chart. Look for drugs that may promote hyperglycaemia, e.g. corticosteroids, thiazide diuretics, beta blockers.

INITIAL INVESTIGATIONS

- Bedside: 12-lead ECG (to rule out cardiac pathology or in the presence of electrolyte imbalance)
- Haematology: FBC (leukocytosis or anaemia)
- Biochemistry: U&Es (acute kidney injury, electrolyte imbalance and calculating serum osmolality). VBG, blood/urine ketones (to assess acid–base status and exclude a diagnosis of DKA) and random glucose
  - Consider further electrolyte testing, CRP, LFTs, amylase or myocardial enzymes (as indicated to look for precipitating causes)
- Microbiology: Blood cultures and urine MSU (if infection suspected)
- Radiology: CXR (if chest infection suspected)

MAKING A DIAGNOSIS

HHS is characterised by hypovolaemia, profound hyperglycaemia (≥ 30 mmol/L), serum osmolality ≥ 320 mosmol/kg and the absence of other features of DKA (blood ketones <3.0 mmol/L, pH > 7.3 and HCO_3^- >15 mmol/L).

SYMPTOMS

- Symptoms of hyperglycaemia (polydipsia and polyuria). Non-specific symptoms include reduced GCS, clinical dehydration, focal neurology or seizures. Symptoms of the precipitating cause.

SIGNS

- Signs of hypovolaemia such as dry mucous membranes, reduced skin turgor, low BP and tachycardia.

MANAGEMENT

This patient has a blood sugar > 30 mmol/L and is hypovolaemic. If capillary ketone testing and VBG exclude DKA we must consider a diagnosis of HHS. Serum osmolality can be requested or calculated from the patient's U&Es using the formula: $2xNa^+$ + glucose + urea. If this is ≥ 320 mosmol/kg the patient has HHS.

FLUID THERAPY

When treating HHS the aim is to normalise the blood glucose and osmolality and restore fluid balance. This is done with IV fluids – 0.9% NaCl is the recommended fluid.

This patient is hypotensive so requires fluid resuscitation. Aggressive fluid replacement is recommended: 1–2 litres within the first hour, then 1 L over 2 hours, another 1 L over 2 hours and 1 L over 4 hours.

The aim is for the patient to be in positive fluid balance and strict input/output monitoring is required to see if this is achieved.

ELECTROLYTE IMBALANCE

After the first hour, consider replacing potassium by giving 1 L of 0.9% NaCl + 40 mmol KCl if the patient's potassium is 3.5–5.5 mmol/L. Some trusts may require cardiac monitoring or a higher level of care, if potassium is given at a rate >20 mmol/hour.

INSULIN THERAPY

Insulin is not routinely given unless the capillary ketones are >1 mmol/L or the blood glucose is not falling with IV fluids, in which case an fixed-rate IV insulin at 0.05 units/kg/hour can be initiated. Insulin therapy should not be given if serum potassium is less than 3.3 mmol/L to avoid precipitating life-threatening hypokalaemia.

MONITORING

Regular monitoring of blood glucose and electrolytes (Na^+, K^+ and calculated osmolality) is required. Hourly for the first 6 hours, reducing to 2-hourly if the patient is responding appropriately to treatment.

The aim is to reduce blood glucose by 4–6 mmol/L/hour and reduce serum osmolality by 3–8 mosmol/kg/hour. It often takes several days to fully correct the metabolic abnormalities present in HHS.

SUPPORTIVE AND ADJUNCTIVE THERAPY

Venous thromboembolism prophylaxis is essential due to the prothrombotic state incurred by severe dehydration.

Clinical Tip

An initial rise in sodium is expected. However, if the serum osmolality is not reducing despite adequate fluid resuscitation then the fluids may be switched to 0.45% NaCl (hypertonic saline).

ESCALATION

Depending on the patient's level of frailty and comorbidity, patients who do not respond to initial medical therapy may be considered for escalation to intensive care. Most commonly, this is to help with fast potassium replacement through central line insertion in the case of severe hypokalaemia, but it could also be for the consideration of renovascular, cardiovascular or airway support if consciousness is fluctuant. It is important to note that often patients with HHS are frail, and may not be fit for any intervention beyond basic medical care. Always escalate to your direct senior and intensive care team when in doubt. You should involve the local endocrine team for input and care for any patient with HHS.

STATION 9.3: HYPOGLYCAEMIA

The Bleep Scenario

A 45 year old male, who has type 1 diabetes (insulin-dependent), has been found unresponsive in his chair. His blood sugar is 2.3 mmol/L. His observations are: HR 60 bpm, BP 113/72 mmHg, RR 16 breaths per minute, SpO_2 96% on room air and temperature 36.5°C. He was admitted directly to the ED, and you have been asked to review him urgently.

DEFINITION

Hypoglycaemia is a low blood glucose level (<4.0 mmol/L).

INITIAL THOUGHTS

This patient has severe hypoglycaemia and requires urgent assessment and treatment. Most hospital trusts have insulin charts where the medical management of hypoglycaemia is pre-prescribed, although it still requires a doctor's signature. This should be administered as soon as possible as hypoglycaemia is a potentially severe and life threatening emergency.

As hypoglycaemia is most commonly a result of overtreatment with diabetic medications or a lack of glucose intake, it is important to consider potential precipitants straightaway.

Risk factors for hypoglycaemia include reduced oral intake, sulfonylurea or insulin therapy, increased exercise, alcohol intake, acute kidney injury, infection, adrenal insufficiency, growth hormone insufficiency or insulin-producing tumours (insulinomas).

DIFFERENTIAL DIAGNOSIS

- Cardiology: myocardial infarction
- Endocrinology: hypoglycaemia, electrolyte imbalance
- Neurology: stroke, head injury, seizures
- Other: alcohol or drug toxicity

INITIAL INSTRUCTIONS OVER PHONE

Ask the referrer to obtain IV access, take bloods and proceed with treatment using the trust's pre-prescribed hypoglycaemia treatment chart whilst you are on your way.

ASSESSMENT AND RESUSCITATION

- End of the bed assessment: the patient has been moved on to the bed and appears unresponsive.
- Airway: the patient is unresponsive and not able to communicate.
  - Check for a carotid pulse, the patency of the airway and signs of breathing. A good volume carotid pulse is palpable, and signs of breathing are noted. He is maintaining his own airway with no added sounds. If he is able to tolerate it, an airway adjunct can be used.
- Breathing: RR 16 breaths per minute, SpO_2 96% on room air. On auscultation, there are vesicular breath sounds with good air entry bilaterally.
- Circulation: CRT <2 s, HR 60 bpm, regular. BP 113/72 mmHg, JVP normal, HS I + II + 0.
  - Administer glucose infusion, e.g. 75–100 mL of 20% glucose over 15 minutes.
- Disability: GCS 9/15 (E2V2M5), PEARL, temperature 36.5°C, CBG 2.3 mmol/L.
- Exposure: abdomen soft and non-tender. Normal bowel sounds. No other significant findings.

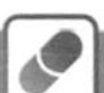

Prescribing Tip

Once the episode of hypoglycaemia has been appropriately managed the drug chart of any diabetic patient needs to be reviewed to ensure the correct dose of the right diabetic medication has been prescribed. It is also useful to review the patient's food chart.

INITIAL INVESTIGATIONS

- Biochemistry: U&Es and LFTs (impaired renal or hepatic function is a hypoglycaemia risk). Random glucose and HbA_{1c} (to assess glycaemic control)

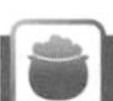

Clinical Tip

Further investigation in a known diabetic is not normally required. However, if a patient who is not known to be diabetic has an episode of hypoglycaemia, further investigation may be warranted. This may include HbA_{1c}, serum glucose, sulfonylurea screen, serum insulin and C-peptide level (taken at the time of the episode) to determine whether it was due to endogenous (e.g. insulinoma) or exogenous insulin.

MAKING A DIAGNOSIS

SYMPTOMS

- Autonomic symptoms such as sweating, anxiety, hunger, tremor, palpitations or dizziness. Neuroglycopenic symptoms such as confusion, drowsiness, visual disturbance, seizures or coma.

MANAGEMENT

This patient is severely hypoglycaemic. As his GCS is low he will be unable to tolerate glucose orally. If already cannulated, or it is easy to get IV access, give IV glucose. These infusions should be readily available on the ward. Equipment and medications needed to treat hypoglycaemia can be found in the hypoglycemia toolkit, normally stored on the crash trolley.

Prescribing Tip

Trust guidelines may differ but usually either 75–100 mL of 20% glucose or 150–200 mL of 10% glucose could be administered over 15 minutes.

If IV access is not present and cannot be gained, 1g intramuscular (IM) glucagon can be given instead. It is important to note that IM glucagon is not normally the first-line treatment as its effect will be dependent on the patient having sufficient glycogen stores and may be less effective.

If a patient is alert, orientated and able to swallow (mild hypoglycaemia), 15–20 g of quick-acting carbohydrate can be given orally, such as 150–200 mL of pure orange juice or 3–4 heaped teaspoons of sugar dissolved in water.

If a patient can swallow, but is confused or agitated (moderate hypoglycaemia), Glucogel can be given instead (two tubes). This is a sugary gel containing 40% glucose, and it can be squeezed into the patient's gums or teeth.

MONITORING

The patient will need close monitoring and the blood glucose rechecking in 10 minutes. If it remains low, treatment can be repeated (up to three times). If a clinical and blood glucose improvement is noted, then long acting glucose can be given orally once the patient is able to swallow, such as two biscuits or a piece of toast. It is important never to omit long acting insulin, especially in patients with type 1 diabetes, as it is important to maintain basal insulin control to avoid an acute surge in blood glucose levels. Remember that hypoglycaemia can recur and thus you should have a low threshold for this.

ESCALATION

If the patient has a low GCS and is unable to maintain their airway, you should put out a medical emergency call for consideration of airway support administered by the anaesthetist and potential escalation to intensive care for further management. Otherwise discuss with your direct senior and, if appropriate, the diabetes team.

STATION 9.4: HYPOCALCAEMIA

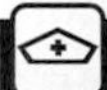

The Bleep Scenario

The biochemistry laboratory has just phoned you with urgent results for a patient with a serum calcium of 1.80 mmol/L. The patient is a 82 year old female, who has been an inpatient for a few days following a fall. She is medically fit and is awaiting a package of care prior to discharge. Her observations are: HR 73 bpm, BP 140/80 mmHg, RR 20 breaths per minute, SpO_2 97% on room air and temperature 37.0°C. You are asked by the nurse to review her.

DEFINITION

Hypocalcaemia is a state of reduced serum calcium (Ca^{2+}) and can be symptomatic or asymptomatic depending on the degree.

INITIAL THOUGHTS

Abnormal blood results, grossly outside the normal range, are generally called through to the ward from the laboratory. This patient has severe hypocalcaemia (Ca^{2+} < 1.90 mmol/L) and will need an urgent IV calcium infusion.

Causes for hypocalcaemia include nutritional deficiencies (e.g. vitamin D deficiency), other electrolyte imbalances including hypomagnesemia, rhabdomyolysis, pancreatitis, post-parathyroidectomy, primary hypoparathyroidism and multiple blood transfusions.

It is imperative therefore to do a full electrolyte screen, including calcium and magnesium, as deficiencies in these may result in hypocalcaemic blood results.

INITIAL INSTRUCTIONS OVER PHONE

Ask the referrer to obtain IV access, take bloods and complete an ECG.

ASSESSMENT AND RESUSCITATION

- End of the bed assessment: the patient looks well.
- Airway: patent.
- Breathing: RR 20 breaths per minute, SpO_2 97% on room air. On auscultation, there are vesicular breath sounds with good air entry bilaterally.
- Circulation: CRT 2 s, 73 bpm, regular. BP 140/80 mmHg, JVP normal, HS I + II + 0.
  - 12-lead ECG: may show signs of hypocalcaemia, prolonged QT interval and any arrhythmias.
- Disability: GCS 15/15, PEARL, temperature 37.0°C, CBG 7.2 mmol/L.
- Exposure: abdomen soft and non-tender. Normal bowel sounds. Positive Chvostek's and Trousseau's sign.

Prescribing Tip

Review the patient's drug chart. Look for drugs that may be precipitating the hypocalcaemia e.g. proton pump inhibitors, bisphosphonates, chemotherapy, chelating agents, gadolinium and glucocorticoids.

INITIAL INVESTIGATIONS

- Haematology: FBC (leukocytosis or anaemia)
- Biochemistry: U&Es (electrolyte imbalance, renal insufficiency), PO_4, Mg^{2+}, parathyroid hormone (PTH)

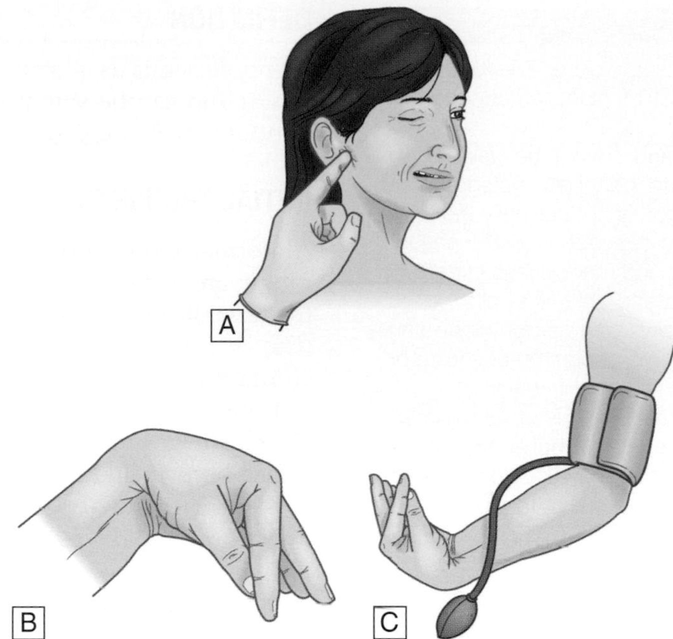

Fig. 9.1 Tests for hypocalcaemia. (A) Chvostek's sign is contraction facial muscles in response to a light tap over the facial nerve in front of the ear. (B) Trousseau's sign is a carpal spasm induced by (C) inflating a blood pressure cuff above the systolic pressure for a few minutes. (Source: Chintamani, M. and Mani, M. [Eds.]. [2021]. *Lewis's medical-surgical nursing, fourth South Asia edition: assessment and management of clinical problems*. Elsevier.)

and vitamin D level (to identify cause for hypocalcaemic state).

 **Clinical Tip**

The majority of calcium is found in the bone. Calcium in the blood is found in its ionised form or is bound to proteins, including albumin. If a patient's albumin is outside the normal reference range this will influence the total serum calcium. The laboratory will report two calcium values – the total calcium and the adjusted calcium, which has adjusted the calcium to the patient's albumin level. Always use the adjusted calcium level: serum Ca^{2+} + [(40 – albumin) × 0.02].

MAKING A DIAGNOSIS

Mild hypocalcaemia is an adjusted serum Ca^{2+} of 1.90–2.19 mmol/L and is usually asymptomatic. Severe hypocalcaemia is an adjusted serum Ca^{2+} <1.90 mmol/L or if the patient is symptomatic with a Ca^{2+} below reference range (2.20–2.60 mmol/L) and is classed as a medical emergency.

SYMPTOMS

- Perioral or peripheral paraesthesia, generalised weakness, carpopedal spasm, seizures, cardiac hyperexcitability, hypotension, tetany, confusion or in extreme cases laryngospasm.

SIGNS

- Chvostek's and Trousseau's sign.

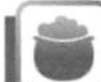 **Clinical Tip**

A positive Chvostek's sign is demonstrated by facial muscle spasm as a result of tapping over cranial nerve VII. Trousseau's sign occurs when inflation of a BP cuff around a patient's arm or leg results in carpopedal spasm (Fig. 9.1).

MANAGEMENT

Acute management of severe hypocalcaemia requires IV administration of 10–20 mL of 10% calcium gluconate (in 50–100 mL of 5% dextrose) over 10 minutes. The patient should have ECG monitoring whilst this is administered, as there is a risk of arrhythmia. Repeat infusions can be given until the patient is asymptomatic (up to three times).

If adjusted calcium remains <1.90 or the patient is still symptomatic, commence an IV infusion to prevent further hypocalcaemia. An infusion of 100 mL of 10% calcium gluconate is mixed with 1 litres of crystalloid (either 0.9% NaCl or 5% dextrose) and given at a rate of 50 mL/hour, although this can later be titrated. Recheck calcium after 6 hours.

Mild hypocalcaemia can be treated with oral calcium supplements, e.g. Adcal-D3.

The underlying cause of the hypocalcaemia needs to be identified and corrected. Patients with concurrent hypomagnesaemia, for example, will need their magnesium correcting as a priority, as calcium levels will generally not normalise until this is done.

ESCALATION

Patients with severe hypocalcaemia should be escalated to your registrar. The patient may need to be moved to a bed where cardiac monitoring can be undertaken.

STATION 9.5: HYPERCALCAEMIA

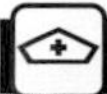

The Bleep Scenario

A 64 year old woman has been admitted to the acute medical unit by her general practitioner (GP) with a serum calcium of 3.30 mmol/L. She reports a history of back pain and weight loss. Her observations are: HR 68 bpm, BP 140/90 mmHg, RR 17 breaths per minute, SpO_2 95% on room air and temperature 36.7°C. You are asked to review the patient.

DEFINITION

Hypercalcaemia is a state of raised serum calcium (Ca^{2+}) levels and can vary in degree from mild to moderate or severe.

INITIAL THOUGHTS

In some instances blood test results may be from a few days ago and will require repeating to ensure accuracy. Hypercalcaemia is often asymptomatic and n incidental finding on blood tests. Whilst there are a number of causes, around 90% of cases are due to malignancy or primary hyperparathyroidism.

Other causes include sarcoidosis, drug related, high levels of vitamin D, thyrotoxicosis and familial hypocalciuric hypercalcaemia.

INITIAL INSTRUCTIONS OVER PHONE

Ask the referrer to obtain IV access, take bloods and obtain an ECG.

ASSESSMENT AND RESUSCITATION

- End of the bed assessment: the patient looks well.
- Airway: patent.
- Breathing: RR 17 breaths per minute, SpO_2 95% on room air. On auscultation, there are vesicular breath sounds with good air entry bilaterally.
- Circulation: CRT <2 s, HR 68 bpm, regular, BP 140/90 mmHg, JVP normal, HS I + II + 0.
  - 12-lead ECG: may see signs of hypercalcaemia: shortening of QT interval and arrhythmias.
- Disability: GCS 15/15, PEARL, temperature 36.7°C, CBG 5.2 mmol/L.
- Exposure: abdomen soft and non tender. Normal bowel sounds. There is some bony tenderness over the lumbar spine.

Prescribing Tip

Review the patient's drug chart; look for drugs that may be precipitating the hypercalcaemia, e.g. thiazide diuretics, lithium or any over-the-counter medications containing calcium.

INITIAL INVESTIGATIONS

- Haematology: FBC (leukocytosis or anaemia)
- Biochemistry: U&Es, bone profile (Ca^{2+}, PO_4^{3-}, alkaline phosphatase, to recheck serum calcium) and PTH (a paired sample, meaning it is taken at the same time as the serum calcium, to look for hyperparathyroidism). Vitamin D levels and magnesium levels (cause for calcium imbalance). Serum protein electrophoresis and urine electrophoresis (multiple myeloma).
- Radiology: bone density (dual-energy X-ray absorptiometry) scan may also be necessary.

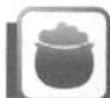

Clinical Tip

There are several cancers that can cause hypercalcaemia, including myeloma (plasma cell malignancy) and primary cancers that metastasise to bone (chiefly breast, lung, thyroid, kidney and prostate). Biochemically they cause a high calcium and low PTH. Hyperparathyroidism (primary or, less commonly, tertiary) causes a high calcium and high PTH.

MAKING A DIAGNOSIS

Mild hypercalcaemia is an adjusted serum Ca^{2+} of 2.60–2.90 mmol/L. Moderate hypercalcaemia is an adjusted serum Ca^{2+} of 3.00–3.50 mmol/L. Severe hypercalcaemia is an adjusted serum Ca^{2+} > 3.50 mmol/L.

SYMPTOMS

- Symptoms of hypercalcaemia generally only present with calcium ≥ 3.00 mmol/L. Symptoms are commonly remembered using the mnemonic 'bones, stones, moans, groans' (and occasionally thrones):
  - Bones: bony pain and fractures
  - Stones: renal stones due to kidney's inability to secrete excess calcium
  - Moans: cognitive dysfunction, depression
  - Groans: generalised abdominal pain (peptic ulceration, pancreatitis), nausea and vomiting
  - Thrones: constipation

Other non-specific symptoms include tiredness, polyuria, polydipsia and in severe cases reduced consciousness or coma (Fig. 9.2).

MANAGEMENT

Acute management of hypercalcaemia involves correcting dehydration with IV fluids. Patients should receive 4–6 L of 0.9% NaCl over 24 hours with daily monitoring of adjusted calcium levels. They will need careful monitoring as they are at risk of fluid overload.

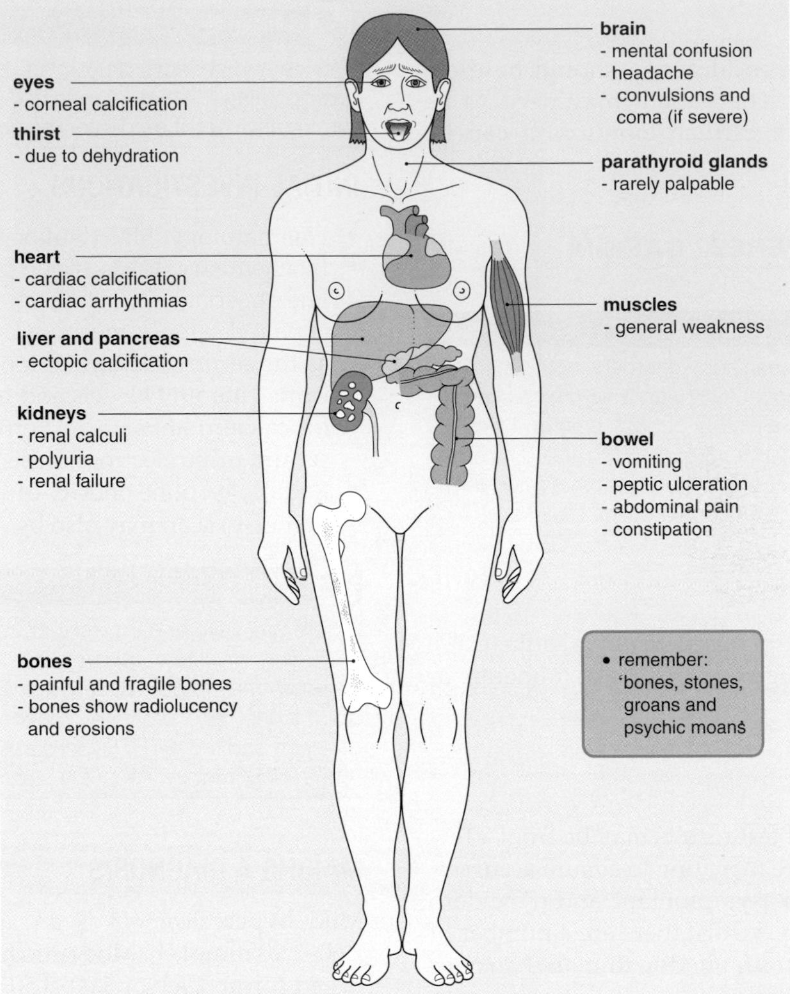

Fig. 9.2 Symptoms and signs of hypercalcaemia. (Source: Murphy, R. et al. [2016]. *Crash course endocrinology*. Elsevier.)

If this occurs it may require treatment with loop diuretics, which also increase calcium secretion.

If calcium levels remain persistently elevated after adequate IV fluids, then consider IV bisphosphonates, which inhibit bone resorption by osteoclasts. A number of IV bisphosphonates may be given, including 30–90 mg pamidronate (at rate of 20 mg/hour) or 4 mg zoledronic acid (given over 15 minutes). It may take a few days before the full effect of the bisphosphonate is seen.

Any further management will depend on the cause of hypercalcaemia. A patient with sarcoidosis may be given oral steroids, for example, whereas a patient with primary hyperparathyroidism may need a surgical parathyroidectomy.

ESCALATION

Patients with severe hypercalcaemia should be escalated to your registrar for review and further management. Patients may require cardiac monitoring for risk of arrhythmias depending on the severity of their metabolic imbalance.

STATION 9.6: HYPERKALAEMIA

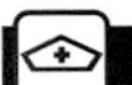

The Bleep Scenario

A 65 year old male has been admitted to the AMU complaining of muscle weakness and paraesthesia. He has previously had issues with raised serum potassium levels. His observations are: HR 90 bpm, BP 135/75 mmHg, RR 17 breaths per minute, SpO_2 95% on room air and temperature 36.5°C. You are asked to review him by one of the nurses.

DEFINITION

Hyperkalaemia is defined as an elevated serum potassium (K^+) level ≥ 5.50 mmol/L and can vary in degree from mild to moderate and severe.

INITIAL THOUGHTS

Potassium is an important electrolyte in our bodies, with the vast majority (~98%) contained in the intracellular fluid. Causes of hyperkalaemia can be divided into three main categories: increased intake, reduced excretion and redistribution of potassium from the intracellular to extracellular compartment. Increased intake may be the result of a massive blood transfusion, administration of IV fluids containing potassium or through diet. Reduced excretion may be seen with acute or chronic renal insufficiency, secondary to medications that compromise the kidney's ability to maintain potassium homeostasis and in low sodium states, as sodium intake influences the ability of the kidney to excrete potassium. Potassium may shift from the intracellular to extracellular compartment in metabolic acidotic states such as rhabdomyolysis and DKA.

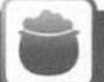

Clinical Tip

Remember to also consider artefact as a cause of hyperkalaemia. This may be secondary to cell lysis, often following traumatic or prolonged venepuncture, delayed centrifugation of the blood sample (>4 hours post-venepuncture) and contamination. A factitiously elevated potassium can occur when sampling from a 'drip arm', where the patient is receiving IV fluids containing potassium or if U&Es have been taken after other blood tests, such as FBC, which is collected in an ethylenediaminetetraacetic acid bottle. When in doubt, repeat the sample using a lithium heparin tube or on a VBG.

DIFFERENTIAL DIAGNOSIS

- Endocrinology: electrolyte imbalances, vitamin deficiencies
- Neurology: neuropathy
- Other: anxiety, drug-related

INITIAL INSTRUCTIONS OVER PHONE

Ask the nurse to obtain IV access, take initial bloods and complete an ECG.

ASSESSMENT AND RESUSCITATION

- End of the bed assessment: the patient looks anxious and sweaty.
- Airway: patent.
- Breathing: RR 17 breaths per minute, SpO_2 95% on room air. On auscultation, there are vesicular breath sounds with good air entry bilaterally.
- Circulation: CRT 2 s, HR 90 bpm, regular. BP 135/75 mmHg, JVP normal, HS I + II + 0.
  - 12-lead ECG: signs of hyperkalaemia such as classically tall tented T waves, small P waves and widening of the QRS, which may become sinusoidal. Arrhythmias such as monomorphic ventricular tachycardia, polymorphic ventricular tachycardia (torsades de pointes) and ventricular fibrillation (Fig. 9.3).
- Disability: GCS 15/15, PEARL, temperature 36.5°C, CBG 5.9 mmol/L.

ECG Changes in Hyperkalaemia

QRS Complex	Approximate Serum Potassium (mmol/l)	ECG Change
P wave T wave	4–5	Normal
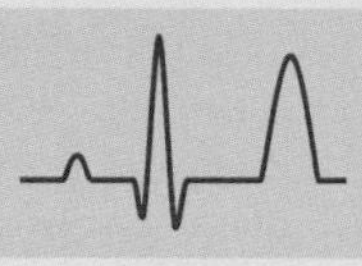	6–7	Peaked T waves
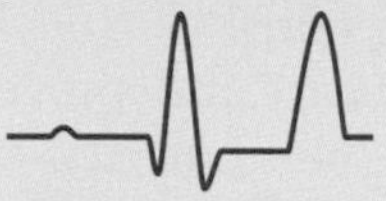	7–8	Flattened P wave, prolonged PR interval, depressed ST segment, peaked T wave
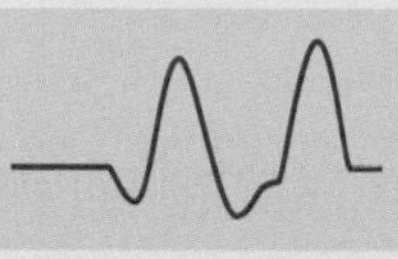	8–9	Atrial standstill, prolonged QRS duration, further peaking T waves
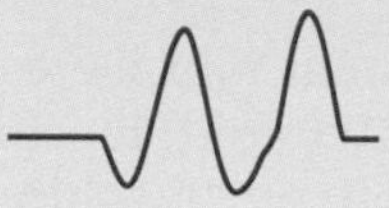	>9	Sinusoid wave pattern

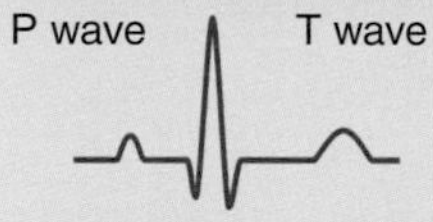

Fig. 9.3 Electrocardiogram (ECG) changes in hyperkalaemia. (Source: Johnson, R.J., Feehally, J. and Floege, J. [2015]. *Comprehensive clinical nephrology*. Elsevier.)

- Exposure: abdomen soft and non tender. Normal bowel sounds. No other significant findings.

Prescribing Tip

Review the patient's drug chart. Look for drugs that may be precipitating the hyperkalaemia, e.g. potassium sparing diuretics (e.g. spironolactone), angiotensin-converting enzyme inhibitors, angiotensin II receptor blockers, non steroidal anti-inflammatory drugs, trimethoprim, heparin, calcineurin inhibitors such as ciclosporin and tacrolimus, beta blockers and digoxin.

INITIAL INVESTIGATIONS

- Haematology: FBC (anaemia)
- Biochemistry: U&Es (serum K^+, other electrolyte imbalances, renal insufficiency). VBG (quick K^+ reading), creatinine kinase (rhabdomyolysis, which is a cause for hyperkalaemia) and blood glucose (cause for hyperkalaemia)

MAKING A DIAGNOSIS

Mild hyperkalaemia is a serum K^+ of 5.50–5.90 mmol/L. Moderate hyperkalaemia is a serum K^+ of 6.00–6.40 mmol/L. Severe hyperkalaemia is a serum of $K^+ \geq$ 6.50 mmol/L.

SYMPTOMS

- Often asymptomatic but may cause palpitations, muscle weakness, paraesthesia, chest pain and light headedness.
- The ECG is a key diagnostic investigation.

MANAGEMENT

Patients with mild hyperkalaemia or asymptomatic, moderate hyperkalaemia without ECG changes do not need immediate medical treatment. Emergency management is needed to treat moderate or severe hyperkalaemia with ECG changes or symptoms.

The priority is to stabilise the heart and prevent fatal arrhythmias by administering 30 mLof 10% calcium gluconate IV over 5–10 minutes (or 10 mL of 10% calcium chloride). If the patient is on digoxin, treatment would need to be diluted and given more slowly.Cardiac monitoring may be required, with senior input.

The next step is to move potassium into the cells by giving soluble insulin (10 units Actrapid) together with 50 mL of 50% glucose or 125 mL of 20% glucose as an IV infusion over 10–20 minutes (to prevent hypoglycaemia). Salbutamol nebulisers (10–20 mg) may also be administered. Again, these shift potassium into the cells.

Cation exchange resins (calcium resonium 15 g orally three or four times daily) is not recommended in the acute treatment of severe hyperkalaemia but may be considered in mild to moderate hyperkalaemia and works slowly. This drug binds potassium in the gastrointestinal tract, and this is then excreted via the faecal route.

MONITORING

The patient's blood glucose will need monitoring regularly for the next 6 hours if receiving insulin treatment for the hyperkalaemia. Repeat bloods and an ECG will be required to check if the treatment is working. Urine output should be monitored in cases of acute kidney injury.

Clinical Tip

Be aware that states of hyperglycaemia induce the movement of potassium from the intracellular to extracellular compartment, resulting in high serum potassium levels. This may hide an underlying state of potassium depletion. Therefore, it is important to correct the hyperglycaemia before being able to assess the potassium balance accurately.

ESCALATION

Always escalate patients with severe hyperkalaemia to your registrar promptly as these patients will require cardiac monitoring. Refractory hyperkalaemia, especially in the context of renal failure, may require renal team input for consideration of haemodialysis or haemofiltration.

STATION 9.7: HYPOKALAEMIA

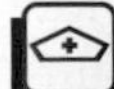

The Bleep Scenario

A 90 year old female patient, on the geriatric ward, presented last week in fast atrial fibrillation, which has settled on beta-blockers and digoxin. She also has a background of congestive cardiac failure, for which she is on furosemide. Her bloods were checked today, and her potassium is 2.4 mmol/L. Her observations are: HR 60 bpm, BP 114/68 mmHg, RR 16 breaths per minute, SpO_2 95% on room air and temperature 36.3°C. You are asked to review the patient.

DEFINITION

Hypokalaemia is defined as a serum potassium (K^+) level < 3.60 mmol/L.

INITIAL THOUGHTS

The patient has severe hypokalaemia, likely a result of diuretic use given her history. Hypokalaemia aetiology can be chiefly divided into insufficient intake, increased loss and cellular redistribution. Hospitalised patients may have insufficient intake due to inadequate potassium being prescribed in IV fluids. Redistribution of potassium into cells may be the result of insulin administration, alkalosis, hypothermia or secondary to drugs. Increased loss may be via the renal tract (from diuretics, hyperaldosteronism or renal tubular acidosis), via the gastrointestinal tract (in diarrhoea and vomiting and excessive laxative use) or via the skin (burns and increased sweat loss).

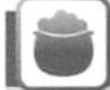

Clinical Tip

It is useful to check if a previous potassium result is available to determine if this is an acute or chronic reduction and whether the patient is symptomatic.

INITIAL INSTRUCTIONS OVER PHONE

Ask the nurse to obtain IV access, take initial bloods and complete an ECG.

ASSESSMENT AND RESUSCITATION

- End of the bed assessment: the patient looks well.
- Airway: patent.
- Breathing: RR 16 breaths per minute, SpO_2 95% on room air. On auscultation, there are vesicular breath sounds with good air entry bilaterally.
- Circulation: CRT 2 s, HR 60 bpm, regular. BP 114/68 mmHg, JVP normal, HS I + II + 0.

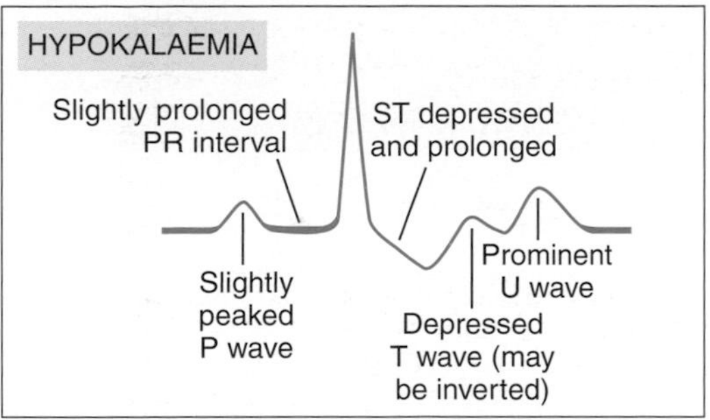

Fig. 9.4 Electrocardiogram (ECG) changes in hypokalaemia. (Source: Harris, P., Nagy, S. and Vardaxis, N. [2019]. *Mosby's dictionary of medicine, nursing and health professions – revised 3rd ANZ edition.* Elsevier.)

- 12 lead ECG: signs of hypokalaemia such as, ST depression, T-wave flattening or inversion, U waves and arrhythmias (Fig. 9.4).
- Disability: GCS 15/15, PEARL, temperature 36.3°C, CBG 4.3 mmol/L.
- Exposure: abdomen soft and non tender. Normal bowel sounds. No other significant findings.

 **Prescribing Tip**

Review the patient's drug chart. Look for drugs that may be precipitating the hypokalaemia, e.g. loop diuretics, corticosteroids, beta-2 agonists (e.g. salbutamol), amphotericin B, chloroquine or theophylline intoxication.

INITIAL INVESTIGATIONS

- Bedside: VBG (quick K^+ reading, pH, HCO_3^- and Cl^+)
- Haematology: FBC (anaemia)
- Biochemistry: U&Es (serum K^+, other electrolyte imbalances, look for renal causes). Magnesium levels (as this can affect potassium balance)

MAKING A DIAGNOSIS

Mild hypokalaemia is a serum K^+ of 3.00–3.50 mmol/L. Moderate hypokalaemia is a serum K^+ of 2.50–3.00 mmol/L. Severe hypokalaemia is a serum K^+ < 2.5 mmol/L or if symptomatic.

SYMPTOMS

- Often asymptomatic but may cause lethargy, weakness, muscle pain or cramps and, in severe cases, palpitations and paralysis

MANAGEMENT

This patient has severe hypokalaemia, which will require IV replacement. IV potassium can be an irritant to veins, therefore should not be given at a concentration >40 mmol/L. In addition, if potassium is replaced too quickly it may precipitate arrhythmias, therefore on a general ward it should not be infused at a rate >20 mmol/L/hour. If faster or a higher concentration of potassium replacement is necessary, the patient will need continuous cardiac monitoring, often in HDU or ICU and a central line.

As the patient takes digoxin the risk of arrhythmia is greater; she will need a digoxin level. This is normally taken 6 hours after her last dose.

Mild and moderate hypokalaemia can generally be treated with oral potassium replacement. This is usually in the form of Sando K, an effervescent tablet that contains 12 mmol potassium and 8 mmol chloride. The dose is 1–2 tablets twice or three times daily. Generally, only a short course of oral replacement is required and this should be reviewed after 3 days. If a patient is nil by mouth or it is thought that the absorption of oral drugs is compromised, IV therapy can be used instead.

MONITORING

Daily monitoring of potassium is recommended while on IV or oral replacement. If not appropriately reviewed, excessive potassium supplementation can result in hyperkalaemia and fatal arrhythmias.

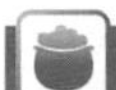 **Clinical Tip**

If a patient has concurrent hypomagnesaemia this needs to be corrected first, before the potassium will improve.

ESCALATION

A senior should be informed of patients with severe hypokalaemia as they will require cardiac monitoring. Your registrar may need to discuss with critical care teams if faster or a higher concentration of potassium replacement is required through insertion of a central line.

STATION 9.8: HYPONATRAEMIA

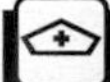 **The Bleep Scenario**

A 69 year old woman is admitted with confusion. The biochemistry team have has just phoned through her biochemistry results, stating her Na^+ is 127 mmol/L. Her observations are: HR 72 bpm, BP 138/66 mmHg, RR 19 breaths per minute, SpO_2 95% on room air and temperature 36.8°C. You are asked to review the patient.

DEFINITION

Acute hyponatraemia is a low sodium (Na^+) level developing in less than 48 hours. Hyponatraemia beyond 48 hours is regarded as chronic. Acute severe hyponatraemia is a medical emergency.

Table 9.2 Causes of hyponatraemia

EXTRACELLULAR VOLUME STATUS		
HYPOVOLAEMIA	**NORMOVOLAEMIA**	**HYPERVOLAEMIA**
Gastrointestinal fluid loss	SiADH	Heart failure
Primary adrenal failure	Hypocortisolism	Cirrhosis
Salt-losing nephritis	Hypothyroidism	Nephrotic syndrome
Cerebral salt wasting	Primary polydipsia	Renal failure
Burns		
Diuretics		

SIADH, syndrome of inappropriate antidiuretic hormone secretion.

INITIAL THOUGHTS

When clerking a patient with a vague history, such as confusion, you may not be certain of the diagnosis. Your history and examination may help to rule out some differentials. However, it may not be until further results come back that you reach a firm diagnosis.

There are many causes of hyponatraemia. These can be separated into groups according to the extracellular volume status, as illustrated in Table 9.2.

DIFFERENTIAL DIAGNOSIS

- Cardiovascular: myocardial infarction
- Endocrinology: electrolyte imbalance
- Neurology: stroke, head injury
- Other: infection

INITIAL INSTRUCTIONS OVER PHONE

Ask the nurse to obtain IV access and take initial bloods.

ASSESSMENT AND RESUSCITATION

- End of the bed assessment: the patient looks well but is fidgeting.
- Airway: patent.
- Breathing: RR 19 breaths per minute, SpO_2 95% on room air. On auscultation, there are vesicular breath sounds with good air entry bilaterally.
- Circulation: CRT 2 s, HR 72 bpm, regular. BP 138/66 mmHg, JVP normal, HS I + II + 0.
- Disability: GCS 14/15 (E4V4M6), PEARL, temperature 36.8°C, CBG 6.1 mmol/L.
- Exposure: abdomen soft and non tender. Normal bowel sounds. Calves are unremarkable with no peripheral leg oedema.

 **Prescribing Tip**

Review the patient's drug chart; look for drugs that may be precipitating the hyponatraemia, e.g. proton pump inhibitors, thiazide diuretics or antidepressants.

INITIAL INVESTIGATIONS

- Bedside: VBG (quick Na^+ result).
- Haematology: FBC (leukocytosis or anaemia)
- Biochemistry: U&Es (electrolyte imbalance, assess for renal causes). CBG (exclude pseudohyponatraemia from hyperglycaemia). Thyroid stimulating hormone (exclude hypothyroidism). Cortisol (exclude adrenal insufficiency). Serum osmolality, urine sodium and osmolality (to classify and manage the hyponatraemia)
- Radiology: CXR (exclude any pulmonary cause of syndrome of inappropriate antidiuretic hormone secretion (SIADH)) and computed tomography (CT) thorax, abdomen and pelvis if indicated (malignancy)

MAKING A DIAGNOSIS

- Mild hyponatraemia is a Na^+ 130–135 mmol/L.
- Moderate hyponatraemia is a Na^+ 125–129 mmol/L.
- Severe hyponatraemia is a Na^+ ≤125 mmol/L.

SYMPTOMS

- These can be non specific and divided into moderately severe and severe. This patient has nausea and confusion, both of which are moderately severe symptoms, along with headache. Severe symptoms include vomiting, cardiorespiratory distress, seizure activity, severe sleepiness and low GCS (≤8).

INVESTIGATIONS

- As well as being classified by severity and chronicity, hyponatraemia can be described as hypotonic (the most common), isotonic and hypertonic. This is based on the serum osmolality: <275 mmol/kg is hypotonic, 275–295 mmol/kg is isotonic and >295 mmol/kg is hypertonic.

MANAGEMENT

Patients with severe hyponatraemia (Na^+ ≤ 125 mmol/L) with seizures or coma are managed as a medical emergency and need to be discussed urgently with a senior to consider an IV infusion of hypertonic NaCl: 150 mL of 3% NaCl over 20 minutes. This patient has moderate hyponatraemia (Na^+ 125–129 mmol/L and moderately severe symptoms marked by confusion). Further management will depend on the results of a paired serum and urine osmolality, as well as the sodium and fluid status of the patient.

A urine osmolality ≤ 100 mosmol/kg suggests primary polydipsia. If urine osmolality is > 100 mosmol/kg and urine sodium ≤ 30 mmol/L consider hypervolaemia (heart failure, cirrhosis, nephrotic syndrome) or hypovolaemia (gastrointestinal losses, diuretics). A urine sodium >30 mmol/L (with a urine osmolality >100 mosmol/kg) may be due to SiADH.

Fluid status can be divided into three categories: hypovolaemic, euvolaemic and hypervolaemic. If a patient is hypovolaemic and hypotensive a fluid challenge should be given. Following this 0.9% NaCl is started at a rate of 0.5–1.0 ml/kg/hour. If a patient is euvolaemic or hypervolaemic her fluid intake is restricted, initially to 1L in 24 hours with daily monitoring of the serum sodium. If fluid restriction alone fails to resolve the hyponatraemia, the endocrine or renal team should be contacted and either demeclocycline or a vasopressin receptor antagonist (tolvaptan) considered. Patients who are profoundly overloaded may require treatment with IV loop diuretics.

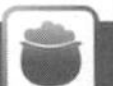

Clinical Tip

If sodium levels are increased too quickly before brain cells have had time to adapt, which usually takes about 48 hours, this can result in a shift of water into the cells, resulting in cerebral oedema and potential cerebral pontine myelinolysis with potentially chronic, debilitating effects. The increase in sodium should be ≤ 10 mmol/L during the first 24 hours of treatment and ≤ 8 mmol/L in the 24 hours following that (until the target of 130 mmol/L is reached).

ESCALATION

Patients with severe hyponatraemia should be escalated to the medical registrar. They may also require input from the endocrinology or renal teams. Critical care will need to be involved if the sodium is very low, there are seizures or the patient is obtunded for airway support and management under sedation and intubation.

STATION 9.9: ADRENAL (ADDISONIAN) CRISIS

The Bleep Scenario

A 43 year old female, known to have Addison's disease, has presented to the AMU feeling generally unwell with a fever of 37.8°C. You have been asked to review her.

Her observations are: HR 100 bpm, BP 85/59 mmHg, RR 22 breaths per minute and SpO_2 98% on room air. You are asked to review her.

DEFINITION

Adrenal crisis (also known as acute adrenal insufficiency) is a life threatening medical emergency. It can occur in patients with known adrenal insufficiency, as a result of inadequate amounts of glucocorticoid production in times of acute stress or illness, or can manifest as a first presentation.

INITIAL THOUGHTS

When asked to see an ill patient with adrenal insufficiency, the possibility of an adrenal crisis should always be considered. Adrenal insufficiency can be primary (a problem with the adrenal glands themselves, most commonly the autoimmune condition Addison's disease) or secondary (a problem outside the adrenal glands; for example, the pituitary gland or hypothalamus).

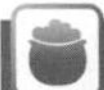

Clinical Tip

An adrenal crisis may be triggered by patients stopping their corticosteroids, prolonged nausea and vomiting or as a result of a stress response (e.g. infection, trauma or childbirth) where an increase in demand of corticosteroids is not met.

DIFFERENTIAL DIAGNOSIS

- Cardiovascular: myocardial infarction
- Endocrinology: adrenal crisis, electrolyte imbalance
- Other: Infection

INITIAL INSTRUCTIONS OVER PHONE

Ask the nurse to obtain IV access, take initial bloods and start IV fluids for resuscitation as required.

ASSESSMENT AND RESUSCITATION

- End of the bed assessment: the patient looks unwell, pale and sweaty.
- Airway: patent.
- Breathing: RR 22 breaths per minute, SpO_2 98% on room air. On auscultation, there are vesicular breath sounds with good air entry bilaterally.
- Circulation: CRT 3 s, HR 100 bpm, regular, BP 85/59 mmHg, JVP normal, HS I + II + 0.
  - 12-lead ECG: to rule out cardiac causes.
- Disability: GCS 15/15, PEARL, temperature 37.8°C, CBG 4.2 mmol/L.
- Exposure: abdomen soft and non-tender. Normal bowel sounds. Calves are unremarkable with no other significant findings.

INITIAL INVESTIGATIONS

- Haematology: FBC (leukocytosis and anaemia)
- Biochemistry: U&Es (electrolyte imbalance; often there is a picture of hyponatraemia and hyperkalaemia). Random glucose (blood glucose imbalance). Consider

a paired serum cortisol (taken in the morning) and plasma adrenocorticotrophic hormone (ACTH) level (if secondary adrenal hypofunction is suspected and the patient does not have known adrenal insufficiency)
- Microbiology: blood cultures and urine MSU (if infection is suspected as a precipitating cause)
- Radiology: CXR (if infection is suspected as a precipitating cause)

MAKING A DIAGNOSIS

SYMPTOMS

- Symptoms tend to be non specific, including fatigue, weight loss, hypotension (including postural hypotension, which may lead to dizziness and collapse), nausea, vomiting and abdominal pain

INVESTIGATIONS

- Bloods tests may show hyponatraemia and hyperkalaemia, low serum cortisol and low glucose. Short ACTH stimulation test (Synacthen test) is a diagnostic test for Addison's disease (positive if cortisol level <500 nmol/L 30 minutes after ACTH administration)

MANAGEMENT

This patient is having an adrenal crisis precipitated by an infection, taking into account the history of fever and circulatory instability. This is a medical emergency. It is not necessary to wait for further investigations; the patient should be treated immediately with corticosteroids and IV fluids.

High dose corticosteroids need to be administered urgently i.e. hydrocortisone IV/IM 100 mg. This is followed by an IV hydrocortisone infusion (200 mg/24 hours) or 50 mg IV or IM four times daily. Patients typically have an 'emergency steroid pack' at home (IM hydrocortisone 100 mg) and clarification is needed to know if this has already been administered. Once the patient has recovered from the crisis the steroid dose can be reduced in a stepwise fashion.

This patient is hypotensive and requires IV fluid resuscitation. Start initially with a fluid challenge (500 mL 0.9% NaCl), reassess the BP and prescribe accordingly. If a patient is hypoglycaemic than IV 5% dextrose may also be given alongside.

Fludrocortisone replacement is not required in the acute setting. If a patient has proven mineralocorticoid deficiency this can be started alongside oral hydrocortisone replacement.

Clinical Tip

Steps are taken to reduce the risk of a crisis developing secondary to a stress response by preemptively doubling the glucocorticoid dose if unwell in known adrenal insufficiency patients, i.e. 'sick day rules.' Steroid doses should be given parenterally if there is protracted nausea and vomiting or the patient is nil by mouth.

ESCALATION

Patients with adrenal crisis need to be escalated to the medical registrar and endocrine team promptly for further review and management.

FURTHER READING

Alfonzo, A., et al. (2020). *The Renal Association clinical practice guidelines. Treatment of acute hyperkalaemia in adults*. Available at: https://ukkidney.org/sites/renal.org/files/RENAL%20ASSOCIATION%20HYPERKALAEMIA%20GUIDELINE%202020.pdf. [Accessed 16 January 2022].

Arlt, W., et al. (2016). Society for Endocrinology endocrine emergency guidance: Emergency management of acute adrenal insufficiency (adrenal crisis) in adult patients. *Endocrine Connections*, *5*(5), G1–G3.

BMJ Best Practice. (2020). *Assessment of hypokalaemia*. Available at: https://bestpractice.bmj.com/topics/en-gb/59. [Accessed 16 January 2022].

BMJ Best Practice. (2021). *Assessment of hypocalcaemia*. Available at: https://bestpractice.bmj.com/topics/en-gb/160. [Accessed 16 January 2022].

BMJ Best Practice. (2021). *Assessment of hyponatraemia*. Available at: https://bestpractice.bmj.com/topics/en-gb/57. [Accessed 16 January 2022].

BMJ Best Practice. (2021). *Diabetic ketoacidosis*. Available at: https://bestpractice.bmj.com/topics/en-gb/3000097. [Accessed 16 January 2022].

BMJ Best Practice. (2018). *Addison's disease*. Available at: http://bestpractice.bmj.com/best-practice/monograph/56/diagnosis/step-by-step.html. [Accessed 16 January 2022].

BMJ Best Practice. *Hyperosmolar hyperglycaemic state*. Available at: https://bestpractice.bmj.com/topics/en-gb/3000124. [Accessed 16 January 2022].

Cooper, M. S., & Gittoes, N. J. (2008). Diagnosis and management of hypocalcaemia. *British Medical Journal*, *336*(7656), 1298–1302.

Dhatariya, K., et al. (2020). Diabetes at the front door. A guideline for dealing with glucose related emergencies at the time of acute hospital admission from the Joint British Diabetes Society (JBDS) for inpatient care group. *Diabetes Medicine*, *37*(9), 1578–1589.

Hassan, Z., Subramonyam, D. M., & Thakore, S. (2003). Venous blood gas in adult patients with diabetic ketoacidosis. *Emergency Medicine Journal*, *20*, 363–364.

Joint British Diabetes Societies Inpatient Care Group. (2018). *The hospital management of hypoglycaemia in adults with diabetes mellitus*. Available at: www.diabetologists-abcd.org.uk/JBDS/JBDS_HypoGuideline_FINAL_280218.pdf. [Accessed 16 January 2022].

Joint British Diabetes Societies Inpatient Care Group. (2012). *The management of hyperosmolar hyperglycaemic state (HHS) in adults*. Available at: www.diabetologists-abcd.org.uk/JBDS/JBDS_IP_HHS_Adults.pdf. [Accessed 16 January 2022].

Joint British Diabetes Societies Inpatient Care Group. (2021). *The management of diabetic ketoacidosis in adults*. Available at: https://abcd.care/sites/abcd.care/files/site_uploads/JBDS_Guidelines_Current/JBDS_02%20_DKA_Guideline_amended_v2_June_2021.pdf. [Accessed 16 January 2022].

Longmore, M., et al. (2014). *Oxford handbook of clinical medicine* (9th ed.). Oxford: Oxford University Press.

Misra, S., & Oliver, N. S. (2015). Diabetic ketoacidosis in adults. *British Medical Journal*, *28*, 351 h5660.

NICE. (2020). *Addison's disease*. Available at: https://cks.nice.org.uk/addisons-disease#!scenario. [Accessed 16 January 2022].

Raine, T., et al. (2011). *Oxford handbook for the foundation programme* (3rd ed.). Oxford: Oxford University Press.

Spasovski, G., et al. (2014). Clinical practice guideline on diagnosis and treatment of hyponatraemia. *Intensive Care Medicine*, *40*(3), 320–331. *Erratum in* Intensive Care Medicine, *40(6), p. 924*.

Turner, J., et al. (2016). *Society for Endocrinology endocrine emergency guidance, Emergency management of acute hypocalcaemia in adult patients*. Available at: www.endocrineconnections.com/content/5/5/G7.full.pdf+html. [Accessed 16 January 2022].

Uptodate. (2022). *Diabetic ketoacidosis and hyperosmolar hyperglycemic state in adults: Epidemiology and pathogenesis*. Available at: www.uptodate.com/contents/diabetic-ketoacidosis-and-hyperosmolar-hyperglycemic-state-in-adults-epidemiology-and-pathogenesis#H10. [Accessed 16 January 2022].

Walsh, J., et al. (2016). Society for Endocrinology endocrine emergency guidance. *Emergency management of acute hypercalcaemia in adult patients*. Available at: http://www.endocrineconnections.com/content/5/5/G9.full. [Accessed 16 January 2022].

10 Neurology

Content Outline

STATION 10.1: STROKE AND TRANSIENT ISCHAEMIC ATTACK

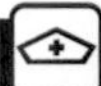
The Bleep Scenario

You are fast-bleeped to a thrombolysis call in accident and emergency (A&E). On arrival, the paramedics hand over a 76 year old woman who developed expressive dysphasia and right-sided upper and lowerlimb weakness during dinner. The time from symptom onset is 70 minutes. She is haemodynamically stable but face, arm, speech test (FAST)-positive. Her physical observations are: temperature 37.4°C, heart rate (HR) 96 bpm, blood pressure (BP) 165/108 mmHg, respiratory rate (RR) 20 breaths per minute, saturations and SpO_2 97% on room air.

DEFINITION

Stroke is defined as an acute neurological deficit lasting more than 24 hours and caused by cerebrovascular aetiology. It is subdivided into ischaemic stroke (caused by vascular occlusion or stenosis) and haemorrhagic stroke (caused by vascular rupture, resulting in intraparenchymal and/or subarachnoid haemorrhage).

INITIAL THOUGHTS

Any patient with acute-onset focal neurology such as new hemiparesis or speech slurring at time of assessment, regardless of onset time, requires a complete stroke assessment.

It is crucial to determine the onset time of the stroke, as any stroke that occurs within a 4.5-hours window will require consideration for thrombolysis by the stroke team. If symptoms have completely resolved by time of assessment and total symptom duration was under 24 hours, this can be considered a transient ischaemic attack (TIA), requiring different investigation and management.

Risk factors strongly associated with ischaemic stroke include older age, family history, hypertension, smoking, diabetes, atrial fibrillation, comorbid cardiac conditions, carotid artery stenosis, sickle cell disease and dyslipidaemia.

DIFFERENTIAL DIAGNOSIS

- Neurology: encephalopathy, seizures (Todd's paresis), hypertensive encephalopathy, cerebral venous thrombosis and hemiparetic migraine
- Psychological: conversion or somatic disorder
- General: hypoglycaemia

ASSESSMENT AND RESUSCITATION

- End of the bed assessment: the patient is leaning to her right side.
- Airway: patent.
- Breathing: SpO_2 97% on room air, RR 20 breaths per minute, no evidence of cyanosis. Chest clear on auscultation.
- Circulation: HR 96 bpm, irregular rhythm, BP 165/108 mmHg, capillary refill time (CRT) 2 s
  - 12-lead electrocardiogram (ECG): atrial fibrillation. No ischaemic changes.
- Disability: glucose 9 mmol/L. Glasgow Coma Scale (GCS) 15/15 (M6V5E4). Temperature 37.4°C.
  - Pupils: right pupil 5 mm non-reactive, left pupil 3 mm reactive.
  - Cranial nerves: II, III, IV and VI intact. V sensory loss right side. VII right facial paralysis. VIII nil. IX, X, XI, XII dysphonia, bulbar weakness.
- Exposure: no significant findings.

INITIAL INVESTIGATIONS

- Haematology: full blood count (FBC) and coagulation profile, especially if the patient is on anticoagulants (this may be a contraindication to thrombolysis)

- Biochemistry: urea and electrolytes (U&Es), serum glucose, HbA_{1c}, serum lipids and cholesterol (to assess cardiovascular risk factors).
- Radiology: computed tomography (CT) head, magnetic resonance imaging (MRI), carotid Doppler ultrasound (US). Please note: many stroke teams may wish to request a CT angiogram of the cerebral and carotid vessels in addition to the above tests to visualise potential aneurysms and vascular thromboses.

A discussion with the on call radiologist may be required for these patients. It is of particular relevance to check U&Es for patients who require CT angiograms as these are contrast-based imaging.

MAKING A DIAGNOSIS

This patient requires an urgent CT head as she meets criteria for thrombolysis: presenting within 4.5 hours of stroke symptom onset. The National Institutes of Health Stroke Scale (NIHSS) score should be used with immediacy, to objectively quantify the impairment caused by the stroke. The most sensitive and specific form of radiological imaging for stroke is an MRI head. The patient should be booked for this as soon as possible, providing there are no contraindications.

If the patient's symptoms have resolved within 24 hours of onset, you should adapt your management to the new diagnosis of a TIA. You should formally assess the patient's risk with the NIHSS score,. a key tool in the clinical diagnosis of stroke; the NIHSS score is displayed in Fig. 10.1.

Clinical Tip

There are a number of different classification systems for ischaemic stroke. The Bamford classification is one of the most common, and divides ischaemic stroke into four distinct anatomic regions. The four types of stroke defined by this system are: total anterior circulation stroke, partial anterior circulation stroke, lacunar stroke and posterior circulation syndrome. Haemorrhagic stroke is divided into the major categories of intracerebral and subarachnoid haemorrhage.

Instructions	Scale Definition	Score
1a. Level of Consciousness: The investigator must choose a response if a full evaluation is prevented by such obstacles as an endotracheal tube, language barrier, orotracheal trauma/bandages. A 3 is scored only if the patient makes no movement (other than reflexive posturing) in response to noxious stimulation.	0 = **Alert;** keenly responsive. 1 = **Not alert**; but arousable by minor stimulation to obey, answer, or respond. 2 = **Not alert**; requires repeated stimulation to attend, or is obtunded and requires strong or painful stimulation to make movements (not stereotyped). 3 = Responds only with reflex motor or autonomic effects or totally unresponsive, flaccid, and areflexic.	____
1b. LOC Questions: The patient is asked the month and his/her age. The answer must be correct - there is no partial credit for being close. Aphasic and stuporous patients who do not comprehend the questions will score 2. Patients unable to speak because of endotracheal intubation, orotracheal trauma, severe dysarthria from any cause, language barrier, or any other problem not secondary to aphasia are given a 1. It is important that only the initial answer be graded and that the examiner not "help" the patient with verbal or non-verbal cues.	0 = **Answers** both questions correctly. 1 = **Answers** one question correctly. 2 = **Answers** neither question correctly.	____
1c. LOC Commands: The patient is asked to open and close the eyes and then to grip and release the non-paretic hand. Substitute another one step command if the hands cannot be used. Credit is given if an unequivocal attempt is made but not completed due to weakness. If the patient does not respond to command, the task should be demonstrated to him or her (pantomime), and the result scored (i.e., follows none, one or two commands). Patients with trauma, amputation, or other physical impediments should be given suitable one-step commands. Only the first attempt is scored.	0 = **Performs** both tasks correctly. 1 = **Performs** one task correctly. 2 = **Performs** neither task correctly.	____
2. Best Gaze: Only horizontal eye movements will be tested. Voluntary or reflexive (oculocephalic) eye movements will be scored, but caloric testing is not done. If the patient has a conjugate deviation of the eyes that can be overcome by voluntary or reflexive activity, the score will be 1. If a patient has an isolated peripheral nerve paresis (CN III, IV or VI), score a 1. Gaze is testable in all aphasic patients. Patients with ocular trauma, bandages, pre-existing blindness, or other disorder of visual acuity or fields should be tested with reflexive movements, and a choice made by the investigator. Establishing eye contact and then moving about the patient from side to side will occasionally clarify the presence of a partial gaze palsy.	0 = **Normal.** 1 = **Partial gaze palsy;** gaze is abnormal in one or both eyes, but forced deviation or total gaze paresis is not present. 2 = **Forced deviation,** or total gaze paresis not overcome by the oculocephalic maneuver.	____

Fig. 10.1 National Institutes of Health Stroke Scale (NIHSS) scoring. (Source: Mythen, M. M., Burdett, E., Stephens, R. C., & Walker, D. [2010]. Anaesthesiology: *Churchill's Ready Reference*. Elsevier.)

3. Visual: Visual fields (upper and lower quadrants) are tested by confrontation, using finger counting or visual threat, as appropriate. Patients may be encouraged, but if they look at the side of the moving fingers appropriately, this can be scored as normal. If there is unilateral blindness or enucleation, visual fields in the remaining eye are scored. Score 1 only if a clear-cut asymmetry, including quadrantanopia, is found. If patient is blind from any cause, score 3. Double simultaneous stimulation is performed at this point. If there is extinction, patient receives a 1, and the results are used to respond to item 11.	0 = **No visual loss.** 1 = **Partial hemianopia.** 2 = **Complete hemianopia.** 3 = **Bilateral hemianopia** (blind including cortical blindness).	____
4. Facial Palsy: Ask – or use pantomime to encourage – the patient to show teeth or raise eyebrows and close eyes. Score symmetry of grimace in response to noxious stimuli in the poorly responsive or non-comprehending patient. If facial trauma/bandages, orotracheal tube, tape or other physical barriers obscure the face, these should be removed to the extent possible.	0 = **Normal** symmetrical movements. 1 = **Minor paralysis** (flattened nasolabial fold, asymmetry on smiling). 2 = **Partial paralysis** (total or near-total paralysis of lower face). 3 = **Complete paralysis** of one or both sides (absence of facial movement in the upper and lower face).	____
5. Motor Arm: The limb is placed in the appropriate position: extend the arms (palms down) 90 degrees (if sitting) or 45 degrees (if supine). Drift is scored if the arm falls before 10 seconds. The aphasic patient is encouraged using urgency in the voice and pantomime, but not noxious stimulation. Each limb is tested in turn, beginning with the non-paretic arm. Only in the case of amputation or joint fusion at the shoulder, the examiner should record the score as untestable (UN), and clearly write the explanation for this choice.	0 = **No drift;** limb holds 90 (or 45) degrees for full 10 seconds. 1 = **Drift;** limb holds 90 (or 45) degrees, but drifts down before full 10 seconds; does not hit bed or other support. 2 = **Some effort against gravity;** limb cannot get to or maintain (if cued) 90 (or 45) degrees, drifts down to bed, but has some effort against gravity. 3 = **No effort against gravity;** limb falls. 4 = **No movement.** UN = **Amputation** or joint fusion, explain: ____ **5a. Left Arm** **5b. Right Arm**	____ ____
6. Motor Leg: The limb is placed in the appropriate position: hold the leg at 30 degrees (always tested supine). Drift is scored if the leg falls before 5 seconds. The aphasic patient is encouraged using urgency in the voice and pantomime, but not noxious stimulation. Each limb is tested in turn, beginning with the non-paretic leg. Only in the case of amputation or joint fusion at the hip, the examiner should record the score as untestable (UN), and clearly write the explanation for this choice.	0 = **No drift;** leg holds 30-degree position for full 5 seconds. 1 = **Drift;** leg falls by the end of the 5-second period but does not hit bed. 2 = **Some effort against gravity;** leg falls to bed by 5 seconds, but has some effort against gravity. 3 = **No effort against gravity;** leg falls to bed immediately. 4 = **No movement.** UN = **Amputation** or joint fusion, explain: ____ **6a. Left Leg** **6b. Right Leg**	____

Fig. 10.1 cont'd

7. Limb Ataxia: This item is aimed at finding evidence of a unilateral cerebellar lesion. Test with eyes open. In case of visual defect, ensure testing is done in intact visual field. The finger-nose-finger and heel-shin tests are performed on both sides, and ataxia is scored only if present out of proportion to weakness. Ataxia is absent in the patient who cannot understand or is paralyzed. Only in the case of amputation or joint fusion, the examiner should record the score as untestable (UN), and clearly write the explanation for this choice. In case of blindness, test by having the patient touch nose from extended arm position.	0 = **Absent.** 1 = **Present in one limb.** 2 = **Present in two limbs.** UN = **Amputation** or joint fusion, explain: ______________	______
8. Sensory: Sensation or grimace to pinprick when tested, or withdrawal from noxious stimulus in the obtunded or aphasic patient. Only sensory loss attributed to stroke is scored as abnormal and the examiner should test as many body areas (arms [not hands], legs, trunk, face) as needed to accurately check for hemisensory loss. A score of 2, "severe or total sensory loss," should only be given when a severe or total loss of sensation can be clearly demonstrated. Stuporous and aphasic patients will, therefore, probably score 1 or 0. The patient with brainstem stroke who has bilateral loss of sensation is scored 2. If the patient does not respond and is quadriplegic, score 2. Patients in a coma (item 1a=3) are automatically given a 2 on this item.	0 = **Normal;** no sensory loss. 1 = **Mild-to-moderate sensory loss;** patient feels pinprick is less sharp or is dull on the affected side; or there is a loss of superficial pain with pinprick, but patient is aware of being touched. 2 = **Severe to total sensory loss;** patient is not aware of being touched in the face, arm, and leg.	______
9. Best Language: A great deal of information about comprehension will be obtained during the preceding sections of the examination. For this scale item, the patient is asked to describe what is happening in the attached picture, to name the items on the attached naming sheet and to read from the attached list of sentences. Comprehension is judged from responses here, as well as to all of the commands in the preceding general neurological exam. If visual loss interferes with the tests, ask the patient to identify objects placed in the hand, repeat, and produce speech. The intubated patient should be asked to write. The patient in a coma (item 1a=3) will automatically score 3 on this item. The examiner must choose a score for the patient with stupor or limited cooperation, but a score of 3 should be used only if the patient is mute and follows no one-step commands.	0 = **No aphasia;** normal. 1 = **Mild-to-moderate aphasia;** some obvious loss of fluency or facility of comprehension, without significant limitation on ideas expressed or form of expression. Reduction of speech and/or comprehension, however, makes conversation about provided materials difficult or impossible. For example, in conversation about provided materials, examiner can identify picture or naming card content from patient's response. 2 = **Severe aphasia;** all communication is through fragmentary expression; great need for inference, questioning, and guessing by the listener. Range of information that can be exchanged is limited; listener carries burden of communication. Examiner cannot identify materials provided from patient response. 3 = **Mute, global aphasia;** no usable speech or auditory comprehension.	______
10. Dysarthria: If patient is thought to be normal, an adequate sample of speech must be obtained by asking patient to read or repeat words from the attached list. If the patient has severe aphasia, the clarity of articulation of spontaneous speech can be rated. Only if the patient is intubated or has other physical barriers to producing speech, the examiner should record the score as untestable (UN), and clearly write an explanation for this choice. Do not tell the patient why he or she is being tested.	0 = **Normal.** 1 = **Mild-to-moderate dysarthria;** patient slurs at least some words and, at worst, can be understood with some difficulty. 2 = **Severe dysarthria;** patient's speech is so slurred as to be unintelligible in the absence of or out of proportion to any dysphasia, or is mute/anarthric. UN = **Intubated** or other physical barrier, explain:______________________	______
11. Extinction and Inattention (formerly Neglect): Sufficient information to identify neglect may be obtained during the prior testing. If the patient has a severe visual loss preventing visual double simultaneous stimulation, and the cutaneous stimuli are normal, the score is normal. If the patient has aphasia but does appear to attend to both sides, the score is normal. The presence of visual spatial neglect or anosagnosia may also be taken as evidence of abnormality. Since the abnormality is scored only if present, the item is never untestable.	0 = **No abnormality.** 1 = **Visual, tactile, auditory, spatial, or personal inattention** or extinction to bilateral simultaneous stimulation in one of the sensory modalities. 2 = **Profound hemi-inattention or extinction to more than one modality;** does not recognize own hand or orients to only one side of space.	______

Fig. 10.1 cont'd

MANAGEMENT

The first step to any assessment in stroke is the completion of NIHSS scoring, which helps determine the pattern and severity. All patients who fall within a 4.5-hours window are required to be considered for thrombolysis in the event of a suspected stroke as an immediate step, before the commencement of any antiplatelet therapy. The contraindications of thrombolysis are listed below. Before any treatment is commenced, it is crucial to exclude an intracerebral bleed by performing a CT head scan (Fig. 10.2).

It is an important point of safety to remember that thrombolysis is not administered to any patient with significant contraindications, those who present outwith the window or those with small strokes with a low NIHSS score (usually considered <8, though this

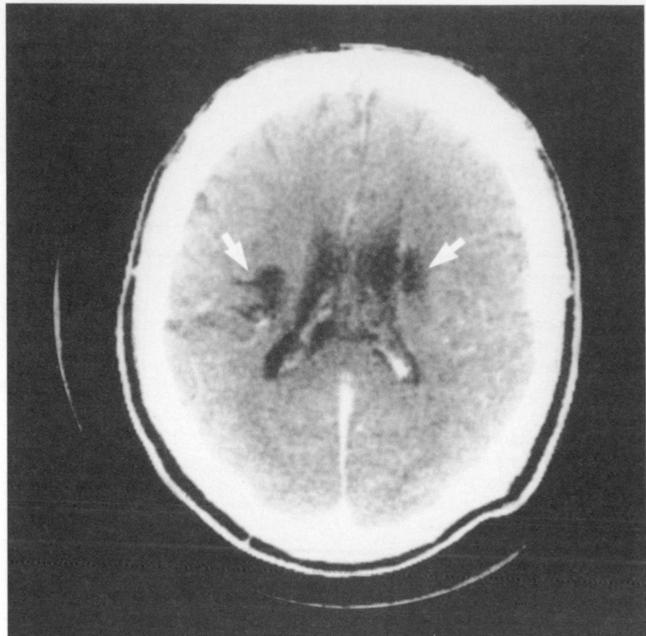

Fig. 10.2 Head computed tomography scan shows relatively small infarcts in the centrum semiovale bilaterally (arrows) that were associated with a severe spastic dysarthria. (Source: Bassert, J. M. [2014]. *McCurnin's Clinical Textbook for Veterinary Technicians.* Elsevier.)

may vary depending on other risk factors the patient presents with), as the risks of an intracerebral bleed outweigh the potential benefits of clot lysis.

THROMBOLYSIS INCLUSION CRITERIA

- Before 4.5 hours of stroke symptom onset
- Intracranial haemorrhage has been ruled out by imaging
- Age ≥ 18 years

THROMBOLYSIS ABSOLUTE CONTRAINDICATIONS

- Intracranial haemorrhage
- Hypertension > 185/110 mmHg despite two attempts to correct
- Significant head trauma or stroke in previous 3 months
- Surgery or trauma within previous 2 weeks
- Active internal bleeding
- Coagulopathy
- Anticoagulant use causing hypocoagulability (shown on laboratory tests)
- International normalised ratio (INR) > 1.7, activated partial thromboplastin time (APTT) > 40 or platelets < 100,000/mm^3

The second step is to assess the need for antiplatelet therapy; this treatment will apply to the majority of stroke patients and many of the TIA patients. Patients who do not undergo thrombolysis with a radiologically confirmed or suspected ischaemic stroke will be commenced on 300 mg aspirin once daily (OD) for 14 days, following which it is stepped down to 75 mg OD long-term. Patients with a TIA should be commenced on 300 mg aspirin OD and referred to the urgent stroke clinic. If the TIA occurred within 7 days, patients should be referred for an assessment within 24 hours. If the TIA occurred more than 7 days ago, the patient should be reviewed within 7 days. The patient flow of stroke and TIA inpatient review and outpatient clinics is different for each trust so ensure you are familiar with local guidelines.

The next step is to address the need for admission, rehabilitation and long-term antiplatelet therapy and risk factor management. The duration and extent of these depend on the severity of the patient's stroke and comorbidity, but generally involve an antiplatelet or anticoagulants in the context of atrial fibrillation for stroke prevention in addition to anticholesterol agents. It is crucial to ensure the patient's blood pressure is well controlled, and any diabetes is appropriately managed.

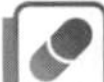

Prescribing Tip

Antiplatelet regimens in the longer term are individualised in the care of stroke patients and should be discussed with a specialist. Although the antiplatelet agent of choice for immediate treatment is almost always aspirin, it is not uncommon to see clopidogrel used instead of aspirin in some instances, particularly in the care of TIA and in long-term stroke prevention. Antiplatelet regimes will also vary depending on the anticoagulation status of the patient. Be mindful of this and remember to discuss every patient with the stroke team.

When patients are under the care of the stroke team, prevention of a deep vein thrombosis will be an important aspect of care. Again, treatment is individualised and depends on the risk factors and needs of the patient but includes heparin-based thromboprophylaxis, intermittent pneumatic compression or anticoagulants, e.g. warfarin or rivaroxaban.

Stroke care is a fine balance of acute and chronic management. It is multidisciplinary in nature and may also involve further tests to determine risk factors, such as an echocardiogram and cardiac monitoring to elucidate the possible cause.

The involvement of the speech and language and physiotherapy teams is key in the management of stroke, and it is important to perform a swallow assessment straight away to determine the best source of feeding for the patient.

ESCALATION

Each case of stroke should be discussed with the on call stroke team which most commonly consists of stroke nurses, junior doctors and a consultant. If unavailable out of hours, the best point of contact is the medical registrar. In the event of any airway instability, immediate discussion with the anaesthetic and intensive care teams should be considered. Patients with cerebral bleeds should be discussed with the on call neurosurgical team.

STATION 10.2: SEIZURES

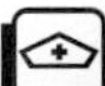

The Bleep Scenario

A ward nurse bleeps you requesting an immediate review for one of his patients. A 54 year old male is having a seizure with witnessed tonic clonic activity, for the last minute.

He was admitted yesterday for treatment of pyelonephritis and is a known epileptic, with poor antiepileptic compliance.

His physical observations are: temperature 37.8°C, HR 86 bpm, BP 156/104 mmHg, RR 18 breaths per minute and SpO_2 99% on air.

DEFINITION

A seizure is a sudden attack of physical manifestations such as convulsions, sensory disturbances or loss of consciousness resulting from abnormal and excessive electrical discharges in the brain.

STATUS EPILEPTICUS

Status epilepticus is a seizure lasting longer than 5 minutes, or multiple shorter seizures with incomplete recovery in between.

REFRACTORY STATUS EPILEPTICUS

Refractory status epilepticus is a persistent seizure despite two adequate doses of intravenous (IV) anticonvulsant agents (>45 minutes).

INITIAL THOUGHTS

In this patient with known epilepsy, it is important to consider medication non-compliance and acute illness as key potential instigators of this acute event.

DIFFERENTIAL DIAGNOSIS

- Neurology: intracranial haemorrhage, space-occupying lesion and encephalitis
- Drugs: poor compliance with epilepsy medications and toxins
- General: seizure provoked by a concomitant illness, hypoglycaemia and non-epileptic seizures

INITIAL INSTRUCTIONS OVER PHONE

You should advise the nurse to ensure that lorazepam, per rectum diazepam or buccal midazolam is available for immediate use. It is crucial to monitor for signs of airway compromise as this would require immediate escalation for potential intubation.

ASSESSMENT AND RESUSCITATION

- End of the bed assessment: the patient demonstrates tonic clonic jerking of both the upper and lower limbs. There is urinary spillage, indicative of incontinence, on the bedsheets.
- Airway: patent.
- Breathing: RR 18 breaths per minute, SpO_2 99% on room air. Chest expansion is symmetrical, there is no tracheal deviation, chest is clear on auscultation.
- Circulation: HR 86 bpm, pulse regular and good volume, BP 156/104 mmHg, CRT 3 seconds. Heart sounds (HS) I + I + 0; cannot assess jugular venous pressure (JVP).
- Disability: pupils dilated to 6 mm bilateral and sluggishly responsive. Blood glucose 6 mmol/L. Temperature 37.8°C.
- Environment: no obvious external injury or rashes.

MAKING A DIAGNOSIS

The most common causes of acute, new-onset seizures are:

- Structural lesions
- Acute provoked illness such as stroke
- Hypoxia
- Toxin-mediated (drug and alcohol withdrawal)

Status epilepticus in patients with known epilepsy is most often due to:

- Treatment non-adherence
- Intercurrent illness
- Polypharmacy

Early identification and treatment are key; the mortality for status epilepticus lies between 7.6 and 39%.

MANAGEMENT

IMMEDIATE

Secure this patient's airway.

Clinical Tip

Upon assessment of the airway, look for signs of head or neck trauma, particularly Battle's sign (mastoid ecchymosis) or raccoon eyes (periorbital ecchymosis), which will guide you to the appropriate airway adjunct to use. If there is no trauma and nasal anatomy looks normal, insert a nasopharyngeal airway into the right nostril. Oropharyngeal airways should be avoided due to risk of trauma in the patient's mouth. If you are unable to stabilise the airway, give high-flow oxygen and call the crash team.

Once the airway has been secured, management of epileptic activity, using a time-based strategy, is optimal.

BY 5 MINUTES

- If patient has no IV access: give 10 mg buccal midazolam or 10–20 mg rectal diazepam.
- Alert your medical registrar.

- Obtain IV access within the next 5 minutes. Intraosseous access may be required: call a crash team for this.
- Treat hypoglycaemia or electrolyte abnormalities if present. If there is concern about alcohol excess or malnutrition, consider giving IV Pabrinex.

BY 15 MINUTES

- Give 4 mg IV lorazepam (or 0.1 mg/kg) if there is IV access, otherwise give a second dose of rectal diazepam or buccal midazolam.
- If seizure activity is persistent, escalate to inform the intensive therapy unit (ITU)/anaesthetic registrar as the patient only has one more treatment trial before intubation and general anaesthetic are required.

BY 25 MINUTES

- Give phenytoin at a dose of 15–18 mg/kg at a rate of 50 mg/minute.
- If the patient takes phenytoin regularly, give phenobarbital instead.
- Await senior support for management of refractory status epilepticus.

AFTER THE SEIZURE HAS TERMINATED

Determine the cause of seizure. If no cause is identified or this is a first seizure, arrange neuroimaging (CT, MRI and CT venogram if risk factors for possible venous thrombosis exist) and refer for neurological opinion – this may be done as an outpatient depending on risk factors and severity.

ESCALATION

Most seizures will be managed by the emergency medical or general medical teams. Escalation to anaesthetics and/or the ITU team should be considered at any point if there is suggestion of airway compromise. Prolonged refractory status will need to be managed in an ITU setting. After termination of the acute episode, patients will need review from neurology to ensure their chronic epileptic management is optimal in the case of known epilepsy, or that they are assessed in first-seizure clinic for new activity.

STATION 10.3: SUBARACHNOID HAEMORRHAGE

The Bleep Scenario

You are bleeped by the ward sister on the acute medical unit. The patient is a 21 year old female who woke with a headache this morning.

The headache was of sudden onset and increased to a severity of 10/10 over one minute.

Her GCS has dropped suddenly and her observations are: temperature 36.7°C, HR 97 bpm, BP 194/98 mmHg, RR 24 breaths per minute and SpO_2 94% on room air.

DEFINITION

The National Institute for Health and Care Excellence (NICE) definition of a subarachnoid haemorrhage is the presence of blood in the fluid-filled subarachnoid space around the brain and spinal cord, most commonly caused by an aneurysmal rupture.

INITIAL THOUGHTS

The acute-onset deterioration in a young patient coupled with the classic history of a sudden onset headache prompts the question of possible subarachnoid haemorrhage and requires urgent review.

MAKING A DIAGNOSIS

- Neurology: tension headache, cluster headache, migraine, meningitis, neoplasm, idiopathic intracranial hypertension, intracranial haemorrhage
- Drugs & Toxins: medication overuse, alcohol consumption

INITIAL INSTRUCTIONS OVER PHONE

You should ask the nurse to repeat the patient's observations, including a formal GCS. Inform the nurse to put out an emergency call if the patient becomes unresponsive or her breathing is compromised.

ASSESSMENT AND RESUSCITATION

Upon assessment, the patient is confused. She is accompanied by her partner, who provides you with a collateral history as you perform a structured ABCDE assessment.

Her partner informs you she woke suddenly with a severe headache and a stiff neck. She was fit and well, and had no other significant medical history.

- End of the bed assessment: patient is drowsy and confused.
- Airway: patent, no stridor or bulbar weakness noted.
- Breathing: RR 24 breaths per minute, SpO_2 100% on room air. On auscultation, there are vesicular breath sounds with good air entry bilaterally.
- Cardiovascular: HR 97 bpm, BP 194/98 mmHg, CRT 3 s, JVP normal, HS I + II + 0.
- Disability: temperature 36.7°C, capillary blood gas 5.3 mmol/L. Pupil 4 mm left eye, 6 mm right eye. No pupillary response to light in the right eye. Left eye normal pupillary light response.
  - Does not follow directions for a full neurological examination, but appears to have 4/5 power on right upper and lower limbs, 5/5 power left limbs. Reflexes are abrupt on the right upper and lower limbs and right plantar is upgoing.
  - GCS: opening eyes to voice (3/4), confused verbal response (4/5), localises to pain (5/6), total 12/15.
- Exposure: no other external findings.

INITIAL INVESTIGATIONS

- Bedside: ECG
- Haematology: FBC (leucocytosis, anaemia, thrombocytopenia), clotting disorders (INR), group and save and cross-match (in case transfusion is required)
- Biochemistry: U&Es (renal dysfunction), C-reactive protein (CRP) (acute inflammatory marker) and blood glucose (risk of hypoglycaemia)

MAKING A DIAGNOSIS

Ultimately, this patient needs urgent brain imaging. The first-line investigation is a CT head. If this is positive for a haemorrhage, move the patient to ITU or stroke unit for continuous monitoring.

The sensitivity of CT decreases with time, so consider an MRI in subacute cases. Most subarachnoid haemorrhages are traumatic; however, 80% of non-traumatic cases are aneurysmal. Aneurysms are diagnosed by CT angiogram and require occlusion through interventional radiologists at specialist centres.

If the imaging is negative and a subarachnoid haemorrhage is clinically suspected, you must arrange for a lumbar puncture. This should occur 12 hours after symptom onset; before this time it is difficult to differentiate blood from a traumatic lumbar puncture and a subarachnoid haemorrhage. After 12 hours, any blood of central origin will have haemolysed and you will detect xanthochromia in the sample, confirming diagnosis. Fig. 10.3 depicts a subarachnoid haemorrhage on CT.

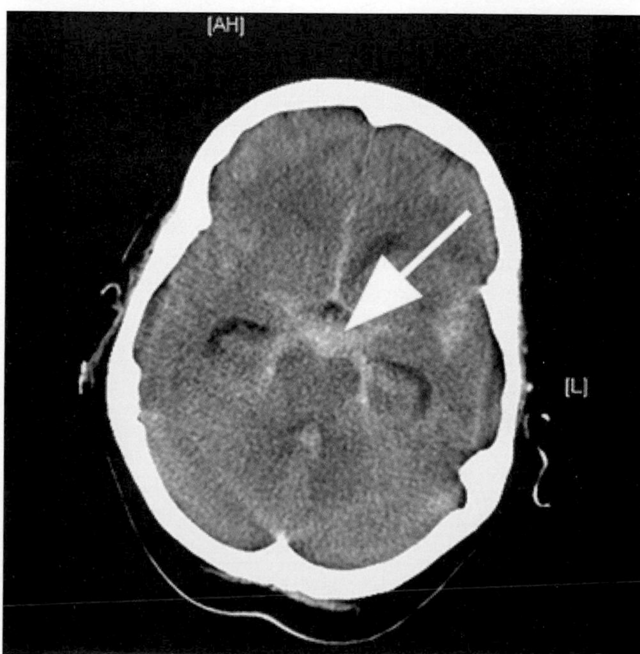

Fig. 10.3 Subarachnoid haemorrhage (arrow). (Source: Naqvi, T. Z. [2021]. *Point-of-Care Echocardiography: A Clinical Case-Based Visual Guide.* Elsevier.)

MANAGEMENT

Monitor GCS, focal neurology, temperature and blood pressure hourly.

Medical management of subarachnoid haemorrhage includes enteral nimodipine, which reduces vasospasm and is thought to decrease the risk of cerebral damage secondary to subarachnoid haemorrhage. Analgesia should be managed cautiously, with paracetamol, codeine and morphine, given in small titrated doses as required. There must be strict avoidance of any agents that may intensify the bleed.

The patient should be discussed with the local neurosurgical team straight away, for transfer if necessary for potential endovascular coiling or neurosurgical clipping.

Some centres may not have a neurosurgical unit, in which case this patient should be urgently discussed with the medical team.

ESCALATION

It is crucial to monitor the patient and ensure she maintains her airway. Patients may require an airway adjunct, and intubation if their GCS < 8. This will involve prompt discussion with the anaesthetic team with consideration of ITU admission.

STATION 10.4: MENINGITIS

The Bleep Scenario

A 19 year old man has presented to A&E with pyrexia and requires immediate assessment. Observations are as follows: temperature is 38.7°C, HR 110 bpm, BP 89/62 mmHg, RR 17 breaths per minute, and SpO_2 98% on room air. He complains of a generalised headache.

DEFINITION

Meningitis is inflammation of the meninges (the surface surrounding the brain). It is most commonly caused by bacterial or viral infection.

INITIAL THOUGHTS

This patient is unwell. A young male should normally be able to maintain his blood pressure and will show signs of sepsis much later than other patients. You should review the patient immediately.

Given his headache and fever, you should think of bacterial meningitis as a key differential. Time is of the essence; mortality and serious morbidity rise if treatment is not initiated promptly.

MAKING A DIAGNOSIS

The presentation of pyrexia and headache is very suspicious of meningitis. The onset of symptoms within

24 hours and the quick escalation in severity point you towards bacterial meningitis.

The presentation can be non-specific with fever, nausea and vomiting, agitation, headache, anorexia, arthralgia or cough. The classic triad of photophobia, phonophobia and neck stiffness may be present, in addition to petechial rash, focal neurological deficit and bulging fontanelle in children.

Chronic symptoms could indicate more unusual infectious disease and differentials include:

- Neurology: subarachinoid haemorrhage, encephalitis, viral/bacterial or fungal meningitis, pyrexia following recent seizure
- Haematology: haematological malignancy e.g. lymphoma

INITIAL DIAGNOSIS

Risk factors for bacterial meningitis include:

- Recent pneumococcal infection: pneumonia, otitis media, trauma, immunocompromised
- Recent *Neisseria meningitidis* infection: children and adolescents, outbreaks in crowded areas
- Recent *Staphylococcus* infection: neurosurgery or skull penetration
- Fungal infections: human immunodeficiency virus (HIV) and transplantation
- *Haemophilus influenzae*: otitis, sinusitis, head trauma with cerebrospinal fluid (CSF) leak
- *Listeria*: neonates and elderly
- Anaerobes: abscess, elderly

INITIAL INSTRUCTIONS OVER THE PHONE

The patient's GCS should be continuously monitored, with other observations closely noted. If possible, the patient should be placed in a side room in case of meningococcal disease. It is important for the team to be conscious of the fact that meningitis, particularly meningococcal disease, is a notifiable disease.

ASSESSMENT AND RESUSCITATION

- End of the bed assessment: the patient looks unwell and flushed. You notice a rash on his limbs.
- Airway: patent.
- Breathing: RR 24 breaths per minute, SpO_2 95%, chest expansion equal and symmetrical, chest clear on auscultation.
- Circulation: CRT 5 s, HR 122 bpm, BP 92/67 mmHg, JVP not visible. Pulse regular, weak volume.
  - ECG: sinus rhythm.
- Disability: temperature 38.9°C, blood glucose 5.8 mmol/L, GCS 12/15 (M5V4E3).
  - Perform a full neurological examination of both the cranial nerves and peripheral neurology.
  - The specific tests for neck rigidity are Kernig's sign and Brudzinski's sign.
- Exposure: violaceous, non-blanching rash on arms and legs.

INITIAL INVESTIGATIONS

- Haematology: FBC (haemoglobin trend, platelets) and coagulation screen (clotting abnormalities in potential sepsis)
- Biochemistry: U&Es (raised urea), liver function tests (LFTs: liver injury) and CRP (acute inflammatory marker)
- Microbiology: blood and urine cultures
- Radiology: CT head to exclude bleeding (non-specific investigation in the context of meningitis) and MRI (for more detailed imaging)

MAKING A DIAGNOSIS

A lumbar puncture should be performed to analyse the CSF. but this should not delay treatment with antibiotics.

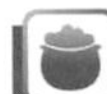

Clinical Tip

It is important to exclude an intracranial mass with CT or MRI, and to monitor for any signs of raised intracranial pressure, such as seizures, as performing a lumbar puncture under either of these situations can result in cerebral coning. Table 10.1 gives a detailed breakdown of lumbar fluid findings in meningitis.

MANAGEMENT

The key priority in managing meningitis is the treatment of potential sepsis. (See Chapter 5 for further details.)

Table 10.1 Lumbar fluid findings in meningitis

	NORMAL	BACTERIAL	VIRAL
WBCs/µL	<5	>100–5000+	5–1000
Cell predominance	None	Neutrophils	Lymphocytes
Protein	<0.5 g/dL	Raised	Mildly raised
Glucose	2.6–4.5 mmol	Very low	Low/normal
CSF/plasma glucose	>0.66	Very low	Low/normal

CSF, cerebrospinal fluid; WBCs, white blood cells.

It is important to give continuous symptomatic support with analgesia and antiemetics.

Trust guidelines vary in the course and choice of antibiotics. Each case should be discussed with a microbiologist immediately, but detailed below are common choices and their associated indications in the context of meningitis:

- Pre-hospital: benzylpenicillin IM (penicillin allergy: cefotaxime)
- Hospital setting: IV ceftriaxone. Immunocompromised patients may require additional cover for *Listeria monocytogenes* with amoxicillin
- Suspicion of viral encephalitis: if the patient has symptoms of encephalitis (typically seizures, personality change or focal neurology), aciclovir is most often prescribed. This can be prescribed along with antibiotics whilst awaiting lumbar puncture results for a clearer aetiology

 **Prescribing Tip**

Corticosteroids are sometimes administered an additional treatment for patients with meningitis in variance with local policy: they do not reduce mortality, but potentially have a role in reducing inflammation in infection. There is some evidence that administering corticosteroids can reduce potential neurological sequelae.

ESCALATION

Falling GCS and loss of airway reflexes require emergency stabilisation with an airway adjunct, and definitively, intubation by the anaesthetic team with potential escalation to intensive care.

Septic shock and disseminated intravascular coagulation are common complications of meningitis that are life threatening. Patients may require organ support in intensive care.

A microbiologist should be consulted for advice in all cases of meningitis. Contact tracing should be initiated following confirmation of meningococcal disease, with vaccination or prophylactic antibiotics, as recommended by secondary care.

STATION 10.5: REDUCED GCS

 **The Bleep Scenario**

ED requests a review of a 68 year old man who has arrived with a GCS of 7. He was found unconscious at home by his wife, and was last seen by her with a preserved GCS 36 hours ago. According to the paramedic notes, he has type 1 diabetes and a GCS of 7. His physical observations are: temperature 35.4°C, HR 90 bpm, BP 103/57 mmHg, RR 12 breaths per minute and SpO_2 92% on 15 L oxygen.

DEFINITION

Reduced GCS is a prolonged state of decreased consciousness.

INITIAL THOUGHTS

This man is in a critical condition; a GCS of 7 requires urgent intubation. Fast-bleep the anaesthetic team for intubation, stabilising the airway with an airway adjunct until they arrive on scene.

MAKING A DIAGNOSIS

- Neurology: ischaemic stroke, intracerebral haemorrhage, subarachnoid haemorrhage, subdural haematoma, malignancy, infection (meningitis, encephalitis, cerebral abscess), trauma, cerebral oedema, encephalopathy, seizures
- Metabolic: hyperglycaemia (diabetic ketoacidosis, hyperosmolar non-ketotic coma), hypoglycaemia, electrolyte abnormalities of K^+ and Na^+, hypercalcaemia, hypothyroidism, sepsis, uraemia, hepatic encephalopathy, hypercapnia, anoxic brain injury, iatrogenic poisoning
- Other: trauma, psychiatric coma

ASSESSMENT AND RESUSCITATION

- End of the bed assessment: patient is unresponsive.
- Airway: snoring sounds can be heard.
- Breathing: RR 12 breaths per minute, SpO_2 93% on high-flow oxygen. Trachea central. Chest expansion equal and symmetrical. Right basal coarse crepitations on auscultation.
- Circulation: HR 90 bpm, BP 103/57 mmHg. Pulse weak and regular. HS I + II + 0, JVP not visible.
  - Get IV access with two wide-bore cannulae in the antecubital fossae if possible.
- Disability: GCS 6/15 (E1V2M3). Blood glucose 7 mmol/L, pupils 5 mm bilaterally, sluggishly reactive. Table 10.2 gives a detailed breakdown of the GCS.
- Exposure: no obvious external injury or rashes.

INITIAL INVESTIGATIONS

- Haematology: FBC (anaemia, leukocytosis, thrombocytosis), coagulation screen and group and save
- Biochemistry: U&Es, including calcium and magnesium (dehydration, deranged electrolytes), LFTs, bone profile, glucose, CRP (inflammatory marker), troponin (cardiac ischaemia) and haematinics (deficiencies), lactate
- Microbiology: blood and urine cultures for microscopy, culture and sensitivity
- Arterial blood gas: pH 7.32, PaO_2 10.7 kPa, $PaCO_2$ 7.5 kPa, HCO_3^- 22 mmol/L
- Radiology: portable chest X-ray to exclude lower respiratory tract infection. Urgent CT head to exclude a bleed and structural causes. An MRI may be required at a later stage.
- Other: lumbar puncture, urine and blood toxicology screen.

Table 10.2 Glasgow Coma Scale

	1	2	3	4	5	6
Eye	Does not open eyes	Opens eyes in response to painful stimuli	Opens eyes in response to voice	Opens eyes spontaneously	N/A	N/A
Verbal	Makes no sounds	Incomprehensible sounds	Utters incoherent words	Confused, disoriented	Oriented, converses normally	N/A
Motor	Makes no movements	Extension to painful stimuli (decerebrate response)	Abnormal flexion to painful stimuli (decorticate response)	Flexion / withdrawal to pain	Localises painful stimuli	Obeys commands

MANAGEMENT

As illustrated in the differential diagnosis list. The aetiology for low GCS varies widely and management will depend on the cause. Many of the conditions above have been covered in further detail in other chapters.

In this patient, the cause is currently unclear so all of the above investigations will needs to be actioned in order to investigate this.

Despite not knowing the cause, which is often the case in a clinical setting, it is imperative that regular ABCDE assessments are performed with cautious monitoring of the airway. Patients should be monitored with regular GCS recordings.

ESCALATION

Any patient with a GCS under 8 will need escalation to an anaesthetist for definitive airway management.

Involve ITU early and particularly if the GCS fails to respond to glucose or if there are marked abnormalities on venous blood gas.

The medical registrar should be notified immediately. Other teams should be involved in accordance with the aetiology.

STATION 10.6: SPINAL CORD COMPRESSION

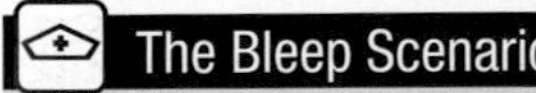

The Bleep Scenario

You are bleeped by a ward nurse to prescribe analgesia for a 92 year old woman admitted with diverticulitis on the surgical ward.

She complains of persistent, increasing back pain with no response to paracetamol and difficulty mobilising.

Her observations are temperature 37.2°C, HR 80 bpm, BP 125/90 mmHg, RR 12 breaths per minute and SpO_2 97% on room air.

DEFINITION

This involves spinal cord or cauda equina compression by external or internal pressure that threatens or causes neurological damage

INITIAL THOUGHTS

This is a very common bleep for an on call junior doctor.

These patients often have chronic joint problems such as osteoarthritis.

It is important, however, to bear in mind a diagnosis of spinal cord compression, particularly as it is most common in elderly patients who are at greater risk of vertebral collapse and malignancy.

INITIAL INSTRUCTIONS OVER PHONE

You should ask the nurse to complete a full set of observations and ensure the patient notes and drug charts are ready for you to review. The patient should not be mobilised until your assessment.

ASSESSMENT AND RESUSCITATION

- End of the bed assessment: appears settled.
- Airway: patent.
- Breathing: RR 14 breaths per minute, SpO_2 98% on room air, trachea central, chest expansion asymmetrical: she has kyphoscoliosis. Chest clear on auscultation.
- Circulation: CRT 3 seconds, pulse irregular, normal volume, HR 75 bpm. HS I + II + ejection systolic murmur.
- Disability: GCS 15/15, CBG 6.2 mmol/L, temperature 36.5°C.
- Exposure: no obvious injury.

Assessing for potential red-flag symptoms is key in the assessment of potential spinal cord compression. Red-flag symptoms to consider in assessment are detailed below:

- Onset age <20 or >55 years
- Non-mechanical back pain
- Thoracic pain
- Severe unremitting lumbar spinal pain
- Localised spinal tenderness
- Previous history of malignancy or HIV
- B symptoms (fever, night sweats, and weight loss)
- Limb weakness
- Difficulty mobilising
- Sensory disturbance, e.g. saddle anaesthesia
- Bladder or bowel dysfunction
- Structural spinal deformity

MAKING A DIAGNOSIS

Apart from assessing for red-flag symptoms, it is important to think through common differentials for back pain. Some examples are listed below:

- Degenerative: osteoarthritis, osteoporosis, spondylolisthesis
- Rheumatological: rheumatoid arthritis, systemic lupus erythematosus, reactive arthritis, ankylosing spondylitis

DIFFERENTIAL DIAGNOSIS

- Infective: abscess, meningitis, pyelonephritis
- Traumatic: fracture, muscle or ligament tear or sprain
- Neoplasm: primary malignancy or metastases

Figure 10.4 illustrates spinal cord compression.

INITIAL INVESTIGATIONS

- Haematology: FBC (anaemia, leukocytosis, thrombocytosis) to exclude acute infection which can cause musculoskeletal discomfort and lethargy.
- Biochemistry: U&Es, including calcium and magnesium (dehydration, deranged electrolytes that may cause muscular pain), LFTs (potential cause of musculoskeletal discomfort), bone profile (malignancy), CRP (possible infective or inflammatory causes) and troponin (cardiac ischaemia)
- Radiology: urgent MRI spine to exclude cord compression.

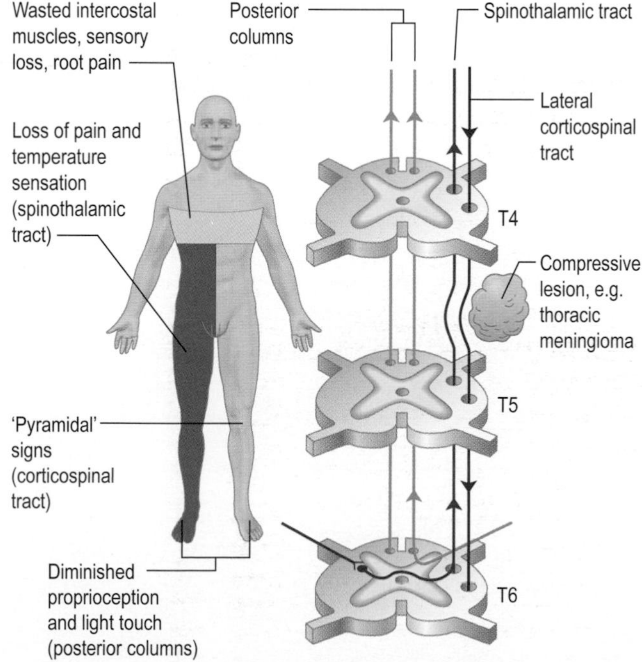

Fig. 10.4 Spinal cord compression: features and anatomy. (Source: Goldberger, A. [2018]. *Goldberger's Clinical Electrocardiography.* Philadelphia: Elsevier.)

MANAGEMENT

Supportive management is key. It is crucial for the patient to remain immobilised until cervical spine injury has been excluded with imaging. A bladder scan is indicated to confirm or refute urinary retention. She will require a catheter if there is greater than 500 mL urine in the bladder.

Treatment will depend on the aetiology and will be decided upon after the urgent MRI is performed. In the event of malignant cord compression, dexamethasone intravenous (IV) is the most important immediate treatment, alongside a thorough multidisciplinary investigation of a primary malignancy.

Teams that may need to be involved include orthopaedics (if traumatic in nature), oncology and medicine, depending on the cause.

ESCALATION

All suspected cord compressions should be discussed with the medical registrar on call if due to suspected malignancy, or the orthopaedic registrar on call if traumatic. A neurosurgeon may be involved after these initial discussions.

In the case of advanced malignant cord compression, the palliative and oncology teams will be pivotal.

FURTHER READING

Bamford J et al. Classification and natural history of clinically identifiable subtypes of cerebral infarction. *Lancet.* 1991: *337*(8756); 1521–1526.

BNF. *Central nervous system infections, bacterial*. Available at: https://bnf.nice.org.uk/treatment-summary/central-nervous-system-infections-antibacterial-therapy.html. [Accessed 17 January 2022].

Brouwer, M. C., et al. (2015). Corticosteroids for acute bacterial meningitis. *Cochrane Database of Systematic Reviews, 9*, CD004405.

Cantu, R. M., & Das, J. (2021). Viral meningitis. In *StatPearls*. Treasure Island, FL: StatPearls. Available at: www.ncbi.nlm.nih.gov/books/NBK545217/figure/article-24970.image.f1/. [Accessed 17 January 2022].

Cooksley, T., Rose, S., & Holland, M. (2018). A systematic approach to the unconscious patient. *Clinical Medicine (London), 18*(1), 88–92.

Jauch, E. C., et al. (2013). Guidelines for the early management of patients with acute ischemic stroke. *Stroke, 44*(3), 870–947.

Johnston, S. C., et al. (2007). Validation and refinement of scores to predict very early stroke risk after transient ischaemic attack. *Lancet, 369*, 283–292.

Kinney, M., & Craig, J. (2015). Grand rounds: An update on convulsive status epilepticus. *Ulster Medical Journal, 84*(2), 88.

Liversedge, T., & Hirsch, N. (2010). Coma. *Anaesthesia and Intensive Care Medicine, 11*(9), 337–339.

NICE. (2004). *Appendix F: Protocols for treating convulsive status epilepticus in adults and children.* NICE clinical guideline. Available at: www.nice.org.uk/guidance/cg137/chapter/appendix-f-protocols-for-treating-convulsive-status-epilepticus-in-adults-and-children-adults-published-in-2004-and-children-published-in-2011. [Accessed 17 January 2022].

NICE. (2012). *Alteplase for treating acute ischaemic stroke.* NICE clinical guideline. Available at: www.nice.org.uk/guidance/ta264. [Accessed 17 January 2022].

NICE. (2016). *Meningitis – bacterial meningitis and meningococcal disease*. Clinical guideline. Available at: https://bnf.nice.org.uk/treatment-summary/central-nervous-system-infections-antibacterial-therapy.html. [Accessed 17 January 2022].

NICE. (2019). *Stroke and transient ischaemic attack in over 16s: Diagnosis and initial management*. NICE clinical guideline. Available at: www.nice.org.uk/guidance/ng128. [Accessed 17 January 2022].

NICE. (2021). *Subarachnoid haemorrhage caused by a ruptured aneurysm: Diagnosis and management*. Draft guideline. Available at: www.nice.org.uk/guidance/GID-NG10097/documents/draft-guideline. [Accessed 17 January 2022].

NICE. (2022). *Metastatic spinal cord compression in adults: Risk assessment, diagnosis and management*. Available at: www.nice.org.uk/guidance/cg75. [Accessed 17 January 2022].

Steiner, T., et al. (2013). European Stroke Organization guidelines for the management of intracranial aneurysms and subarachnoid haemorrhage. *Cerebrovascular Diseases*, *35*(2), 93–112.

Suarez, J. I., Tarr, R. W., & Selman, W. R. (2006). Aneurysmal subarachnoid hemorrhage. *New England Journal of Medicine*, *354*(4), 387–396.

Teasdale, G., & Jennett, B. (1974). Assessment of coma and impaired consciousness. A practical scale. *Lancet*, *2*, 81–84.

Waterhouse, E., & Kaplan, P. (2011). The causes of convulsive status epilepticus in adults. In S. E. Shorvon, F. Andermann, & R. Guerrini (Eds.), *The causes of epilepsy: Common and uncommon causes in adults and children* (p. 735). Cambridge: Cambridge University Press.

WHO. (2021). *Meningitis fact sheet*. Available at: www.who.int/gho/epidemic_diseases/meningitis/suspected_cases_deaths_text/en/. [Accessed 17 January 2022].

Elderly Care Medicine

11

Content Outline

STATION 11.1: COMPREHENSIVE GERIATRIC ASSESSMENT

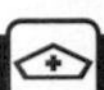 **The Bleep Scenario**

You are bleeped by your consultant from the elderly care ward. An 82 year old woman has arrived in the ward following step down from the intensive care unit. The patient has been treated for urinary sepsis requiring inotropic support. You are asked to complete a comprehensive geriatric assessment (CGA).

INITIAL THOUGHTS

As a junior doctor, you will be looking after many geriatric patients. Patients in this population often have multiple comorbidities, frailty and polypharmacy.

Previously, the 'geriatric giants' were thought to be immobility, instability, incontinence and impaired memory. Now, new terminology is used, i.e. frailty, sarcopenia, anorexia of ageing and cognitive impairment. These factors are closely linked to falls, hip fracture and delirium – therefore it is important to identify these factors to prevent and treat the resultant conditions effectively.

A CGA allows you to do this and organise appropriate support.

WHAT IS THE COMPREHENSIVE GERIATRIC ASSESSMENT?

Geriatricians, in the hospital/community setting, are often at the core of this assessment, and they should cover the five Ms: *mind, mobility, medications, multicomplexity* and *matters* most. The key features are patient-centred medicine and decision making. It is important to take a global clinical view, and not to focus solely on one condition the patient has. This will help alleviate risks of polypharmacy and adverse outcomes.

A hospital admission can offer a good opportunity to undertake a CGA, but it can also be performed in the community and be led by a general practitioner (GP) or social worker. It is an iterative process, with a patient being continuously assessed during admission, and beyond.

The key principles include a thorough multidisciplinary assessment, initiation of interventions and review of progress. Evidence suggests that CGAs improve outcomes, including reducing mortality and improving independence, compared to standard medical care, during hospital admission. A full CGA can take up to 2 hours.

THE FOUR KEY COMPONENTS OF THE CGA

1. Physical assessment, including sensation, feet and footwear, gait and balance, postural hypotension, assessment of joints and any pain, weight and nutrition, per rectum examination and external genitalia, as well as non-pathological age-related changes
2. Functional, social and environmental assessment
3. Psychological components, including mood and cognition
4. Medication review: one approach is to use the STOPP-START model (Screening Tool of Older People's Prescriptions and Screening Tool to Alert to Right Treatment)

The purpose is to create a comprehensive plan that accommodates the patient's individual goals, including a problem list, care and support planning and goal setting.

Care plans may address mobility and balance, bone health, fall and fracture risk, depression, mental capacity issues, incontinence, weight loss and end-of-life care.

Thus doing a proper assessment can minimise poor management, including inappropriate diagnoses or treatments, resulting in better outcomes for patients.

SUMMARY

The CGA is a multidisciplinary diagnostic process intended to identify an elderly person's medical, psychosocial and functional capabilities and limitations in order to address issues of concern of patient or their next of kin.

The CGA process is known to improve outcomes for older people. Your involvement as a junior doctor may be to review the patient's medications or perform a full history and examination (possibly with collateral information). It is important to recognise that the needs of elderly patients are often complex and multidimensional. The multidisciplinary team (MDT) plays a crucial role in this process.

STATION 11.2: FRAILTY

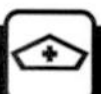

The Bleep Scenario

You are bleeped by a nurse on the elderly care ward. A 78 year old man has been admitted with a chest infection, on a background of COPD. He is on home oxygen. You are asked to review the patient.

INITIAL THOUGHTS

As a junior doctor, you should be aware that frailty is a medical syndrome with multiple causes and contributors including reduced strength, endurance and physiological function that increase an individual's vulnerability to morbidity and mortality. Signs of frailty include falls, reduced mobility, incontinence and delirium. When assessing patients aged 65 or over, you should calculate and document their clinical frailty score. This score will help you to determine where they should be cared for, and how to care for them appropriately; this includes seeking support from MDT members and initiation of the CGA.

FRAILTY AND ITS RELEVANCE TO CLINICAL PRACTICE

As a junior doctor, particularly in your first year, you are unlikely to be the patient's main decision maker, but you should be aware that patients with higher frailty scores (i.e. 7, 8 or 9), are likely to have poorer outcomes, i.e. to including length of admission, readmission rates and inpatient mortality. Therefore, it is important to try and avoid hospital admission possible. This could be done by effectively utilising community services.

The idea of managing frailty includes importance of discussing patient preferences, not only around resuscitation, but also advanced care planning. Frail patients may have a Coordinate My Care (CMC) record which has been created by a doctor well known to them; for example, a specialist they see regularly or their general practitioner (GP). Finding out if the patient has a CMC record (or any other form of advanced directive or decision to refuse treatment) will enable you to understand their previously discussed and documented wishes.

It is also important to consider what level of support patients will require once they have recovered from their acute illness. For example, frail patients may need community multidisciplinary team (MDT) involvement. Patients in the middle ranges may need 'flagging up' to their GP so they are aware to monitor and refer for appropriate support if needed. Getting this right helps to ensure patients can live independently and healthily for as long as possible.

ROCKWOOD'S CLINICAL FRAILTY SCALE (CFS)

HOW TO USE THE CFS (FIG. 11.1)

The CFS is used for patients aged 65 and above, apart from patients with learning disabilities. You can obtain information from carers and/or next of kin if the patient cannot give an accurate picture. It is important to be open and honest with patients and next of kin.

Consider how the patient was 2 weeks before this interaction and consider to elicit through a thorough history from the patient if able or next of kin to determine changes in function.

You should base your assessment on their current level of function; note that patients may fluctuate between stages quite significantly – for example, a dying patient can suddenly progress to stage 9.

Other tests include: the gait speed test, the timed up and go test and the electronic frailty index – used in the community by GPs.

SUBSEQUENT ACTIONS

Further actions may include medication reviews with a view to stopping any long term medications that do not add clinical or prognostic value. A common example is reviewing the need for anti-hypertensive medications. Every patient should be considered for calcium and vitamin D replacement. They should also be screened for postural hypotension and falls as part of a comprehensive geriatric.

MDT members are crucial. They may help with the assessment of the patient's mobility and skin integrity. You may make referrals for dietician reviews, and strength and balance exercises. Social services may be involved in arranging care and community MDTs will be involved in managing patients post-discharge. The patient may also need an onward referral to community geriatricians or old-age psychiatrists (memory clinic).

Consider holistic needs, including spiritual needs as well as support for the family, including any relevant financial support, such as fast-track or continuing healthcare funding. Advanced-care planning and end-of-life discussions are also an iterative process, which should be started in these situations.

SUMMARY

The CFS should be used to assess all patients aged 65 or over to identify common signs of frailty such as

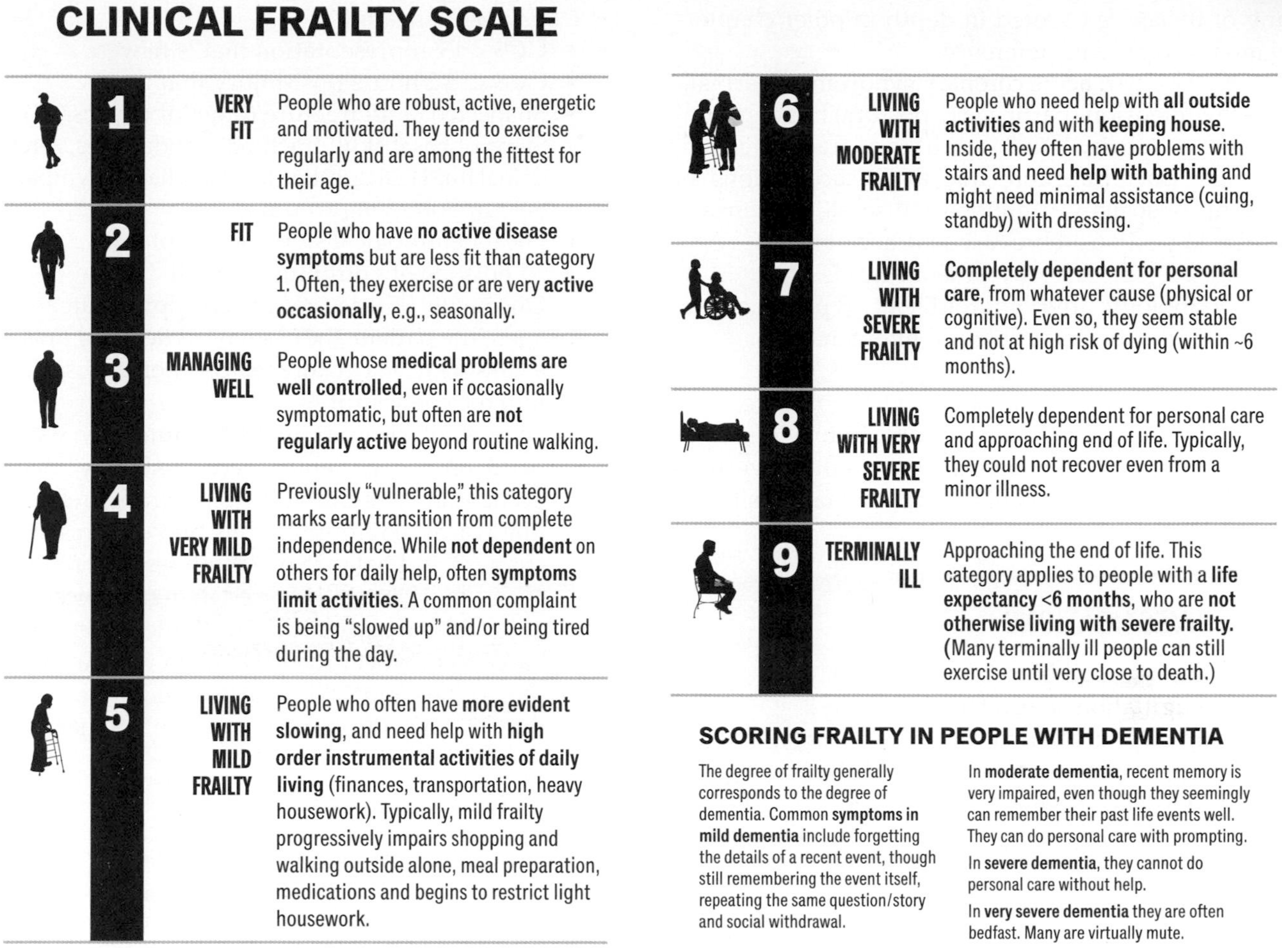

CLINICAL FRAILTY SCALE

1	**VERY FIT**	People who are robust, active, energetic and motivated. They tend to exercise regularly and are among the fittest for their age.
2	**FIT**	People who have **no active disease symptoms** but are less fit than category 1. Often, they exercise or are very **active occasionally**, e.g., seasonally.
3	**MANAGING WELL**	People whose **medical problems are well controlled**, even if occasionally symptomatic, but often are **not regularly active** beyond routine walking.
4	**LIVING WITH VERY MILD FRAILTY**	Previously "vulnerable," this category marks early transition from complete independence. While **not dependent** on others for daily help, often **symptoms limit activities.** A common complaint is being "slowed up" and/or being tired during the day.
5	**LIVING WITH MILD FRAILTY**	People who often have **more evident slowing**, and need help with **high order instrumental activities of daily living** (finances, transportation, heavy housework). Typically, mild frailty progressively impairs shopping and walking outside alone, meal preparation, medications and begins to restrict light housework.
6	**LIVING WITH MODERATE FRAILTY**	People who need help with **all outside activities** and with **keeping house.** Inside, they often have problems with stairs and need **help with bathing** and might need minimal assistance (cuing, standby) with dressing.
7	**LIVING WITH SEVERE FRAILTY**	**Completely dependent for personal care**, from whatever cause (physical or cognitive). Even so, they seem stable and not at high risk of dying (within ~6 months).
8	**LIVING WITH VERY SEVERE FRAILTY**	Completely dependent for personal care and approaching end of life. Typically, they could not recover even from a minor illness.
9	**TERMINALLY ILL**	Approaching the end of life. This category applies to people with a **life expectancy <6 months**, who are **not otherwise living with severe frailty.** (Many terminally ill people can still exercise until very close to death.)

SCORING FRAILTY IN PEOPLE WITH DEMENTIA

The degree of frailty generally corresponds to the degree of dementia. Common **symptoms in mild dementia** include forgetting the details of a recent event, though still remembering the event itself, repeating the same question/story and social withdrawal.

In **moderate dementia**, recent memory is very impaired, even though they seemingly can remember their past life events well. They can do personal care with prompting.

In **severe dementia**, they cannot do personal care without help.

In **very severe dementia** they are often bedfast. Many are virtually mute.

Fig. 11.1 Clinical Frailty Scale. IADLs, instrumental activities of daily living. (Source: Dalhousie University, Geriatric Medicine Research, © 2007–2009, Halifax Canada.)

falls, reduced mobility, incontinence and delerium. You should be aware that patients with higher scores are likely to have poorer outcomes.

STATION 11.3: FALLS REVIEW

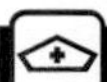

The Bleep Scenario

You are bleeped to the geriatrics rehabilitation ward to review an elderly patient. An 83 year old patient, who was admitted 2 weeks ago with a chest infection and is now medically stable, has had a witnessed fall whilst trying to get back into bed.

INITIAL THOUGHTS

Falls are a very common reason for hospital admission in the elderly and they represent a diagnostic challenge due to the wide range of underlying conditions that can present this way.

You must ensure the patient is clinically stable before taking a careful history of pre- and post-fall symptoms to guide your differential diagnosis. In the case of the witnessed fall, collateral history from the bystander is key.

ASSESSMENT AND RESUSCITATION

- End of the bed assessment: patient appears stable and comfortable once helped up.
- Airway: patent, speaking in full sentences.
- Breathing: respiratory rate (RR) 34 breaths per minute, SpO_2 92% on air, trachea central, air entry symmetrical. Left basal coarse crepitations on auscultation.
- Circulation: capillary refill time (CRT) 5 s, heart rate (HR) 106 bpm, blood pressure (BP) 95/50 mmHg. Jugular venous pressure (JVP) not visible. Heart sounds (HS) I + II + 0.
- Disability: Glasgow Coma Scale (GCS) 14/15 (E4V4M6), temperature 38.2°C, capillary blood glucose (CBG) 6 mmol/L.
- Exposure: erythematous area over left hip, no broken skin.

MAKING A DIAGNOSIS

In this case, it is evident that the patient has most likely had a mechanical fall.

Potential differential diagnoses of falls are wide, with some listed below to consider depending on the history and other symptoms the patient complains of.

Many of these are covered in depth in other chapters and are listed here for reference.

- Cardiovascular: acute coronary syndrome, heart failure, hypotension (particularly postural hypotension)
- Infective: sepsis, lower respiratory tract infection, urinary tract infection, infective exacerbations of chronic obstructive pulmonary disease, influenza
- Neurological: Cerebrovascular accidents (CVA's), Parkinson's disease, myasthenia gravis
- Endocrinology: hypothyroidism, hypoglycaemia, adrenal insufficiency, postural hypotension
- Haematological: anaemia
- Metabolic: dehydration, electrolyte imbalances
- Renal: acute kidney injury, chronic kidney disease
- Others: depression, medication side effects, vertigo, particularly BPPV (benign paroxysmal positional vertigo)

INITIAL INVESTIGATIONS

- Haematology: full blood count (leukocytosis, anaemia), coagulation screen (coagulopathy)
- Biochemistry: urea and electrolytes (U&Es), including calcium and magnesium (acute kidney injury, electrolyte abnormalities), liver function tests (hypoalbuminaemia, deranged liver function tests), C-reactive protein (infection marker), creatine kinase (rhabdomyolysis)
- Microbiology: blood cultures, urine microscopy, culture and sensitivities if any indication to any suspicion of infection
- Radiology: chest X-ray (if evidence of chest symptoms or hypoxia)

MANAGEMENT

The management involves a full physical examination to exclude any of the causes above that may need further investigation, and a falls review, as detailed below:

- Check for scalp lesions and bony tenderness. Look in the eyes, ears, nose and mouth. Palpate bony prominences of the face and jaw.
- Palpate the cervical spine; if there is bony tenderness, apply a hard collar and arrange an X-ray or computed tomography (CT) spine as per local protocol. If there is no bony tenderness, ask the patient to move the neck in all axes of movement. Consider imaging if pain is elicited.
- Specifically palpate all ribs, anteriorly and posteriorly, for tenderness.
- Inspect and palpate the abdomen, focusing on liver, spleen, kidneys and bladder.
- Palpate and test movement in limbs and joints for evidence of soft-tissue or bony tenderness. Particularly focus on examining the hips and pelvis in elderly patients.
- Arrange X-rays of any areas flagged by the secondary survey.
- Consider CT head if:
  - GCS < 13 at presentation that is new
  - GCS <15 2 hours post-injury that is new
  - Suspected skull fracture (open or depressed)
  - Signs of basal skull fracture: 'panda' eyes, cerebrospinal fluid leakage, Battle's sign, haemotympanum
  - Seizure following trauma
  - Focal neurological signs or symptoms
  - >1 episode of vomiting after fall
  - Once acute injuries have been appropriately managed, the patient should have a detailed falls risk assessment, especially before being discharged into the community
  - Sources of support in the community will depend on the patients needs and may include: occupational therapy, physiotherapy, rehabilitation wards, community falls prevention services, strength and balance programmes, carer input or even a move into supported living. Services available will vary according to the location you are based in however the MDT team will be aware of the options and will be instrumental in ensuring the patient is discharged in a safe manner.

ESCALATION

Escalation will depend on the cause as well as the wishes of the patient, but a frailty assessment and CGA are key components of the ongoing management of patients who experience falls.

FURTHER READING

BGS. (2018). *Good practice guide. Frailty: What's it all about?* Available at: www.bgs.org.uk/resources/frailty-what%E2%80%99s-it-all-about. [Accessed 17 January 2022].

BGS. (2019). *Comprehensive geriatric assessment toolkit for primary care practitioners.* Available at www.bgs.org.uk/sites/default/files/content/resources/files/2019-02-08/BGS%20Toolkit%20-%20FINAL%20FOR%20WEB_0.pdf. [Accessed 17 January 2022].

Hughes, L. D. (2018). *Geriatric Medicine Journal blog. The geriatric 5Ms: An important new construct in geriatric medicine.* Available at: www.gmjournal.co.uk/the-geriatric-5ms-an-important-new-construct-in-geriatric-medicine. [Accessed 17 January 2022].

NHS England (n.d.) *NHS resources on identifying frailty.* Available at: www.england.nhs.uk/ourwork/clinical-policy/older-people/frailty/frailty-risk-identification/. [Accessed 17 January 2022].

NICE. (2014). *Head injury: Assessment and early management.* NICE clinical guideline. Available at: www.nice.org.uk/guidance/cg176/chapter/1-recommendations. [Accessed 17 January 2022].

Rockwood, K., et al. (2005). A global clinical measure of fitness and frailty in elderly people. *Canadian Medical Association Journal, 173*(5), 489–495.

Rockwood, K., & Theou, O. (2020). Using the clinical frailty scale in allocating scarce health care resources. *Canadian Geriatric Journal, 23*(3), 210–215.

World Health Organization. (2008). Ageing, life course unit. WHO global report on falls prevention in older age. Available at: www.who.int/publications/i/item/9789241563536. [Accessed 17 January 2022].

Haematology and Oncology

12

Content Outline

STATION 12.1: ANAEMIA

 **The Bleep Scenario**

You are bleeped by the emergency department (ED) about a 70 year old man admitted with shortness of breath and light-headedness on exertion. He is now reporting chest pain after getting up to go to the toilet. His haemoglobin is 70 g/L. He has a background of gout and allergic rhinitis.

His observations are: heart rate (HR) 110 bpm, blood pressure (BP) 140/60 mmHg, respiratory rate (RR) 20 breaths per minute, SpO_2 95% on room air and temperature 36.8°C. You are asked to review him.

DEFINITION

Anaemia is a condition in which either the number of red blood cells or their oxygen-carrying capacity is insufficient to meet physiological needs. Anaemia is defined as a haemoglobin level <120 g/L in females and <130 g/L in males.

INITIAL THOUGHTS

This patient's history is suggestive of symptomatic anaemia. It is important to consider the current haemoglobin level in the context of previous readings to determine the patient's baseline.

The acuity of the drop should be determined to classify the anaemia as acute, chronic or acute-on-chronic; each category has different implications for differential diagnosis. Causes of anaemia are classified as microcytic, normocytic or macrocytic.

It is paramount to establish if the patient is bleeding and whether there is evidence of haemodynamic compromise. If there is any sign of acute compromise, activation of the major haemorrhage protocol requires immediate consideration.

His chest pain may be related to cardiac ischaemia. Additional risk factors include personal or family history of coronary artery disease, hypertension, obesity, hyperlipidaemia and lifestyle factors such as smoking.

DIFFERENTIAL DIAGNOSIS

- Microcytic: iron deficiency, thalassaemia, anaemia of chronic disease, sideroblastic anaemia or lead poisoning
- Normocytic: acute haemorrhage, haemolytic anaemias, anaemia of chronic disease, bone marrow failure, drugs or endocrine causes (hypopituitarism, Addison's disease)
- Macrocytic (megaloblastic): vitamin B_{12} deficiency, folate deficiency or drugs
- Macrocytic (non-megaloblastic): liver disease, alcoholism, drugs, reticulocytosis or hypothyroidism

INITIAL INSTRUCTIONS OVER PHONE

Ask the nurse to obtain an electrocardiogram (ECG), intravenous (IV) access and bloods, including a group and save, cross-match and a troponin measurement in account of the chest pain.

Early pain relief with IV morphine plus an antiemetic should be given if the patient is in pain or distressed.

As the patient's risk factors suggest the possibility of cardiac ischaemia, sublingual glyceryl trinitrate should be administered immediately.

ASSESSMENT AND RESUSCITATION

- End of the bed assessment: patient appears pale and is having ongoing chest discomfort.
- Airway: patent.
- Breathing: RR 20 breaths per minute, SpO_2 95% on room air. On auscultation, there are vesicular breath sounds with good air entry bilaterally.
- Circulation: capillary refill time (CRT) 4 s peripherally, CRT 2 s centrally, HR 120 bpm, regular, BP 110/56 mmHg in both arms, jugular venous pressure (JVP) not raised, heart sounds (HS) I + II + 0.
  - 12-lead ECG: sinus tachycardia.

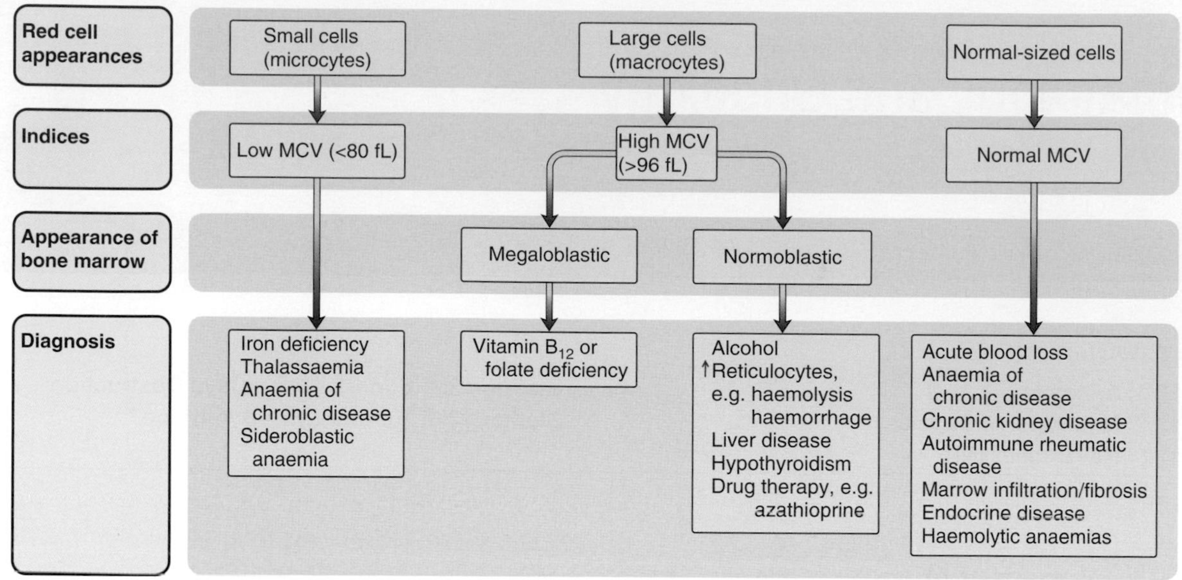

Fig. 12.1 Classification of anaemia. MCV, mean corpuscular volume. (Source: Kumar, P. and Clark, M.L. [2021]. *Kumar & Clark's cases in clinical medicine*. London: Elsevier.)

- Insert a wide-bore IV cannula into each antecubital fossa to obtain blood tests.
- Prescribe and administer a fluid challenge of 250–500 mL crystalloid over 10 minutes as the patient is showing signs of haemodynamic compromise, and there is no evidence of fluid overload.

- Disability: Glasgow Coma Scale (GCS) 15/15, pupils equal and reactive to light (PEARL), temperature 36.8°C, capillary blood glucose (CBG) 6.8 mmol/L.
- Exposure: abdomen is soft, but there is tenderness on palpation in the left iliac fossa, with no evidence of peritonism. Rectal examination reveals melaena in the rectum.

INITIAL INVESTIGATIONS

- Haematology: full blood count (FBC: haemoglobin trend, mean corpuscular volume, platelets), reticulocyte count (bone marrow function), haematinics (iron studies, vitamin B_{12}, folate), peripheral blood film (haemoglobinophathies), cross-match and coagulation studies (bleeding or coagulopathy)
- Biochemistry: troponin (myocardial ischaemia), urea and electrolytes ((U&Es): raised urea), liver function tests (LFTs: underlying liver disease), troponin (myocardial ischaemia) and thyroid function tests (lethargy or anaemia)
- Radiology: endoscopy (if suspicion of upper gastrointestinal bleed (UGIB)), chest X-ray (CXR: evidence of heart failure or respiratory pathology)

MAKING A DIAGNOSIS

The urgency with which anaemia is evaluated depends on the severity at presentation. However, any patient presenting with haemodynamic compromise requires immediate work-up to identify any source of acute bleeding.

Signs suggestive of acute bleeding include hypotension, pallor, cold clammy skin, thready pulse, tachycardia and altered mental status.

In this scenario, the most likely cause of the patient's anaemia is an acute gastrointestinal bleed. For more on UGIB, see chapter on Upper Gastrointestinal Bleed (UGIB).

- Symptoms: fatigue, headache, light-headedness, weakness, decreased exercise tolerance, dyspnoea, palpitations, tinnitus, syncope or menorrhagia.
- Signs: conjunctival pallor, angular stomatitis, glossitis, jaundice, tachycardia, postural hypotension, systolic flow murmur, wide pulse pressure, signs of congestive heart failure, ecchymosis, petechiae, jaundice (if due to haemolysis), koilonychia, splenomegaly or lymphadenopathy. Fig. 12.1 illustrates the classification of anaemia.

MANAGEMENT

This patient has symptomatic anaemia with ischaemic chest pain. Haemoglobin measurements showed a drop from 70 to 62 g/L, necessitating a blood transfusion. Once the patient is stabilised, you should be sure to examine all orifices for bleeding and inspect any site of trauma or recent surgery. You should ask the patient about recent nose bleeds and bleeding from gums. Melaena and coffee-ground vomiting suggest UGIB, as would an isolated rise in urea.

The patient's drug chart should be reviewed to stop any non-steroidal anti-inflammatory drugs (NSAIDs), antiplatelet agents and anticoagulants, such as warfarin or direct oral anticoagulants – these may require reversal however, this is an individualised decision that should be discussed with the haematology team for optimal management.

If the cause of the anaemia is uncertain, further investigations may be indicated depending upon the clinical context. This might include haemoglobin electrophoresis, haematinics, antibody tests (anti-IgA tissue transglutaminase, anti-intrinsic factor), erythropoietin levels, direct Coombs test (for autoimmune haemolytic anaemia) or bone marrow biopsy.

The most common cause of anaemia is iron-deficiency anaemia, for which iron supplements (either oral or IV transfusion) can be prescribed.

Prescribing Tip

Blood transfusion cut-offs vary from one trust guideline to another, but the general rule is that red blood cell transfusion is for counts <70 g/L, with a slightly higher threshold for patients with cardiac failure. Each unit is prescribed over 2–3 hours in duration.

Clinical Tip

It is imperative to group and save your patients as soon as possible after their admission. Usually, this involves two separate samples.

ESCALATION

In the first instance, you should involve a senior within your own team, for example, the medical registrar or consultant, who will be able to advise you on transfusion, including the urgency and quantity of blood products required.

As the most likely cause of the anaemia, in this case, is an UGIB, the gastrointestinal team should be involved with immediate endoscopy arranged to look for the bleeding source and cauterisation or banding of bleeding vessels as relevant.

If profound anaemia continues, or if any advice on reversal of anticoagulation is required, the local haematology team should be consulted. Some trusts may require discussion with he haematology team to sanction the administration of certain blood products; it is important to familiarise yourself with local protocol to ensure timely and effective treatment.

STATION 12.2: NEUTROPENIC SEPSIS

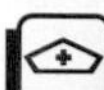

The Bleep Scenario

You are bleeped by a nurse on the haematology ward about a 38 year old woman who is complaining of a productive cough and right-sided chest pain. She completed a course of chemotherapy for non-Hodgkin's lymphoma 5 days ago.

Her observations are: HR 120 bpm, BP 90/60 mmHg, RR 26 breaths per minute, SpO_2 93% on room air and temperature 39.2°C. You are asked to review her.

DEFINITION

Neutropenia is defined as a neutrophil count less than 0.5×10^9, or a count that is less than 1.0×10^9 and falling. Neutropenic sepsis occurs in patients who demonstrate a pyrexia of greater than 38°C, or in those who display concrete clinical signs and symptoms consistent with sepsis.

INITIAL THOUGHTS

This patient has recently had chemotherapy and is therefore at significant risk of neutropenia. Pyrexia, tachycardia, tachypnoea and hypotension in a patient with known immunocompromise and infective symptoms (productive cough and possible pleuritic chest pain) imply neutropenic sepsis until proven otherwise. You need to check her FBC to confirm the neutropenia, but this should not delay treatment.

DIFFERENTIAL DIAGNOSIS

CAUSES OF NEUTROPENIA

- Congenital: disorders of neutrophil production (e.g. Kostmann's syndrome, X-linked agammaglobulinaemia), cyclical neutropenia or ethnic variation
- Decreased or ineffective neutrophil production: bone marrow infiltration/bone marrow cancers, aplastic anaemia, vitamin B_{12}/folate/iron deficiencies, chemotherapy, radiotherapy, drugs (phenytoin, chloramphenicol, alcohol excess), infection (Epstein–Barr virus, hepatitis B, hepatitis C human immunodeficiency virus (HIV) or cytomegalovirus)
- Increased neutrophil turnover: Felty's syndrome, hypersplenism, malaria or acute bacterial infection
- Combination mechanisms: toxoplasmosis, drugs (analgesics, antiepileptics, antidepressants), thyroid dysfunction or autoimmune neutropenia

Other potential causes of fever in patients with malignancy include drug-induced fever, tumour progression, paraneoplastic syndromes and venous thromboembolism due to their procoagulant state.

INITIAL INSTRUCTIONS OVER PHONE

Ask the nurse to commence initial supportive measures, including supplementary oxygen and IV fluid resuscitation. Request an ECG to be completed and bloods to be taken. Ask for the patient to be moved to a monitored side room as quickly as possible in view of the possibility of sudden deterioration and her immunocompromised state.

ASSESSMENT AND RESUSCITATION

- End of the bed assessment: patient appears slightly breathless and flushed.
- Airway: patent.

- Breathing: RR 26 breaths per minute, SpO_2 92% on room air. On auscultation, there are coarse crackles at the right lung base.
  - Arterial blood gas (ABG: pH 7.32, PaO_2 7.0 kPa, $PaCO_2$ 4.0 kPa, HCO_3^- 21 mmol/L.
  - Give high-flow oxygen 15 L/minute. Aim for saturations of 94–98%.
- Circulation: CRT < 2 s, HR 120 bpm, regular, BP 88/58 mmHg, JVP not visible, HS I + II + 0.
  - 12-lead ECG: sinus tachycardia.
  - Prescribe IV fluid resuscitation (500 mL crystalloid bolus over 10 minutes and assess response, repeat bolus(es) if necessary).
- Disability: GCS 15/15, PEARL, temperature 39.2°C, CBG 5.3 mmol/L.
- Exposure: peripherally inserted central catheter (PICC) line situated above the right antecubital fossa. Abdomen soft and non-tender, with normal bowel sounds.

INITIAL INVESTIGATIONS

- Haematology: FBC (neutropenia, leukocytosis), coagulation screen, including fibrinogen and D-dimer (disseminated intravascular coagulation (DIC)) and cross-match
- Biochemistry: U&Es (dehydration, renal dysfunction), LFTs (hypoalbuminaemia) and (CRP (acute inflammatory marker)
- Microbiology: blood cultures (1× peripheral set, 1× set from PICC line), urine microscopy, culture and sensitivity (MCS: to exclude urinary sepsis), stool MCS and sputum MCS
- Radiology: urgent CXR is required in most cases (consolidation, effusion, collapse, pulmonary oedema); consider imaging according to the most likely infective source

MAKING A DIAGNOSIS

Neutropenic sepsis is the most common life-threatening complication of cancer therapy and is an oncological emergency. Patients with neutropenic sepsis are often significantly unstable with the classic features of sepsis and/or septic shock: tachypnoea, tachycardia, hypotension and pyrexia. Other symptoms and signs will depend upon the site of infection.

A thorough systematic examination should be used to evaluate all possible sources of infection, including the gastrointestinal tract, respiratory system, genitourinary system, skin and, importantly, any indwelling devices such as intravascular lines, catheter and shunts.). Thorough history and examination will identify the most likely infection source in most cases.

It is also important to establish the patient's underlying malignancy, the type of chemotherapy, duration, most recent treatments and any adjuvant or neoadjuvant therapy along with the most recent administrations.

MANAGEMENT

This patient is clearly unwell and should immediately be commenced on broad-spectrum IV antibiotics in addition to supportive measures, including oxygen, fluid resuscitation and urinary catheterisation for fluid balance monitoring. You should refer to local protocols for guidance on an appropriate antibiotic regimens and remember to check for drug allergies before any antibiotics are prescribed or administered.

If neutropenic sepsis is suspected, you should not wait for the blood results before treating. Of note, the patient's PICC line is a potential source of sepsis. This should be discussed with both the microbiology and haematology teams with regard to removal, but it should not be removed until initial management has been implemented.

You should also ensure the 'sepsis six' protocol is completed:

1. Oxygen: aim for oxygen saturations of 94–98%.
2. Cultures: blood, urine, stool, sputum, wound swabs as relevant and swabs of PICC line as relevant.
3. Antibiotics: broad-spectrum IV antibiotics according to local guidelines within an hour of diagnosis (most commonly, piperacillin-tazobactam 4.5 g three times a day IV).
4. Fluids: IV resuscitation (250–500 mL crystalloid over 10–15 minutes depending on cardiovascular and renal function), repeating boluses according to the BP, then prescribe maintenance fluids as required.
5. Lactate: a reading >2 mmol/L indicates tissue hypoperfusion and ischaemia.
6. Urine output: catheterise the patient and target a urine output of >0.5 ml/kg/hour.

ESCALATION

The medical registrar and the patient's haematology team should be informed of the new admission. If they are unavailable, the on call haematologist will be the next port of call. If the patient is deteriorating despite treatment, she may require admission to the high dependency unit or intensive care unit (ICU) for organ support that may include inotropes, invasive ventilation or haemofiltration if required.

STATION 12.3: REVERSAL OF INR

 The Bleep Scenario

You are bleeped by the ED about a 75 year old man who has presented with bruising with an unclear history and spontaneous in nature. He is otherwise systemically well.

He has a background of atrial fibrillation and normally takes 5 mg warfarin once a day with a target INR of 2–3. He recently completed a 7 day course of ciprofloxacin for a urinary tract infection. His INR today is 9.

His observations are: HR 80 bpm, BP 140/90 mmHg, RR 14 breaths per minute, SpO_2 96% on room air and temperature 37.0°C. You are asked to review him for admission to the acute medical unit (AMU).

DEFINITION

The international normalised ratio or INR is defined as the ratio of a patient's prothrombin time to a standardised 'normal' prothrombin time.

INITIAL THOUGHTS

An INR of 9 is concerning, and the spontaneous bruising suggests spontaneous bleeding. His observations demonstrate that he is currently stable. You will need to review the patient to ensure that there is no major bleeding resulting in haemodynamic compromise.

Comprehensive haematological and biochemical profiles are needed to be certain of the cause of the coagulopathy.

You should consider why this patient's INR has suddenly increased and familiarise yourself with your local protocol on INR reversal.

DIFFERENTIAL DIAGNOSIS

- Congenital disorders: von Willebrand's disease, haemophilia or platelet dysfunction disorders
- Acquired disorders: liver disease and cirrhosis, vitamin K deficiency, vitamin C deficiency, DIC, renal disease, autoimmune diseases (e.g. systemic lupus erythematosus, idiopathic thrombocytopenic purpura) or amyloidosis
- Drugs: anticoagulants, antiplatelets, thrombolytic agents, NSAIDs, serotonin-noradrenaline reuptake inhibitors or selective serotonin reuptake inhibitors (SSRIs)
- Enzyme inhibitors (reduce the metabolism of warfarin, therefore potentiate its effect): metronidazole, ciprofloxacin, steroids, thyroxine, alcohol, cranberry juice, sodium valproate, isoniazid, fluconazole, erythromycin or omeprazole
- Enzyme inducers (reduce the metabolism of warfarin, therefore attenuate its effect): rifampicin, carbamazepine, phenytoin, St John's wort or chronic alcohol use

INITIAL INSTRUCTIONS OVER PHONE

In this scenario, the patient's INR is dangerously high. Ask the nurse to complete a further set of observations to check for haemodynamic instability due to major bleeding.

Ask the nurse to ensure that no anticoagulant or antiplatelet medications are administered before you attend to review the patient.

ASSESSMENT AND RESUSCITATION

- End of the bed assessment: patient appears well.
- Airway: patent.
- Breathing: RR 14 breaths per minute, SpO_2 96% on room air. On auscultation, there are vesicular breath sounds with good air entry bilaterally.
  - Venous blood gas (VBG): pH 7.35, PaO_2 5.0 kPa, $PaCO_2$ 5.5 kPa, HCO_3^- 26 mmol/L
- Circulation: CRT <2 s, HR 85 bpm, regular, BP 140/90 mmHg in both arms, JVP not raised, HS I + II + 0.
  - Cautiously obtain IV access, remembering that the patient is at high risk of bleeding.
- Disability: GCS 15/15, PEARL, temperature 37.0°C, CBG 6.1 mmol/L.
- Exposure: there is widespread superficial bruising on all four limbs, worse on the left side and over the left hip. There is no evidence of head injury or bleeding from any orifice. Abdomen is soft and nontender, with normal bowel sounds.

INITIAL INVESTIGATIONS

- Haematology: FBC (haemoglobin, platelets), coagulation screen (INR, activated partial thromboplastin time, prothrombin time), fibrinogen and D-dimer (DIC)
- Biochemistry: U&Es and LFTs (hepatic coagulopathy)
- Radiology: consider imaging if indicated in the clinical context, e.g. computed tomography (CT) head if preceding head injury

MAKING A DIAGNOSIS

Once the patient is stabilised in terms of any haemodynamic compromise and major haemorrhage has been excluded, you should focus on reversing the patient's INR according to local protocol.

It is important to check the patient has no history of recent trauma that might lead to significant covert bleeding.

A patient with a deranged INR may present with nose bleeds, bleeding gums, spontaneous bruising, petechiae, ecchymoses, haematuria, rectal bleeding and prolonged bleeding time after minor injuries.

It is important to elicit a careful history to establish any precipitants of the patient's increase in INR.

Given his longstanding use of warfarin for atrial fibrillation, the patient is likely known to the local anticoagulation service who can provide further information on appointments, dosages and recent changes to administration if the patient is unable to do so. In this case, the patient's recent course of ciprofloxacin most likely precipitated the sudden increase in INR. Other triggers are discussed above.

MANAGEMENT

Your initial priority is to ensure the patient is haemodynamically stable; if not, commence resuscitation and call for help immediately. If there is any sign of haemodynamic compromise, the major haemorrhage protocol may need to be activated.

In this scenario, the patient is systemically well and haemodynamically stable. The main concern is his raised INR and evidence of spontaneous bleeding. His INR is >8, and therefore needs to be reversed with vitamin K. Give 0.5–1 mg vitamin K by slow IV injection for immediate effect. Warfarin should be stopped until INR < 5, and can then be restarted with daily monitoring. If there was evidence of a major bleed, you should stop warfarin and treat with IV vitamin K and/or dried prothrombin complex concentrate, or fresh frozen plasma. However, in this circumstance you should seek urgent advice from the haematology department.

If the INR is 6–8, with no or minor bleeding, you should stop warfarin and restart when INR < 5.

 **Clinical Tip**

There are a number of clinical factors to consider in this patient's continual treatment with warfarin. The anticoagulant service are very useful in giving you information about patient compliance. In this context of the drug interaction, the patient should be carefully counselled about potential common drug interactions and about letting the anticoagulant team know if there are any significant medication changes.

Given the man's age, it is important to assess if he has a significant falls risk, which would be a risk factor for intracerebral bleeds on warfarin.

If there is any doubt as to the risk–benefit ratio of long-term warfarin in an elderly patient, a comprehensive geriatric assessment and discussion with a haematologist should be completed.

 **Prescribing Tip**

Both the CHADsVasc and HASBLED scores are useful in calculating bleeding risk. It is also important to consider and discuss the benefits of switching warfarin to a new oral anticoagulant such as rivaroxaban or apixaban, which are seen to be more practical alternatives as INR based monitoring is not required. These are more complex to reverse and require discussion with the haematology team if the scenario arises. See Chapter 3 for further information.

ESCALATION

Patients requiring blood products to correct their clotting should be discussed urgently with the medical registrar and haematologist on call. In cases of complex INR reversal such as in a patient with a metallic valve, or haemodynamic compromise, discuss this with a haematologist immediately to ensure appropriate doses are given and an appropriate plan is made for monitoring the patient. A monitored bed is important if there are any signs of haemodynamic compromise. Ensure the patient is grouped and saved and cross-matched, notifying the lab that blood may be requested in the event of further deterioration.

STATION 12.4: SUPERIOR VENA CAVA OBSTRUCTION

 **The Bleep Scenario**

You are bleeped from ED about a 66 year old man who has been admitted with headache, facial swelling and shortness of breath. He has a background of chronic obstructive pulmonary disease (COPD) and is a lifelong smoker.

His observations are: HR 110 bpm, BP 135/80 mmHg, RR 30 breaths per minute, SpO_2 86% on room air and temperature 37.0°C. You are asked to review him.

DEFINITION

The superior vena cava (SVC) blood flow may be obstructed by external compression, thrombosis or direct invasion of the SVC.

INITIAL THOUGHTS

There are many potential causes for the patient's shortness of breath. However, in conjunction with the history of headache and facial swelling, you should be particularly concerned about SVC obstruction (SVCO). Given that the patient has a history of COPD and is a lifelong smoker, it is very possible that he has an underlying malignancy. Other risk factors to consider are known malignancy, ICD or pacemaker insertion or previous radiotherapy to the chest.

SVCO is a medical emergency because laryngeal oedema can cause acute airway obstruction. The patient's signs of respiratory distress alert you that he is unstable and needs urgent review.

DIFFERENTIAL DIAGNOSIS

- Cardiovascular: cardiac tamponade, constrictive pericarditis, right-sided heart failure or cardiac tumour
- Respiratory: acute COPD exacerbation, pneumonia, pneumothorax, pleural effusion, pulmonary embolism or malignancy
- Malignant causes of SVCO: non-small-cell lung cancer (50%), small-cell lung cancer (25%), lymphoma, thymoma or metastatic disease (commonly breast cancer)

- Benign causes of SVCO (25%): pacemaker/implantable cardioverter defibrillator (ICD) insertion or central venous catheter insertion or mediastinal fibrosis due to chest irradiation

INITIAL INSTRUCTIONS OVER PHONE

This patient is showing signs of respiratory distress (dyspnoea, tachypnoea and hypoxia). You should ask the nurse to ensure the patient is sat upright and to give supplemental oxygen.

IV access, bloods and CXR should be obtained as a matter of urgency. Observations should be repeated, and the patient should be moved to a monitored area as soon as possible.

ASSESSMENT AND RESUSCITATION

- End of the bed assessment: patient appears distressed and is visibly short of breath.
- Airway: patent.
- Breathing: RR 34 breaths per minute, SpO_2 85% on room air. On auscultation, there are vesicular breath sounds with good air entry bilaterally.
  - ABG: pH 7.25, PaO_2 5.5 kPa, $PaCO_2$ 4.0 kPa, HCO_3^- 16 mmol/L.
  - Give high-flow oxygen 15 L/minute. Aim for saturations of 88–92%.
- Circulation: CRT <2 s, HR 110 bpm, regular, BP 130/80 mmHg, JVP raised, HS I + II + 0.
  - 12-lead ECG: sinus tachycardia.
  - Ensure IV access and keep constant watch on any fluctuations in HR and BP that may warrant cautious fluid resuscitation.
- Disability: GCS 15/15, PEARL, temperature 37.0°C, CBG 5.5 mmol/L.
- Exposure: facial swelling with visible venous distension in the face and neck – worsens when arms are raised above the head. Abdomen soft and non-tender, with normal bowel sounds.

INITIAL INVESTIGATIONS

- Haematology: FBC (possible bleed or infection)
- Biochemistry: U&Es, LFTs, troponin (if suspicion of myocardial ischaemia) and CRP (raised in infection/inflammatory disorders)
- Radiology: urgent CXR (widened mediastinum, visible mass), CT chest with contrast (extent of obstruction, visible mass) and ultrasound of the upper limbs. A contrast CT chest will help establish the diagnosis and give more information about the location and severity of the obstruction.
- Microbiology: sputum MCS (organism if infective, malignant cells on cytology)
- Histology: invasive investigations if tissue diagnosis is required such as lymph node biopsy, mediastinoscopy or bronchoscopy.

MAKING A DIAGNOSIS

The diagnosis of SVC syndrome is usually clinical and requires a high degree of clinical suspicion. The most important diagnostic test is a chest CT with contrast to confirm the diagnosis and to evaluate the underlying cause.

- History: known malignancy, smoking history, COPD, previous radiation to the chest, pacemaker/ICD insertion
- Symptoms: dyspnoea, visual disturbance, headache (worse on bending forwards), swelling of face, neck and arms or hoarseness
- Signs: conjunctival / periorbital oedema, facial plethora, dilated non-pulsatile neck veins, dilated collateral veins (arms, anterior chest wall), oedema of hands or arms, Pemberton's sign, papilloedema or stridor

Fig. 12.2 shows SVC compression in a patient with Hodgkin's lymphoma.

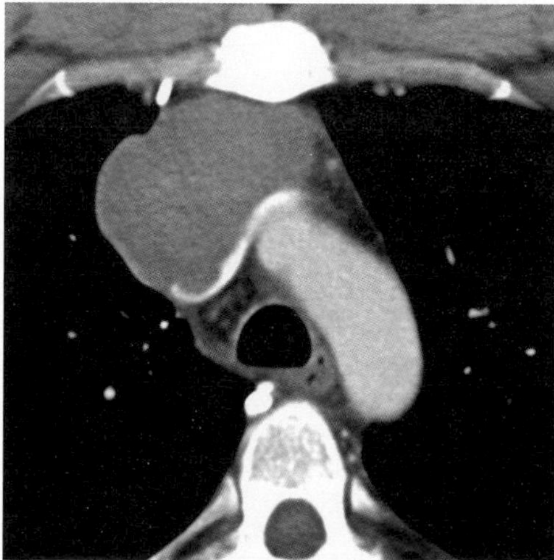

Fig. 12.2 Axial contrast-enhanced computed tomography (CECT) of a patient with nodular sclerosis Hodgkin lymphoma. This image shows a right prevascular mediastinal mass with compression and endoluminal involvement of the superior vena cava (SVC). Patients with Hodgkin lymphoma may present with signs and symptoms of SVC syndrome. (Source: Rosado-de-Christenson, M.L. and Carter, B.W. [2016]. *Specialty imaging: Thoracic neoplasms*. Elsevier.)

MANAGEMENT

Once initial measures have been implemented and you have assessed the patient, you should discuss with the medical registrar or consultant as soon as possible. In case of any airway compromise, the anaesthetic team should be notified.

Further treatment options may include steroids, endovascular stenting, radiotherapy or chemotherapy.

Corticosteroids may be used to treat SVCO, although there is little evidence to support their use. You should seek advice from a palliative care consultant before commencing dexamethasone.

In patients with small-cell lung cancer, systemic anticancer therapy or radiotherapy may be considered the first line, with endovascular stent insertion for relapse or persistent obstruction. For patients with non-small-cell lung cancer, stent insertion may be considered the first line.

In the absence of a need for urgent intervention, the next steps in management should focus on establishing the underlying diagnosis. You should discuss this patient with the respiratory and oncology teams for further guidance.

Symptomatic relief can be offered with a cool flow of air on the patient's face, loosening any tight clothing and ensuring the arms are supported on pillows. You can also consider prescribing opiates or benzodiazepines, respectively, for pain relief and dyspnoea.

ESCALATION

If there is evidence of airway compromise, anaesthetic support may be required. Ensure the patient's escalation status has been reviewed according to their preferences and clinical status.

STATION 12.5: TUMOUR LYSIS SYNDROME

The Bleep Scenario

You are bleeped by the ED about a 45 year old man who was referred by his general practitioner for deranged blood results: serum potassium level is 7.2 mmol/L and creatinine is 190 mmol/L. The patient is asymptomatic. He has just started chemotherapy for non-Hodgkin's lymphoma and is taking allopurinol with his chemotherapy.

His observations are: HR 80 bpm, BP 120/80 mmHg, RR 18 breaths per minute, SpO_2 99% on room air and temperature 37.1°C. You are asked to review him for admission to the AMU.

DEFINITION

Tumour lysis syndrome (TLS) is a severe metabolic and electrolyte disturbance caused by the abrupt release of large quantities of cellular components into the blood following the rapid lysis of malignant cells. It occurs spontaneously or following the initiation of cytotoxic treatment in patients with cancer.

It is characterised by hyperuricaemia, hyperkalaemia, hyperphosphataemia and hypocalcaemia.

INITIAL THOUGHTS

A potassium level of 7.2 mmol/L is a medical emergency, and this man needs an urgent ECG to look for cardiac arrhythmias. While treating his hyperkalaemia, you a need to consider the cause of the abnormal biochemistry. In a patient with biochemical derangements, a known haematological malignancy or high grade tumour and who has recently commenced chemotherapy, TLS should be a top differential.

DIFFERENTIAL DIAGNOSIS

CAUSES OF HYPERKALAEMIA

- Drugs: angiotensin-converting enzyme inhibitors, angiotensin receptor blockers, ciclosporin, beta-blockers or digoxin toxicity
- Endocrine: adrenal insufficiency or insulin deficiency
- Renal: acute kidney injury, chronic kidney disease, urinary obstruction or metabolic acidosis
- Increased K^+ intake: iatrogenic (K supplementation oral/IV), blood transfusion or total parenteral nutrition
- Increased K^+ release from cells: TLS, acute intravascular haemolysis, burns or rhabdomyolysis

INITIAL INSTRUCTIONS OVER PHONE

Ask the nurse to perform an ECG immediately. The patient should be moved to a monitored area for cardiac monitoring. Defibrillator pads should be applied if this is not possible. Ask the nurse to ensure that the patient has IV access with 2 wide bore cannula into each antecubital fossa and to take initial bloods, including a VBG, before your arrival.

ASSESSMENT AND RESUSCITATION

- End of the bed assessment: patient appears comfortable.
- Airway: patent.
- Breathing: RR 18, SpO_2 99% on room air. On auscultation, there are vesicular breath sounds with good air entry bilaterally.
  - VBG: pH 7.40, PaO_2 5.0, $PaCO_2$ 5.5, HCO_3^- 23 mmol/L.
- Circulation: CRT <2 s, HR 80 bpm, regular, BP 120/76 mmHg, JVP not visible, HS I + II + 0, no peripheral oedema.
  - Apply defibrillator pads to allow continuous cardiac monitoring. This may show 'tall tented T waves', flattened P waves, broad QRS. It is currently normal.
- Disability: GCS 15/15, PEARL, temperature 37.1°C, CBG 5.0 mmol/L.
- Exposure: abdomen soft and non-tender, with normal bowel sounds. No renal angle tenderness.

INITIAL INVESTIGATIONS

- Haematology: FBC (raised white cell count increases the risk of TLS)

- Biochemistry: U&Es (raised urea and creatinine, raised K^+), hypocalcaemia, hyperphosphataemia, uraemia and raised lactate dehydrogenase (LDH).

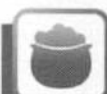
Clinical Tip

Excessive cell lysis results in hyperuricaemia, hyperkalaemia, hypocalcaemia and hyperphosphataemia.

MAKING A DIAGNOSIS

TLS most commonly develops in haematological malignancies, particularly in non-Hodgkin's lymphoma, acute lymphocytic leukaemia and acute myeloid leukaemia. It is infrequently associated with solid tumours, but cases have been reported in patients with breast cancer, small-cell lung cancer and testicular cancer. Further risk factors include pre-existing high white cell count, high lactate dehydrogenase, pre-existing renal impairment and raised levels of uric acid.

- Symptoms: nausea, vomiting, anorexia, diarrhoea, muscle weakness, muscle cramps, lethargy, paraesthesia or chest pain
- Signs: lymphadenopathy, splenomegaly, tetany, Trosseau's sign, Chvostek sign, peripheral oedema, anuria, oliguria, haematuria, seizures or cardiac arrhythmias

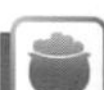
Clinical Tip

Laboratory TLS is defined as a combination of any two of hyperuricaemia, hyperphosphataemia, hyperkalaemia or hypocalcaemia.

MANAGEMENT

The ECG for this patient is normal; if there were ECG features of hyperkalaemia, full treatment for this electrolyte abnormality (see Station 9.6, Chapter 9) would be required.

Initial management includes IV fluid resuscitation (without potassium), cardiac monitoring and supportive management with analgesia and venous thromboembolism prophylaxis. The patient may require IV calcium gluconate for symptomatic hypocalcaemia.

Further management requires a multidisciplinary approach with the involvement of haematologists, nephrologists and ICU doctors. The patient may require rasburicase infusion (in which case allopurinol should be stopped) and haemofiltration or haemodialysis as appropriate.

ESCALATION

Once the patient is stable and you have commenced management of severe hyperkalaemia, you should speak to the medical registrar and further teams which may include the following: haematology regarding rasburicase infusion and ongoing management, nephrology regarding renal failure and need for haemofiltration/dialysis, and ICU regarding intensive monitoring and ongoing management if required.

FURTHER READING

BMJ Best Practice. (2017). *Assessment of neutropenia*. Available at: http://bestpractice.bmj.com/best-practice/monograph/893/overview/aetiology.html. [Accessed 25 July 2022].

BMJ Best Practice. *Superior vena cava syndrome*. Available at: http://bestpractice.bmj.com/best-practice/monograph/848/basics/aetiology.html. [accessed 16 January 2022].

BMJ Best Practice. (2017). *Tumour lysis syndrome*. Available at: http://bestpractice.bmj.com/best-practice/monograph/936.html. [Accessed 16 January 2022].

Jones, G., et al. (2015). Guidelines for the management of tumour lysis syndrome in adults and children with haematological malignancies on behalf of the British Committee for Standards in Haematology. *British Journal of Haematology, 169*(5), 661–671.

NICE. (2012). *Neutropenic sepsis: Prevention and management in people with cancer*. Guideline CG151. Available at: www.nice.org.uk/guidance/cg151/chapter/1-Guidance. [Accessed 16 January 2022].

NICE. (2013). *Clinical knowledge summaries. Anaemia – iron deficiency*. Available at: https://cks.nice.org.uk/anaemia-iron-deficiency#!scenario. [Accessed 16 January 2022].

NICE. (2015). *Clinical knowledge summaries. Neutropenic sepsis. Scenario: Management*. Available at: https://cks.nice.org.uk/neutropenic-sepsis#!scenariorecommendation. [Accessed 16 January 2022].

NICE. (2016). *Clinical knowledge summaries. Anticoagulation – oral. Scenario: Warfarin*. Available at: https://cks.nice.org.uk/anticoagulation-oral#!scenario:4. [Accessed 25 July 2022].

NICE. (2021). *Clinical knowledge summaries. Palliative care – dyspnoea*. Available at: https://cks.nice.org.uk/palliative-care-dyspnoea#!scenario:2. [Accessed 16 January 2022].

Oxford University Press. (2007). *Oxford concise medical dictionary* (7th ed.). Oxford: Oxford University Press, 370.

Philips, R., et al. (2012). Prevention and management of neutropenic sepsis in patients with cancer: summary of NICE guidance. *BMJ, 345*, e5368.

Scottish Palliative Care Guidelines. (2014). *Superior vena cava obstruction*. Available at: www.palliativecareguidelines.scot.nhs.uk/guidelines/palliative-emergencies/Superior-Vena-Cava-Obstruction.aspx. [Accessed 16 January 2022].

SIGN. (2014). *Management of lung cancer*. Guidelines SIGN 137. Available at: www.sign.ac.uk/media/1075/sign137.pdf. [Accessed 25 July 2022].

Snook, J., et al. (2021). *Guidelines for the management of iron deficiency anaemia in adults*. Available at: www.bsg.org.uk/clinical-resource/guidelines-for-the-management-of-iron-deficiency-anaemia/. [Accessed 16 January 2022].

World Health Organization (n.d.) *Anaemia*. Available at: www.who.int/topics/anaemia/en/. [Accessed 16 January 2022].

13 Toxicology

Content Outline

STATION 13.1: TRICYCLIC ANTIDEPRESSANT TOXICITY

 The Bleep Scenario

You are bleeped by an acute medical unit (AMU) nurse to review a patient. A 29 year old man, who admitted having taken an overdose of his regular amitriptyline medication. His observations are: Heart rate (HR) 155bpm, temperature 36.9°C, blood pressure (BP) 130/65 mmHg, respiratory rate (RR) 18 breaths per minute, SpO_2 99% on room air.

DEFINITION

Tricyclic antidepressant toxicity is the intentional or accidental consumption of more than the recommended dose of a tricyclic antidepressant.

INITIAL THOUGHTS

Antidepressant overdoses are associated with supraventricular tachycardia and this is an important differential to exclude. A rate above 120 bpm is unlikely to be sinus tachycardia. If the patient is hypotensive or demonstrates a fluctuant Glasgow Coma Scale (GCS) in the context of this tachycardia, this would call for immediate action through a periarrest call. You should escalate this immediately to the medical registrar or consultant and, after assessing and stabilising the patient, consult Toxbase to help with definitive assessment and management.

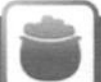 Clinical Tip

It is important to be watchful of autonomic symptoms such as tachycardia, hypotension, fixed and dilated pupils, and urinary retention. It is also crucial to be vigilant of cardiac arrhythmias, a fluctuance in acid–base status and neurological sequelae (including convulsions and hypoactive delirium) which may require complex medical care.

ASSESSMENT AND RESUSCITATION

- End of the bed assessment: the patient is drowsy and unkempt.
- Airway: the patient is talking in short sentences.
- Breathing: RR 18 breaths per minute and SpO_2 99% on room air. On auscultation, vesicular breath sounds are heard. No evidence of cyanosis.
- Circulation: HR 155 bpm, BP 130/65 mmHg. Capillary refill time (CRT) <2 s. Heart sounds (HS) I + II + 0.
  - 12-lead electrocardiogram (ECG): supraventricular tachycardia.
- Disability: GCS is 13, apyrexial 36.9°C and pupils are equal and reactive. Capillary blood glucose (CBG) 4.8 mmol/L.
- Exposure: abdomen is soft, with some suprapubic tenderness. There is a palpable bladder.
  - Bladder scan shows 675 mL in the bladder.

INITIAL INVESTIGATIONS

- Haematology: full blood count (FBC: leukocytosis or anaemia)
- Biochemistry: urea and electrolytes (U&Es: hyponatraemia should be considered in patients on antidepressants who develop convulsions, confusion

or drowsiness), bone profile (Ca^{2+}, PO_4^{3-}, ALP) to recheck serum calcium, C-reactive protein (CRP: inflammation) evidence of infection and liver function tests (LFTs: evidence of hepatic failure) and venous blood gas (VBG: to determine lactate)

- Toxicology: full urine and blood toxicology

MANAGEMENT

Given the significance of the tachycardia, this patient needs immediate medical management. The initial treatment is 50 mmol of 8.4% sodium bicarbonate over 20 minutes intravenously to manage his tachycardia, even in the absence of acidosis. This is the definitive treatment for tricyclic overdose.

It is imperative that the patient remains on a cardiac monitor and should be moved to a high dependency setting, with the involvement of a senior doctor. As he is also in urinary retention, a urinary catheter for close monitoring of fluid status is required.

It is crucial to be watchful of his cardiac rhythm and any neurological sequelae such as seizures. At least initially, seizures can be managed with benzodiazepines, most commonly lorazepam.

Patients with an overdose should have 2–4-hourly VBGs to check for fluctuations in acid–base status, lactate levels and any electrolyte abnormalities that may occur.

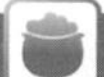

Clinical Tip

Selective serotonin reuptake inhibitors generally have low toxicity; however, citalopram and escitalopram may cause QTc interval prolongation. Serotonin syndrome, characterised by neuromuscular hyperactivity, autonomic dysfunction and altered mental state, is uncommon. Symptoms can occur within hours or days of initiation, dose escalation or overdose, the addition of a new serotonergic drug, or switching serotonergic drugs without an adequate washout period.

Clinical Tip

Be aware that patients can also develop withdrawal symptoms when stopping antidepressant medication. These usually settle in a couple of weeks or earlier with reintroduction of medication.

ESCALATION

If the patient has refractory tachycardia, this requires immediate consultation by the toxicology and cardiology teams to work towards a safe management plan to help with rate, and potentially rhythm, control. Involvement of anaesthetic and intensive care teams is important in the context of neurological sequelae and airway compromise, or in the case of severe abnormalities of electrolyte levels or acid–base status.

STATION 13.2: BENZODIAZEPINE TOXICITY

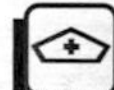

The Bleep Scenario

A ward nurse bleeps you urgently. A 39 year old man who had been treated for alcohol withdrawal and was awaiting discharge has experienced a sudden drop in his RR. His observations are: temperature 37°C, HR 63 bpm, BP 110/65 mmHg, RR 6 breaths per minute, saturations 96% on 2 L oxygen.

DEFINITION

Benzodiazepine toxicity is the intentional or accidental consumption of more than the recommended dose of a benzodiazepine.

INITIAL THOUGHTS

Respiratory depression requires immediate review. As you are on your way to assess this man you should be thinking of common causes of respiratory depression, such as opioids, benzodiazepines, barbiturates or stroke. The history given to you was that of alcohol withdrawal which is commonly treated with benzodiazepines. You should be aware of the antidotes such as naloxone and flumazenil. If there is any concern regarding his ability to maintain his airway then ask the nursing staff to put out a periarrest call.

ASSESSMENT AND RESUSCITATION

- End of the bed assessment: the patient is extremely drowsy but rousable. You elicit from his notes that he was found with packets of diazepam.
- Airway: mild inspiratory stridor corrected with an airway adjunct (Guedel airway).
- Breathing: RR 6 breaths per minute and SpO_2 96% on 2 L via nasal cannula. On auscultation, vesicular breath sounds are heard.
- Circulation: HR 63 bpm, with BP 110/65 mmHg. CRT <2 s. Heart sounds I+II+0. Obtain intravenous (IV) access.
  - 12-lead ECG: sinus rhythm with no acute changes.
- Disability: GCS 8/15, pupils equal and reactive to light (PEARL), temperature 37°C. CBG 5 mmol/L.
- Exposure: abdomen is soft and non-tender. There is no palpable organomegaly.

INITIAL INVESTIGATIONS

- Haematology: FBC (leukocytosis or anaemia)
- Biochemistry: U&Es, bone profile (Ca^{2+}, PO_4^{3-}, ALP) (electrolyte imbalance), CRP (inflammation), LFTs (evidence of hepatic failure) and ABG (to assess oxygenation)
- Toxicology: full urine and blood toxicology

MANAGEMENT

This patient has a compromised airway and requires urgent input from the anaesthetic and periarrest teams. The initial medical treatment after stabilisation of the airway is flumazenil, an antagonist of benzodiazepines (0.5–1 mg), which patient should respond to within 3 minutes and can be repeated if necessary. The patient will need care in an intensive therapy unit if he has ongoing respiratory depression.

You should consult Toxbase to confirm the appropriate dose of Flumazenil.

Clinical Tip

Benzodiazepine overdoses can be managed successfully with flumazenil:

- It is an imidazobenzodiazepine derivative.
- It is a competitive inhibitor of benzodiazepine at the benzodiazepine recognition site on the gamma-aminobutyric acid (GABA)/benzodiazepine receptor complex.
- It's half life is 40–80 minutes.

Patients on alcohol withdrawal treatment need to be reviewed on a daily basis, and their withdrawal regimens should be tapered to reduce the risk of toxicity. This patient should be monitored if he does respond to flumazenil for up to 24 hours until his observations are consistently safe.

Prescribing Tip

It is important to note that, in patients who may require flumenazil in the context of a mixed overdose with epilepsy or with acute seizures, flumazenil can precipitate status epilepticus. In this scenario, it is crucial to consult a toxicologist before treating the patient, as this could be life threatening.

ESCALATION

The anaesthetic and intensive care team should be consulted in cases of airway compromise or respiratory depression. In cases of mixed overdose, especially with haemodynamic instability, the toxicologist can help guide management.

STATION 13.3: OPIATE TOXICITY

The Bleep Scenario

You receive a call from the orthopaedics ward. A patient has had a total hip replacement 2 days ago and has been complaining of significant, persistent pain. He is now very drowsy and has poor respiratory effort. His observations are: temperature 36.5°C, HR 63 bpm, BP 130/65 mmHg, RR 8 breaths per minute, O_2 90% on room air.

DEFINITION

Opiate toxicity is the intentional or accidental consumption of more than the recommended dose of opiate medication, e.g. morphine, tramadol, co-codamol.

INITIAL THOUGHTS

This patient needs an urgent review. On your way to assessing this man, you should be considering the various causes of drowsiness, e.g. delirium, hypovolaemic shock, opiates and hyponatraemia. You should consider a periarrest call if his breathing is significantly affected. Alert the nurse to do so if this is the case before you arrive.

ASSESSMENT AND RESUSCITATION

- End of the bed assessment: you see a man who is slumped over.
- Airway: some snoring, which is corrected with basic airway manoeuvres and using a Guedel airway adjunct.
- Breathing: RR 8 breaths per minute and SpO_2 90% on room air. He has no history of chronic obstructive pulmonary disease. On examination, there are vesicular breath sounds.
    - ABG: pH 7.33, PaO_2 11 kPa, $PaCO_2$ 6.5 kPa, HCO_3^- 30 mmol/L.
- Circulation: heart rate is 63 bpm, with BP 130/65 mmHg. CRT is <2 s. Heart sounds I+II+0.
    - 12-lead ECG: sinus rhythm.
- Disability: the patient is only responsive to pain. Apyrexial 36.5°C. CBG 4.3 mmol/L. Pupils are pinpoint and sluggishly reactive.
- Exposure: abdomen is soft and non-tender. There is no palpable organomegaly.

INITIAL INVESTIGATIONS

- Haematology: FBC (leukocytosis or anaemia)
- Biochemistry: U&Es, bone profile (Ca^{2+}, PO_4^{3-}, ALP) (electrolyte imbalance), CRP (inflammation), LFTs (evidence of hepatic failure) and ABG (to determine oxgenation)
- Toxicology: full urine and blood toxicology

Clinical Tip

Symptoms of opiate toxicity include respiratory depression, drowsiness, constricted pupils, and in some situations, coma. It is important to assess the underlying cause. Monitor the patient's bloods for acute kidney injury, and review bowel charts to ensure patients are not constipated. It is also important to be aware of withdrawal symptoms such as profuse sweating, tachycardia, dilated pupils, vomiting and diarrhoea.

MANAGEMENT

Once the patient has been stabilised, you should take a more detailed history. Postoperative patients often require large doses of opiates to control their pain, but their intake may also be minimal. It is not uncommon to develop an acute kidney injury or constipation in these circumstances. This patient has likely developed opiate toxicity. This needs to be treated with naloxone (0.4–2 mg), repeated every 2 minutes, until breathing is adequate. A continuous naloxone infusion may be required. He also requires IV fluids, accurate fluid balance charts and a thorough medication review if he has developed an acute kidney injury. His opiate doses need to be adjusted according to his renal function.

ESCALATION

This case would have resulted in a periarrest call. Early senior input and anaesthetician input are crucial.

STATION 13.4: ORGANOPHOSPHATE TOXICITY

The Bleep Scenario

You are asked to review a 54 year old gardener who has been admitted, having ingested insecticide. She is nauseous and bradycardic with a heart rate of 35 bpm with recurrent episodes of diarrhoea. The rest of her observations are: temperature 36.7°C, BP 110/65 mmHg, RR 18 breaths per minute, O_2 100% on room air.

DEFINITION

Organophosphate toxicity is the intentional or accidental consumption of organophosphates.

INITIAL THOUGHTS

Organophosphate poisoning is rare. The mechanism by which organophosphate poisoning works is by inactivation of acetylcholinesterase. Anticholinergic symptoms can include salivation, lacrimation, urination and diarrhoea. This can also be accompanied by bradycardia, respiratory distress, small pupils and coma. Toxbase should be consulted after the patient has been stabilised for definitive assessment and management.

ASSESSMENT AND RESUSCITATION

- End of the bed assessment: the patient is settled.
- Airway: patent and self-maintained.
- Breathing: RR 18 breaths per minute and SpO_2 100% on room air. On examination there are vesicular breath sounds.
- Circulation: heart rate is 35 bpm, with BP 110/65 mmHg. CRT is <2 s. Heart sounds I+II+0.
  - 12-lead ECG : sinus bradycardia.
- Disability: patient is alert. GCS is 15. She is apyrexial, temperature 36.7°C, but sweating. CBG 5.4 mmol/L. Pupils are small, but equally reactive.
- Exposure: abdomen is soft and non-tender and there is no organomegaly.

INITIAL INVESTIGATIONS

- Haematology: FBC (leukocytosis or anaemia)
- Biochemistry: U&Es, bone profile (Ca^{2+}, PO_4^{3-}, ALP) (electrolyte imbalance), CRP (inflammation), and LFTs (evidence of hepatic failure) and VBG (to determine lactate)
- Toxicology: full urine and blood toxicology

MANAGEMENT

The bradycardia needs immediate treatment. An additional priority is to wash this patient thoroughly and remove all traces of insecticide.

Organophosphate poisoning is managed with atropine to reverse the effects of cholinergic blockade. The atropine dose would start at 2mg and can be increased incrementally. If the patient does not respond, the next line of treatment is pralidoxime, which reactivates acetylcholinesterase. It is crucial that the toxicology and poisons team are involved. If the bradycardia remains unresolved, cardiology should be consulted.

This patient will require cardiac monitoring. This may be in an AMU, high dependency unit (HDU) or intensive care.

Clinical Tip

Pralidoxime is a commonly used antidote in organophosphate poisoning. It works by reactivating the acetylcholinesterase, by cleaving a bond formed between the organophosphate and acetylcholinesterase. It needs to be given within 24 hours to be effective. You would not be expected to initiate this without clear instructions from the toxicology team.

ESCALATION

Cardiac monitoring is key; the patient may require escalation to HDU, coronary care unit or the intensive care unit depending how they respond to medical treatment or if they have significant cardiac or neurological sequelae.

STATION 13.5: PARACETAMOL TOXICITY

The Bleep Scenario

You are requested to review a 40 year old woman who was admitted yesterday with a headache. She has just been found collapsed in the toilet with a couple of empty packets of paracetamol in her hand. She has a history of depression. She is slightly drowsy and her observations are: temperature 36.6°C, HR 63 bpm, BP 110/65 mmHg, RR 18 breaths per minute, O_2 96% on 2 L.

DEFINITION

Paracetamol toxicity is the intentional or accidental consumption of paracetamol in excess of its recommended dose.

INITIAL THOUGHTS

As you are on your way to assess this patient, you should think about the management of paracetamol overdose. You should remember the importance of assessing for hepatotoxicity, and the use of the nomogram. You should consider involving psychiatry to review the patient when they are stable.

ASSESSMENT AND RESUSCITATION

- End of the bed assessment: the patient is drowsy but easily rousable and lying in bed.
- Airway: she is communicating in full sentences.
- Breathing: RR is 18 breaths per minute and SpO_2 96% on 2 L via nasal cannula. Vesicular breath sounds.
  - ABG: pH 7.30, PaO_2 10.2 kPa, $PaCO_2$ 5.0 kPa, HCO_3^- 19 mmol/L.
- Circulation: HR 63 bpm, with BP 110/65 mmHg. CRT is <2 s. HS are I+II+0.
  - 12-lead ECG: sinus rhythm, with no acute changes.
- Disability: GCS is 13–14, apyrexial 36.6°C and pupils are equal and reactive. CBG 5.2 mmol/L.
- Exposure: abdomen is soft; however there is mild right upper quadrant discomfort on deep palpation. No guarding and rebound tenderness. There is no palpable organomegaly.

INITIAL INVESTIGATIONS

- Haematology: FBC (leukocytosis or anaemia) and a full coagulation profile (to assess clotting factors for signs of hepatic compromise)
- Biochemistry: U&Es, bone profile (Ca^{2+}, PO_4^{3-}, ALP) (electrolyte imbalance), CRP (inflammation), LFTs (evidence of hepatic failure) and VBG (to determine lactate)
- Toxicology: full urine and blood toxicology

MANAGEMENT

This patient needs immediate assessment for early signs of fulminant hepatic failure.

The patient is drowsy, and is maintaining a GCS of 14. The emergency department notes suggest her ingestion time is around 5 hours prior, but this may not be accurate as they could not get a clear history. She will therefore need to be treated as a staggered overdose of indeterminate time frame.

Patients who have taken a paracetamol overdose are managed with *N*-acetylcysteine as per the paracetamol treatment nomogram (Fig 13.1). If it is less than or equal to 1 hour since ingestion then activated charcoal can be given, though patients rarely fall into this category. Referral to psychiatry for management is important.

N-ACETYLCYSTEINE TREATMENT

- Given intravenously:
  - 150 mg/kg in 200 mL of 5% dextrose over 15 minutes then
  - 50 mg/kg in 500 mL of 5% dextrose over 4 hours then
  - 100 mg/kg in 1 L of 5% dextrose over 16 hours

ESCALATION

Given the patient's fluctuant level of consciousness, a low threshold for specialist airway support from the anaesthetic and intensive care teams would be prudent. The other major consideration is her suitability for liver transplant.

High-risk features mandating review for admission to a liver transplant centre are:

- International normalised ratio (INR) >3.0 at 48 hours or >4.5 at any time
- Oliguria or creatinine > 200 µmol/L
- Acidosis with pH < 7.3 after resuscitation
- Systolic hypotension with BP < 80 mmHg
- Hypoglycaemia
- Severe thrombocytopenia
- Encephalopathy of any degree

Clinical Tip

King's College criteria is used to determine which patients should be referred for liver transplantation in paracetamol hepatotoxicity. The criteria are:

- Blood pH < 7.3 or all of the below:
- Grade 3 or 4 encephalopathy
- INR > 6.5
- Renal impairment – creatinine > 300 µmol/L

Remember that there are two different assessment criteria for paracetamol-induced and non-paracetamol-induced acute liver failure.

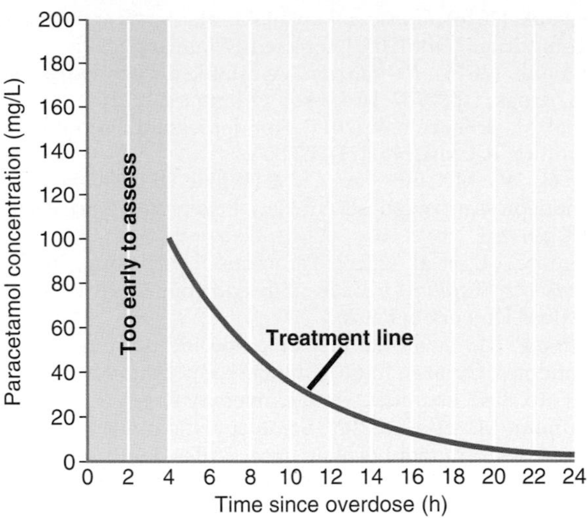

Fig. 13.1 Paracetamol treatment normogram. (Source: Innes, J.A. [2021]. *Davidson's essentials of medicine*. Elsevier.)

STATION 13.6: SALICYLATE TOXICITY

The Bleep Scenario

You are asked to review a ward patient. A 45 year old woman known to have migraines has taken a lot of tablets to try and get rid of the pain from her headache. She feels nauseated, and has ringing in her ears. Her observations are: temperature 36.9°C, HR 103 bpm, BP 110/65 mmHg, RR 25 breaths per minute, O_2 98% on room air.

DEFINITION

Salicylate toxicity is the intentional or accidental consumption of more than the recommended dosage of any salicylate, such as aspirin.

INITIAL THOUGHTS

You should consider the common migraine treatments and their effects in overdose. These medications include aspirin, triptans and beta-blockers. Consult Toxbase accordingly.

ASSESSMENT AND RESUSCITATION

- End of the bed assessment: the patient is sweaty and holding a sick bowl. The patient tells you that she took twenty 300-mg tablets of aspirin over a few hours due to her constant migraine. She says it has been around 3 hours since she took these tablets.
- Airway: patent.
- Breathing: RR 25 breaths per minute and SpO_2 98% on room air. On examination, there are vesicular breath sounds.
- Circulation: HR is 103 bpm, with BP 110/65 mmHg. CRT is <2 s. HS: I + II + 0.
  - 12-lead ECG: sinus rhythm, with no acute changes.
- Disability: GCS is 15. She is apyrexial at 36.9°C and CBG 5.3 mmol/L. PEARL.
- Exposure: abdomen is soft and non-tender. There is no palpable organomegaly.

INITIAL INVESTIGATIONS

- Haematology: FBC (leukocytosis or anaemia)
- Biochemistry: U&Es, bone profile (Ca^{2+}, PO_4^{3-}, ALP) (electrolyte imbalance), CRP (inflammation), LFTs (evidence of hepatic failure) and ABG (to assess oxygenation and lactate level)
- Toxicology: full urine and blood toxicology screen

MANAGEMENT

You should identify and correct any electrolyte abnormalities as a priority and ensure the patient is well hydrated.

Activated charcoal can be used if the patient presents less than 1 hour after the ingestion of aspirin unless contraindicated (e.g. by altered mental status) and may be repeated every 4 hours until charcoal appears in the stool.

After any volume and electrolyte abnormalities are corrected, alkaline diuresis with sodium bicarbonate can be used to increase urine pH, ideally to ≥ 8. Alkaline diuresis is indicated for patients with any symptoms of poisoning and should not be delayed until salicylate levels are determined. This intervention is usually safe and exponentially increases salicylate excretion.

Patients should be given additional potassium supplementation alongside the sodium bicarbonate because hypokalaemia may interfere with alkaline diuresis. Drugs that increase urinary bicarbonate (e.g. acetazolamide) should be avoided because they can worsen metabolic acidosis and decrease blood pH. Drugs that decrease respiratory drive should be avoided because they may impair the hyperventilation response and thus respiratory alkalosis, which can lead to decreasing blood pH.

If there is hypoprothrombinaemia (i.e. prolonged prothrombin time) then vitamin K may be required in addition to the treatment above.

ESCALATION

Haemodialysis is required if plasma salicylate level are greater than 700 mg/L or 5.07 mmol/L. These patients require HDU or intensive care input. If there is a fluctuance of GCS, the patient may require airway and cardiorespiratory support.

Clinical Tip

Salicylate overdose leads to respiratory centre stimulation, causing respiratory alkalosis, and the compensatory mechanisms lead to metabolic acidosis. A fall in pH is an indicator of serious poisoning.

FURTHER READING

Ballinger, A. (2012). Drug therapy, poisoning, and alcohol misuse: Aspirin. In *Kumar and Clark's essentials of clinical medicine* (5th ed.) (pp. 595–597). London: Elsevier.

Ballinger, A. (2012). Drug therapy, poisoning, and alcohol misuse: Opioids. In *Kumar and Clark's essentials of clinical medicine* (5th ed.) (pp. 601–602). London: Elsevier.

Ballinger, A. (2012). Drug therapy, poisoning, and alcohol misuse: Other drugs. In *Kumar and Clark's essentials of clinical medicine* (5th ed.) (p. 600). London: Elsevier.

BMJ Best Practice. (2019). *Opiate overdose*. Available at: https://bestpractice.bmj.com/topics/en-gb/339. [Accessed 17 January 2022].

BMJ Best Practice. (2020). *Salicylate poisoning*. Available at: https://bestpractice.bmj.com/topics/en-gb/3000177. [Accessed 17 January 2022].

BMJ Best Practice. (2021). *Benzodiazepine overdose*. Available at: https://bestpractice.bmj.com/topics/en-gb/3000222. [Accessed 17 January 2022].

BMJ Best Practice. (2021). *Organophosphate poisoning*. Available at: https://bestpractice.bmj.com/topics/en-gb/852. [Accessed 17 January 2022].

BNF. (2021). *Antidepressant drugs*. Available at: https://bnf.nice.org.uk/treatment-summary/antidepressant-drugs.html. [Accessed 17 January 2022].

BNF. (2021). *Poisoning, emergency treatment*. Available at: https://bnf.nice.org.uk/treatment-summary/poisoning-emergency-treatment.html. [Accessed 17 January 2022].

Drugbank. (2016). *Flumazenil*. Available at: https://go.drugbank.com/drugs/DB01205. [Accessed 17 January 2022].

Drugbank. (2016). *Pralidoxime*. Available at: www.drugbank.ca/drugs/DB00733. [Accessed 17 January 2022].

Gabriel, M., & Sharma, V. (2017). Antidepressant discontinuation syndrome. *CMAJ*, *189*(21), E747.

Kerr, G. W., McGuffie, A. C., & Wilkie, S. (2001). Tricyclic antidepressant overdose: A review. *Emergency Medicine Journal*, *18*, 236–241.

Longmore, M., et al. (2010). Paracetamol poisoning. In *Oxford handbook of clinical medicine* (8th ed.) (pp. 856–857). Oxford: Oxford University Press.

Longmore, M., et al. (2010). Some specific poisons and their antidotes: Opiates. In *Oxford handbook of clinical medicine* (8th ed.) (p. 854). Oxford: Oxford University Press.

Longmore, M., et al. (2010). Some specific poisons and their antidotes: Organophosphate insecticides. In *Oxford handbook of clinical medicine* (8th ed.). Oxford: Oxford University Press.

NICE. (2021). *Depression: how toxic are antidepressants in overdose?*. Available at: https://cks.nice.org.uk/topics/depression/prescribing-information/toxicity-in-overdose/. [Accessed 17 January 2022].

Runde, T. J., & Nappe, T. M. (2022). Salicylates toxicity. In *StatPearls*. Treasure Island, FL: StatPearls.

Dermatology

14

Content Outline

STATION 14.1: CUTANEOUS DRUG REACTIONS

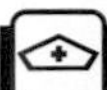

The Bleep Scenario

You are bleeped by the nurse asking you to review a patient newly admitted to the acute medical unit (AMU). He is a 67 year old man presenting with a spotted rash all over his body (Fig. 14.1). His face now appears swollen and he is in severe discomfort. He is normally fit and well.

His observations are: heart rate (HR) 80 bpm, blood pressure (BP) 130/80 mmHg, respiratory rate (RR) 16 breaths per minute, SpO_2 99% on room air and temperature 38.0°C. You are asked to review him.

DEFINITION

A cutaneous drug reaction is an unexpected reaction to a medicine and can be categorised as mild to moderate (the majority of drug eruptions), severe (urticaria, angio-oedema, anaphylaxis, Stevens–Johnson syndrome (SJS)/toxic epidermal necrolysis (TEN), drug hypersensitivity/drug reaction with eosinophilia and systemic symptoms (DRESS) syndrome and erythroderma) and photosensitive drug reactions.

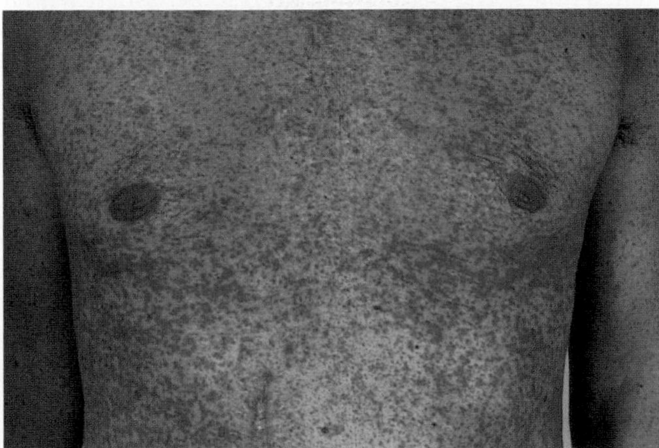

Fig. 14.1 Morbilliform rash. (Source: Kumar, P. and Clark, M.L. [2021]. *Kumar and Clark's clinical medicine*. London: Elsevier.)

INITIAL THOUGHTS

At this point, you should consider the likely differential diagnoses. There are multiple causes of morbilliform (spotted) rashes, and it can be difficult to make a diagnosis based on a very brief history and no examination. However, you have been informed that the patient has developed facial swelling, which should make you suspect potential anaphylaxis. This patient needs urgent review.

You should also consider the patient's risk of skin failure which can result in secondary infection, loss of temperature control, high-output heart failure, fluid and electrolyte imbalances and hypoalbuminaemia.

DIFFERENTIAL DIAGNOSIS

- Morbilliform rash: drug eruptions, erythroderma, vasculitis, folliculitis or exanthems
- Facial swelling: angio-oedema, acute inflammatory dermatosis of face, infectious facial swelling or anaphylaxis

INITIAL INSTRUCTIONS OVER PHONE

If there is a high suspicion of anaphylaxis, inform the nurse to put out a call to the medical emergency team. You should ask the nurse to complete a further complete set of observations to check for haemodynamic instability and the sequelae of skin failure. You can ask for a swab of the skin to be taken to assess for any superimposed infection.

ASSESSMENT AND RESUSCITATION

- End of the bed assessment: the patient has a widespread morbilliform rash and mild facial swelling.
- Airway: patent, no evidence of airway compromise.
- Breathing: RR 16 breaths per minute, SpO_2 99% on room air. No evidence of respiratory distress. On

auscultation, there is equal and bilateral air entry with vesicular breath sounds.
- Circulation: capillary refill time (CRT) <2 s, HR 83 bpm, regular, BP 130/80 mmHg, jugular venous pressure (JVP) normal, heart sounds (HS) I + II + 0.
- Disability: Glasgow Coma Scale (GCS) 15/15, pupils equal and reactive to light (PEARL), temperature 38.0°C, capillary blood glucose (CBG) 5.7 mmol/L.
- Exposure: there is a widespread morbilliform rash with mild generalised facial swelling. There is bilateral cervical and inguinal lymphadenopathy. Abdomen is soft and non-tender, with normal bowel sounds.

INITIAL INVESTIGATIONS

- Haematology: full blood count (FBC: thrombocytopenia, eosinophilia, abnormal lymphocyte count, underlying infection).
- Biochemistry: C-reactive protein (CRP: inflammation), urea and electrolytes (U&Es: electrolyte imbalance, acute kidney injury (AKI)) and liver function tests (LFTs: liver function derangement).
- Microbiology: blood cultures (bacteraemia), skin swabs (superimposed infection).

 **Clinical Tip**

A diagnosis of DRESS is supported by the presence of eosinophilia, abnormal lymphocyte count, thrombocytopenia and deranged LFTs.

MAKING A DIAGNOSIS

Once the patient is stable, a thorough history and examination are essential.

You should ask specifically about recent drug or medicine use; the most common drugs which cause these reactions are antibiotics, antiepileptic drugs, allopurinol and olanzapine. This is by no means an exhaustive list, and you will need to have a thorough look at the BNF for possible precipitants beforehand.

Patients with DRESS often present with a widespread skin rash, fever, facial swelling and may have further organ involvement, including lymphadenopathy, haematological disorders, deranged liver and renal function, pulmonary and cardiovascular involvement, myositis, neurological disturbances, gastrointestinal, endocrine abnormalities and ocular involvement. Fig. 14.2 shows an example of facial swelling associated with DRESS syndrome.

According to the RegiSCAR criteria for DRESS syndrome, potential cases require at least three of the following:
- Hospitalisation
- A suspected drug-related reaction
- Acute rash
- Fever >38°C

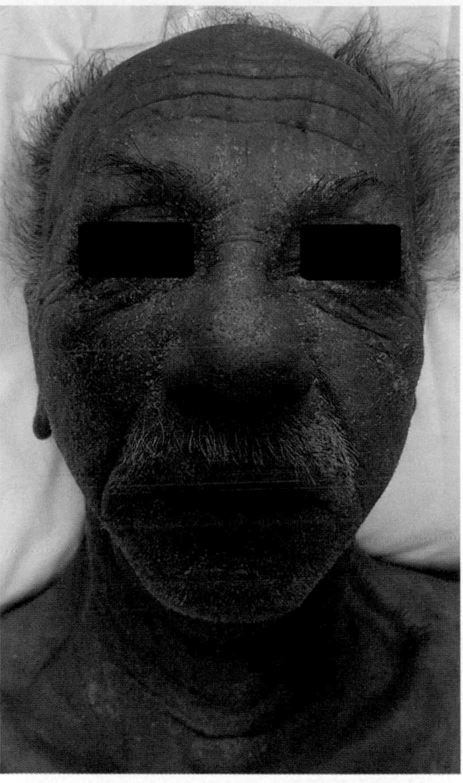

Fig. 14.2 Facial swelling associated with drug reaction with eosinophilia and systemic symptoms (DRESS). (Source: Chan, L., Chan, C. and Cook, D.K. [2018]. Drug reaction with eosinophilia and systemic symptoms [DRESS] syndrome: Case report of severe multiorgan involvement to perindopril/amlodipine combination antihypertensive. *JAAD Case Reports*, *4*(2), pp. 170–174.)

- Enlarged lymph nodes at a minimum of two sites
- Involvement of at least one internal organ
- Eosinophilia or abnormal lymphocytosis
- Thrombocytopenia

MANAGEMENT

Immediate treatment consists of adequate resuscitation as required and immediate cessation of all suspect medicines. Ensure this is clearly documented in the patient's notes. The patient will need to be issued with a MedicAlert bracelet.

Systemic steroids are frequently used in DRESS and severe cutaneous drug reactions, especially if there is significant dermatitis or other organ involvement. A dermatologist should be consulted for prescribing decisions about systemic steroids.

The patient will also require careful monitoring of fluid balance and body temperature given the risk of skin failure. Appropriate intravenous (IV) access will is required, along with catheterisation for strict input and output monitoring.

Supportive treatment for the skin rash may include dressings, topical corticosteroids, topical emollients and oral antihistamines. Secondary infections may require antibiotics. Further general supportive measures include appropriate analgesia, venous thromboembolism (VTE) prophylaxis and referral to the dietetics team to ensure daily calorific and nutritional requirements are met.

ESCALATION

The patient should be referred to dermatology at the earliest opportunity to ensure appropriate management of the skin rash and related complications. He may also require discussion with other specialist teams if there is other organ involvement.

If appropriate, the patient should also be discussed with the medical registrar and the intensive care unit (ICU) if there is any evidence of skin failure that can lead to thermodysregulation, electrolyte abnormalities, dehydration, high-output heart failure, secondary infection, acute respiratory distress syndrome (ARDS) and hypoalbuminaemia. Be aware that the patient may require transfer to ICU or the burns unit for further specialist care depending on the extent of skin involvement and/or multi-organ involvement.

STATION 14.2: ERYTHRODERMA

The Bleep Scenario

You are bleeped by the emergency department senior house officer about a 28 year old man who is being admitted to the AMU. He has red discoloration of his skin covering a large surface area of his body; however, the oromucosal areas are spared (Fig. 14.3). He has recently been diagnosed with psoriasis; his general practitioner suspects that he is noncompliant with his medications. He is now reporting shortness of breath.

His observations are: HR 80 bpm, BP 120/80 mmHg, RR 20 breaths per minute, SpO_2 95% on room air and temperature 35.8°C. You are asked to review him.

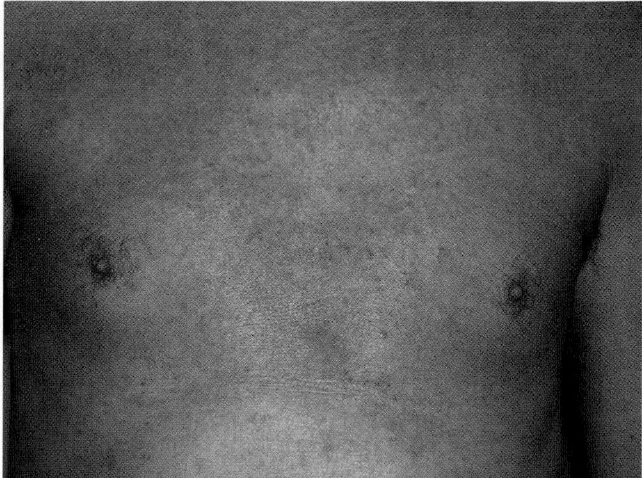

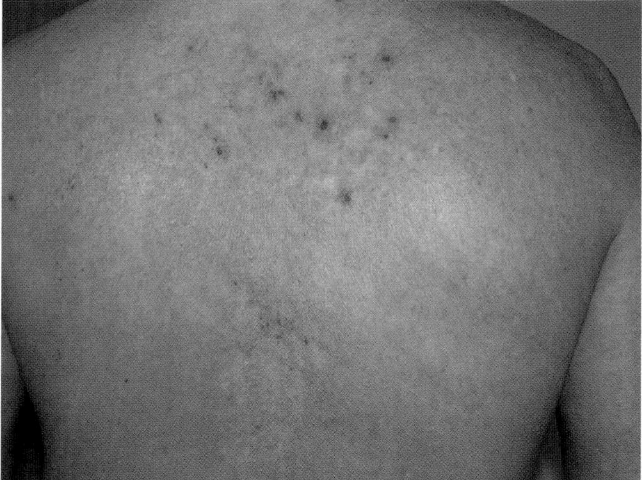

Fig. 14.3 (A, B) Patient with erythroderma. (Source: Micheletti, R.G. et al. [2022]. *Andrews' diseases of the skin clinical atlas*. Elsevier.)

DEFINITION

Erythroderma is the term used to describe an extensive reddening of the skin, usually due to widespread inflammation. There are multiple names for erythroderma; in the common scenario in which erythroderma is preceded by exfoliation (peeling of the skin), it is referred to as dermatitis. Idiopathic erythroderma is sometimes referred to as 'red-man syndrome'. Generalised erythema affects more than 90% of the skin surface.

INITIAL THOUGHTS

From the description given by the nurse, you can be fairly certain that the diagnosis is erythroderma associated with an exacerbation of psoriasis. Your major concern given his shortness of breath is a coexisting pneumonia or ARDS.

Other red flags to consider in the emergency setting include secondary infection and skin failure resulting in loss of temperature control, high-output heart failure, fluid and electrolyte imbalances and hypoalbuminaemia.

DIFFERENTIAL DIAGNOSIS

- Drug eruptions: penicillin, sulfonamides, isoniazid, phenytoin, barbiturates, angiotensin-converting enzyme inhibitors, allopurinol, antiarrhythmics, anticonvulsants, non-steroidal anti-inflammatory drugs and omeprazole
- Pre-existing skin disease: Contact dermatitis, venous eczema, seborrhoeic dermatitis, psoriasis, pityriasis rubra pilaris, and ichthyosis
- Malignancy: Sézary syndrome and mycosis fungoides (cutaneous T-cell lymphomas), haematological malignancies (lymphoma, leukaemia) and solid tumours (rectum, lung, colon, fallopian tubes)
- Infection: staphylococcal scalded-skin syndrome and human immunodeficiency virus (HIV) infection
- Other: graft-versus-host disease, and idiopathic disease

INITIAL INSTRUCTIONS OVER PHONE

The patient should be sat upright and given supplemental oxygen. Observations should be repeated to monitor for clinical deterioration and you can ask the nurse to swab any areas of the skin that are indicative of superimposed infection.

ASSESSMENT AND RESUSCITATION

- End of the bed assessment: the patient's skin is obviously erythematous and the patient appears distressed.
- Airway: patent.
- Breathing: RR 20 breaths per minute, SpO_2 95% on room air. On auscultation, there are diffuse bilateral crackles.
- Circulation: CRT 2 s, HR 82 bpm, regular, BP 120/79 mmHg, JVP not visible, HS I + II + 0.
- Disability: GCS 15/15, PEARL, temperature 35.5°C, CBG 4.5 mmol/L.
- Exposure: the erythema is covering >90% of the patient's body surface area and there is sparing of the oromucosal surfaces. Of note, there are scaly psoriatic plaques throughout the body surface, particularly over the extensor surfaces.

INITIAL INVESTIGATIONS

- Haematology: FBC (underlying infection, baseline haemoglobin (Hb) and eosinophilia)
- Biochemistry: U&Es and LFTs (electrolyte imbalance, metabolic derangements and hypoalbuminaemia)
- Radiology: chest X-ray (assess for consolidation, effusions, or signs of ARDS)
- Microbiology: blood cultures (bacteraemia) and skin swabs (superimposed skin infection)

MAKING A DIAGNOSIS

The diagnosis of erythroderma is by history and examination.

Once the patient is stable, you should elicit a careful history to try and establish the underlying cause. You should focus on recent medication use, pre-existing skin disease, history of any malignancy and conditions causing immunocompromise.

- Symptoms: red skin, pruritus, malaise, chills
- Signs: erythema initially occurs in patches but spreads to involve all, or nearly all, of the body surface area. Skin is warm and tender to touch; there is skin scaling 2–6 days after onset, onycholysis and lymphadenopathy

MANAGEMENT

The initial priority is to manage the systemic effects of skin failure. In this case, the bilateral crackles and respiratory distress are most likely due to ARDS, which is a known complication of erythroderma. Along with the hypothermia, this will require immediate escalation to the ICU.

The patient's medications should be reviewed and any unnecessary medications discontinued. The patient will also require careful monitoring of fluid balance and body temperature. Skin moisture can be maintained with wet wraps and emollients.

It is imperative to note that in the context of erythroderma due to psoriasis, corticosteroids should be avoided. Once the cause has been identified then specific treatment should be initiated after consultation with the on call dermatologist. If you suspect a new drug allergy then this should be clearly documented in the patient's notes and the patient will need to be issued with a MedicAlert bracelet.

The patient will also require careful monitoring of fluid balance and body temperature given the risk of skin failure. Appropriate IV access will need to be ensured, with catheterisation for strict input and output monitoring.

You should ensure that the patient has adequate regular and as-needed (PRN) analgesia and that low-molecular-weight heparin (LMWH) is prescribed for VTE prophylaxis. The patient will require daily review of his fluid requirements; this will depend upon oral intake, any loss of thermoregulation and consideration of insensible losses plus urine output.

If the patient has oromucosal involvement, he will need referral to the dietetics team for consideration of nasogastric feeding and to ensure daily calorific and nutritional requirements are met (approximately 25–30 kcal/kg/day).

ESCALATION

The patient should be referred to dermatology to ensure appropriate management of the erythroderma and any underlying skin disease. The patient should also be discussed with the medical registrar and ICU as there is the potential for sudden deterioration due to skin failure. Complications include thermodysregulation, electrolyte abnormalities, dehydration, high-output heart failure, secondary infections, ARDS and hypoalbuminaemia. The patient may require transfer to the burns unit for specialist care.

STATION 14.3: STEVENS–JOHNSON SYNDROME (SJS) AND TOXIC EPIDERMAL NECROLYSIS (TEN)

The Bleep Scenario

You are bleeped by the nurse to review a patient newly admitted to the AMU. He is a 36 year old man presenting with an extensive rash covering his arms, legs and face. He is also complaining of severe pain and is unable to eat or drink. He is normally fit and well (Fig. 14.4).

His observations are: HR 78 bpm, BP 110/850 mmHg, RR 17 breaths per minute, SpO_2 98% on room air and temperature 37.0°C.

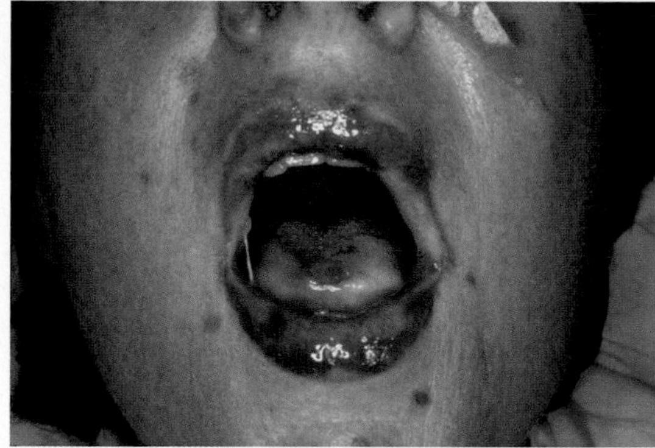

Fig. 14.4 Stevens-Johnson syndrome. (Source: Micheletti, R. G., James, W. D., Elston, D. M., & McMahon, P. J. (2023). *Andrews' Diseases of the Skin Clinical Atlas*. Elsevier Inc.)

DEFINITION

SJS and TEN are severe mucocutaneous reactions, usually to drugs, characterised by blistering and epithelial sloughing. SJS and TEN are both phenotypes of the same disease, the key difference being that SJS is the less extensive form of TEN.

INITIAL THOUGHTS

When presented with a rash, as with any emergency it is imperative to consider emergency skin dermatoses, hence SJS and TEN are important initial differentials.

In this scenario, even from the outset, there are factors pointing towards a skin emergency, which should trigger the need for your assessment:

- The extensive nature of the rash
- The severity of pain
- The patient's inability to eat and drink, indicating spread to the oromucosal surfaces

You should remember that most cases of SJS and TEN are drug-related

DIFFERENTIAL DIAGNOSIS

In a dermatological context, visual inspection is of major importance. However, you may wish to think about some of the other common differentials:

- Drug eruptions
- Immunobullous disease: pemphigus/pemphigoid
- Urticaria
- Eczema
- Psoriasis
- Rashes of an infectious origin

INITIAL INSTRUCTIONS OVER PHONE

You should ask the nurse to complete a further complete set of observations to check for haemodynamic instability due to insensible losses and loss of thermoregulation. You can ask for a swab of the skin to be taken to assess for any superimposed infection.

ASSESSMENT AND RESUSCITATION

- End of the bed assessment: patient appears to be in severe pain with extensive erosion of the mucosal surfaces covering the face, arms and legs.
- Airway: patent.
- Breathing: RR 17 breaths per minute, SpO_2 98% on room air. On auscultation, there is equal and bilateral air entry with vesicular breath sounds.
- Circulation: CRT 2 s, HR 78 bpm, regular, BP 100/80 mmHg, JVP normal, HS I + II + 0.
- Disability: GCS 15/15, PEARL, temperature 37.0°C, CBG 5.4 mmol/L.
- Exposure: erosive mucocutaneous rash covering the anterior and posterior surfaces of the arms and legs, and on examination completely covering the oromucosal region. Abdomen soft and non-tender, with normal bowel sounds.

INITIAL INVESTIGATIONS

- Haematology: FBC (underlying infection, baseline Hb)
- Biochemistry: U&Es (to exclude renal failure), magnesium and phosphate
- Radiology: chest X-ray (to exclude underlying infection)
- Microbiology: blood cultures (bacteraemia), skin swabs (superimposed infection) and mycoplasma serology (commonly associated infection)

MAKING A DIAGNOSIS

Once the patient is adequately resuscitated, a thorough history is essential.

You should ask specifically about recent drug or medicine use, recent bacterial or viral infection and vaccinations. Common comorbidities associated with SJS and TEN include seizures, systemic lupus erythematosus, acquired immunodeficiency syndrome (AIDS), collagen vascular disease and cancer.

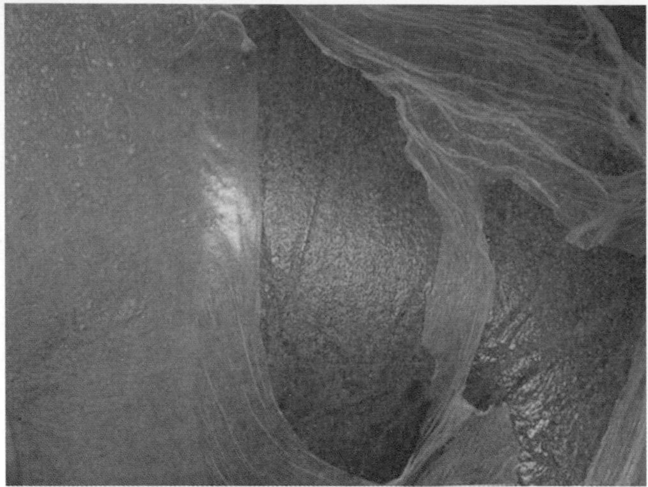

Fig. 14.5 Patient with toxic epidermal necrolysis. (Source: Micheletti, R.G. et al. [2022]. *Andrews' diseases of the skin clinical atlas*. Elsevier.)

Early on in the disease course, signs and symptoms may appear relatively mild. However, the extent of mucosal involvement typically progresses over several days. Patients who present with severe disease may also have mucosal involvement of the upper and lower respiratory tract that may lead to laryngeal stridor, along with oedema of the larynx and nasopharynx. Mucosal involvement may also involve erosions/ulceration of the eyes, lips, gastrointestinal, hepatobiliary and urogenital tract. Fig. 14.5 is an example of a patient with TEN.

- Symptoms: fever, diarrhoea, vomiting, dysuria, arthralgia and shortness of breath (depending on mucosal involvement of body systems)
- Signs: sudden rash (blisters / macules / flat atypical target lesions), diffuse erythema, Nikolsky's sign (epidermal layer sloughs off when pressure is applied), tongue swelling, enlarged lymph nodes, wheeze and signs of dehydration

MANAGEMENT

In this scenario, the most important initial step is to stop the causative agent, ensure it is clearly crossed off the drug chart and documented in the patient's notes. The patient should not be exposed to the causative agent again in the future. If there is suspicion of superimposed infection, you can initiate broad-spectrum IV antibiotics and consider topical antibiotics to any sloughy areas of skin. You should ensure that an emollient is prescribed for the entire skin surface; for example, 50/50 would be a reasonable option. The patient will also require a proton pump inhibitor to prevent gastrointestinal ulceration.

The patient will require careful monitoring of fluid balance and body temperature given the risk of skin failure. Appropriate IV access will need to be ensured, with catheterisation for strict input and output monitoring.

If the patient has oromucosal surface involvement, you should prescribe liquid paraffin for oral lubrication and consider benzydamine hydrochloride. The patient will also need referral to the dietetics team for consideration of nasogastric feeding and to ensure daily calorific and nutritional requirements are met (approximately 25–30 kcal/kg/day).

For patients with ocular involvement, you can prescribe an ocular lubricant such as sodium hyaluronate or carmellose eye drops. These patients should be discussed with opthalmology as they may require topical antibiotics.

For patients with urogenital surface involvement, you should prescribe white liquid paraffin for eroded surfaces and consider prescribing topical steroids for non-eroded areas.

Ensure that the patient has adequate regular and PRN analgesia and that LMWH is prescribed for VTE prophylaxis. The patient will require daily review of his IV fluid requirements; this will depend upon oral intake, any loss of thermoregulation and consideration of insensible losses plus urine output.

ESCALATION

Involve the on call dermatologist as soon as SJS/TEN is suspected. Additionally, any signs of ocular involvement must be discussed with an ophthalmologist. The patient may need transfer to an ICU or burns unit for further specialist care depending on the extent of skin involvement and/or the involvement of other organ systems.

FURTHER READING

Creamer, D., et al. (2016). UK guidelines for the management of Stevens–Johnson syndrome/toxic epidermal necrolysis 2016. *British Journal of Dermatology*, *174*, 1194–1227.

Dermnetz. (2008). *Dermatological emergencies: Erythroderma*. Available at: www.dermnetnz.org/cme/emergencies/erythroderma/. [Accessed 16 January 2022].

Dermnetz. (2016). *Drug hypersensitivity syndrome*. Available at: https://dermnetnz.org/topics/drug-hypersensitivity-syndrome/. [Accessed 16 January 2022].

Dermnetz (n.d.). *Drugs reported to cause erythroderma*. Available at. www.dermnetnz.org/topics/drugs-reported-to-cause-erythroderma. [Accessed 16 January 2022].

Reuler, J. B., Jones, S. R., & Girard, D. E. (1977). Hypothermia in the erythroderma syndrome. *Western Journal of Medicine*, *127*, 243–244.

Umar, S. H. (2020). *Erythroderma (generalized exfoliative dermatitis) treatment and management*. Available at: https://emedicine.medscape.com/article/1106906-treatment. [Accessed 16 January 2022].

Psychiatry

15

Content Outline

STATION 15.1: ACUTE ALCOHOL WITHDRAWAL

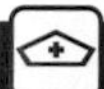

The Bleep Scenario

A ward sister bleeps you about a 52 year old man. He had surgery this afternoon, which was uncomplicated. He has since become extremely distraught, describing seeing snakes all over his bed. His observations are: heart rate (HR) 106 bpm, blood pressure (BP) 129/78 mmHg, respiratory rate (RR) 25 breaths per minute, SpO_2 98% on room air and temperature 38.1°C. You are asked to review the patient.

DEFINITION

Acute alcohol withdrawal is a set of physical and psychological symptoms experienced upon sudden reduction in alcohol intake in someone who has been drinking heavily for a prolonged period of time.

INITIAL THOUGHTS

You should consider causes of new visual hallucinations. This presentation may suggest an acute decompensation of a previously unknown psychotic disorder. Alternatively, this could be a postoperative delirium or secondary to withdrawal from drugs or alcohol.

DIFFERENTIAL DIAGNOSIS

- Medical: delirium, sepsis, postoperative and post-traumatic states, or hallucinogenic medication.
- Neurological: cerebral vascular disease, stroke, contusion, subdural haematoma, meningitis, encephalitis, ophthalmic disorders, or inner- or middle-ear disorders
- Psychiatric: alcohol withdrawal or intoxication, drug withdrawal or intoxication, schizophrenia, mood disorders, dementia, mania, or personality disorders
- Transient: sleep, food or sensory disturbances or deprivation, fatigue, prolonged isolation, chemical stimulation, or bereavement

INITIAL INSTRUCTIONS OVER PHONE

You should ask the nurse to reassure and orient the patient. Request observations if possible whilst being mindful of their own safety.

ASSESSMENT AND RESUSCITATION

- End of the bed assessment: The patient is sweating profusely and has a notable hand tremor.
- Airway: patent
- Breathing: RR 25 breaths per minute, SpO_2 98% on room air. On auscultation, there is equal and bilateral air entry with vesicular breath sounds.
- Circulation: capillary refill time (CRT) < 2 s, HR 106 bpm, BP 129/78 mmHg, heart sounds (HS) I + II + 0, no signs of dehydration
- Disability: Glasgow Coma Scale (GCS) 15/15, pupils equal and reactive to light (PEARL), temperature 38.1°C. Capillary blood glucose (CBG) 5.0 mmol/L
- Exposure: Abdomen is soft and non-tender, with normal bowel sounds. The patient has a catheter in situ.

INITIAL INVESTIGATIONS

- Bedside: electrocardiogram (ECG: tachycardic)
- Haematology: full blood count (FBC: anaemia or infection)
- Biochemistry: urea and electrolytes (U&Es), liver function tests (LFTs: alcoholic liver derangement), thyroid function tests (TFTs: myxoedema madness), C-reactive protein (CRP: infection), ethanol level (inebriation or withdrawal) and glucose (hypoglycaemia)

- Radiology: chest X-ray (CXR: infection)
- Urine sample: toxicology screen and infection

MAKING A DIAGNOSIS

It is important to take a meticulous social history, to ascertain the patient's alcohol intake. Along with the notable nausea and vomiting, the hallucinations are typical of alcohol withdrawal. The onset could be delayed by the anaesthesia from surgery. The diagnosis may be supported by findings such as abnormal LFTs or blood test results suggestive of malnutrition.

MANAGEMENT

You should obtain a thorough alcohol history. Failing that, try to get permission to gain a collateral history from the family. Use the Clinical Institute Withdrawal Assessment for Alcohol - Revised (CIWA-Ar) as an adjunct tool. Prescribe chlordiazepoxide (or another benzodiazepine, or carbamazepine, according to local policy) to be given four times a day (as well as, as needed) depending on the patient's CIWA-Ar score. A symptom triggered administration approach can also be used if the ward has the facilities for this.

- CIWA-Ar 10–14: give 25 mg.
- CIWA-Ar >15: give 50 mg.

Alcohol acts as a central nervous system suppressant via action on the GABAergic system. Therefore, in the absence of alcohol, the brain becomes hyperexcitable. For this reason, dose-reducing regimes of benzodiazepines allow control over dynamic changes in brain excitability and symptom control.

This state of increased excitability introduces a risk of epileptiform seizures, usually within 12–48 hours of abstinence. If this occurs, quick-acting benzodiazepines such as lorazepam help reduce the likelihood of further seizures. If this occurs while the patient is already receiving withdrawal treatment, escalate to a psychiatrist for review.

The patient may be at risk of Wernicke's encephalopathy and therefore prophylactic Pabrinex (B vitamins) is required: one pair of ampoules three times daily for 1 day. Ampoules should be dissolved in 100 mL NaCl 0.9% and infused over 30 minutes.

You should orient the patient in time with a clock in direct view, as well as appropriate lighting. Aim to attend to the patient at least three times a day for observations (or more frequently if concerned), even if he is asleep, including withdrawal scale, BP, pulse and RR.

Once the patient becomes stable, you should explain the withdrawal process and offer referral to alcohol services such as Alcoholics Anonymous.

Clinical Tip

Alcohol withdrawal begins 6–8 hours after the last drink and can occur before blood alcohol levels reach zero.

ESCALATION

You should escalate to the liaison psychiatry team under the following circumstances:

- If the urinary drug screen reveals the patient has taken other psychotropic drugs
- If the blood tests reveal hypokalaemia or hypocalcaemia
- If >300 mg chlordiazepoxide is required over the course of 24 hours
- If de-escalation methods are not able to control behavioural difficulties

The liaison team may wish to add antipsychotic medication.

STATION 15.2: ACUTE PSYCHOSIS

The Bleep Scenario

You are bleeped by the accident and emergency (A&E) department to review a young man. A friend has brought him in after he accused someone at a party of putting spiders under his skin. He is agitated and seems to be very paranoid. His observations are: HR 106 bpm, BP 148/101 mmHg, RR 22 breaths per minute, SpO_2 98% on room air and temperature of 38.4°C. You are asked to review the patient.

DEFINITION

Psychosis is a disorder of perception and thinking where sufferers do not usually attribute their symptoms to a mental disorder.

INITIAL THOUGHTS

The spiders under the skin indicate a tactile hallucination. The patient is also paranoid and may be experiencing persecutory delusions since he believes that someone has done this to him. A psychiatric history will reveal whether or not this is a first episode or a decompensating existing disorder.

Given the demographic of the patient and the fact that this began at a 'party', one could suspect amphetamine-induced psychosis. Lower on the list of differentials would be a first manifestation of schizophrenia or a delusional disorder. However, this is less likely as schizophrenia is usually characterised by auditory hallucinations, delusions and disorganised speech and behaviour.

DIFFERENTIAL DIAGNOSIS

- Medical: delirium, sepsis, postoperative and post-traumatic states, or hallucinogenic medication.
- Neurological: cerebral vascular disease, stroke, contusion, subdural haematoma, meningitis and encephalitis, ophthalmic disorders, or inner- or middle-ear disorders
- Psychiatric: alcohol withdrawal or intoxication, drug withdrawal or intoxication, schizophrenia, mood disorders, dementia, mania, or personality disorders

- Transient: sleep, food or sensory disturbances or deprivation, fatigue, prolonged isolation, chemical stimulation, or bereavement

INITIAL INSTRUCTIONS OVER PHONE

The patient is agitated and paranoid so whilst it is important to ask for observations, you should tell the nurse to use de-escalation methods and be mindful of their own safety.

ASSESSMENT AND RESUSCITATION

- End of bed assessment: The patient is clammy & sweating profusely.
- Airway: patent
- Breathing: RR 22 breaths per minute, SpO_2 98% on room air
- Circulation: CRT < 2 s, HR 106 beats per minute, BP 148/101 mmHg, HS I + II + 0
- Disability: GCS 15/15, pupils are equal but significantly dilated, temperature 38.4°C, CBG 5.3 mmol/L
- Exposure: abdomen is soft and non tender, with normal bowel sounds

INITIAL INVESTIGATIONS

- Bedside: ECG (myocardial infarction/arrhythmias)
- Haematology: FBC (anaemia or infection)
- Biochemistry: U&Es, LFTs (alcoholic liver derangement), TFTs (myxoedema madness), CRP (infection) and glucose (hypoglycaemia)
- Radiology: CXR (infection)
- Microbiology: urine for microscopy, culture and sensitivity (MCS: infection) and toxicology screen

MAKING A DIAGNOSIS

The history is suggestive of acute psychosis. The examination and test results are consistent with drug-induced psychosis.

MANAGEMENT

Amphetamine induced psychosis can persist or carry an increased risk of further psychosis for some time. As such, you should offer the patient an antipsychotic at the lowest therapeutic dose. Olanzapine and haloperidol are recommended. Olanzapine has been found to have the best outcome with the fewest extrapyramidal side effects. In the short term, however, the patient needs to be sedated. It is much safer to do this with benzodiazepines than with antipsychotics as a highly sedating antipsychotic can impede later discharge.

The patient requires regular observations, such as BP, temperature and pulse rate, as well as a fluid balance chart.

Once the patient is stable you need to discuss their drug use. It is also important that you refer the patient to the Early Intervention Service at the beginning of his admission to ensure adequate follow up.

Evidence suggests that this first episode may be followed by relapses and as such it is recommended that the patient continues on low dose olanzapine post-discharge. Furthermore, research has revealed that amphetamine induced psychosis produces a 'kindling' phenomenon whereby, after the first episode of psychosis, further use of substances carries a progressively increasing risk of additional psychotic episodes. For this reason, psychoeducation and engagement with the Early Intervention Service is vital.

ESCALATION

If the patient refuses treatment or is violent, you will need to escalate this to a liaison psychiatrist to consider a Mental Health Act assessment.

Furthermore, the urine drug screen may indicate polydrug intoxication. Crack cocaine and heroin are often used together; this is called snowballing or speedballing and requires escalation for expert intervention.

Clinical Tip

Acute psychosis due to amphetamine abuse is more likely to occur in males and with particular types of amphetamine. Crack cocaine carries a greater risk than intravenous (IV) or insufflated cocaine.

STATION 15.3: CAPACITY ASSESSMENT

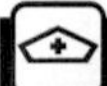

The Bleep Scenario

You are bleeped to the ward to review a 71 year old woman who has become aggressive and refused further IV antibiotics for hospital acquired pneumonia. She was originally admitted for radiotherapy for leptomeningeal disease. Her observations are: HR 88bpm, BP 139/84 mmHg, RR 22 breaths per minute, SpO_2 94% on 15L of oxygen and temperature 38.6°C. You are asked to review her.

DEFINITION

Capacity describes the ability to make decisions for yourself. It involves four main aspects:

- Understanding the information that is relevant to the decision to be made
- Retaining the information for long enough to be able to make the decision
- Weighing up the information available to make the decision
- Communicating the decision by any possible means. This may include talking, using sign language or through simple muscle movements such as blinking an eye or squeezing a hand

INITIAL THOUGHTS

The patient's decision to end treatment contravenes medical advice. This will prompt you to question if she lacks capacity at this time. In this case, the patient is known to have leptomeningeal disease. The aggression and fever in this context is suggestive of delirium, which may be impairing the patient's capacity.

DIFFERENTIAL DIAGNOSIS

- Medical: delirium, sepsis, postoperative and post-traumatic states, or hallucinogenic medication.
- Neurological: cerebral vascular disease, stroke, tumour, contusion, subdural haematoma, meningitis and encephalitis, ophthalmic disorders, inner or middle ear disorders
- Psychiatric: alcohol withdrawal or intoxication, drug withdrawal or intoxication, schizophrenia, mood disorders, dementia, mania, or personality disorders
- Transient: sleep, food or sensory disturbances or deprivation, fatigue, prolonged isolation, chemical stimulation, or bereavement.

INITIAL INSTRUCTIONS OVER PHONE

You should ask the nurse to contact the patient's next of kin to see if it will aid the patient's understanding. If the patient is still aggressive, you should ask the nurse to try to de-escalate the situation and if possible to repeat a full set of observations.

ASSESSMENT AND RESUSCITATION

- End of bed assessment: The patient is sweating profusely.
- Airway: patent.
- Breathing: RR 22 breaths per minute, SpO_2 94% on 15 L O_2, auscultation reveals crackles throughout the right lung field.
- Circulation: CRT < 2 s, HR 88 bpm, BP 139/84 mmHg, HS I + II + 0.
- Disability: GCS 15, PEARL, CBG 5.8 mmol/L, temperature 38.6°C.
- Exposure: abdomen is soft and non-tender, with normal bowel sounds.

INITIAL INVESTIGATIONS

- Haematology: FBC (leukocytosis)
- Biochemistry: U&Es, CRP (inflammatory marker), LFTs (biochemical baseline), arterial blood gas (respiratory failure)
- Microbiology: sputum for MCS, blood cultures, urinary antigens (*Legionella*, pneumococcal antigens), urine for MCS and toxicology
- Radiology: CXR (lobar or multilobar infiltrates)

MANAGEMENT

You should conduct a capacity assessment on the patient to determine if she is able to make this decision. The first stage determines if there is disturbance in the functioning of the person's mind or brain. We can reasonably assume that this is the case because of the history of leptomeningeal disease and the indications for possible delirium. The second stage involves determining if the impairment is sufficient enough to prevent her from making this particular decision. You should consider four factors when assessing this stage:

1. Is she able to understand information relevant to the decision to stop treatment?
2. Is she able to retain this information?
3. Can she weigh up the information and consider the risks of all courses of action in making the decision?
4. Is she able to communicate her decision back to you, by whatever means?

If she is deemed to lack capacity, you should employ methods that may encourage capacity, including presenting the information in a different way, inviting someone the patient knows and trusts to help or trying to discuss the matter at a time or place where the patient will be most likely to understand. You have called for the next of kin. In the meantime you should stabilise the patient and offer as much treatment as she will agree to.

The Mental Capacity Act (2005) has five key principles:

1. We must assume by default that an individual has capacity.
2. We cannot treat someone as lacking capacity unless all reasonable measures have been taken to help them make a decision, with no success.
3. Our judgement of a decision as irrational does not mean a patient lacks capacity.
4. Decisions made on the patient's behalf must be made in their best interest.
5. Decisions made for a patient must be the least restrictive of freedom as possible.

ESCALATION

All doctors should be able to assess capacity. You should escalate if you require assistance to assess capactity or to optimise a factor that may be inhibiting capacity.

If the lack of capacity is accompanied by aggression or risks to others or self, you should consider sedation or a Deprivation of Liberty Act as appropriate, if the patient cannot be treated under the Mental Capacity Act or the Mental Health Act. This decision will require multidisciplinary input.

Patients can be treated under the Mental Capacity Act if there is restriction to, rather than deprivation of, their liberty. If a patient lacks capacity, you should seek the views of their next of kin, or consult the lasting power of attorney for healthcare decisions and/or respect previously expressed views made in advance directives.

 Clinical Tip

Capacity assessments are time-specific and only apply to a specific decision. Capacity should therefore be reassessed separately for each decision to be made.

STATION 15.4: DELIRIUM

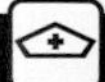 The Bleep Scenario

The nurse on your ward calls you about a 67 year old man who requires a review. He was admitted yesterday to be treated for CURB-65 score 3 community acquired pneumonia. He has ripped out his cannula and became disoriented and aggressive when the nursing staff attempted to replace it. His observations are: HR 89 bpm, BP 136/92 mmHg, RR 21 breaths per minute, SpO_2 95% on room air and temperature 38.1°C. You are asked to review the patient.

DEFINITION

Delirium is an acute state of global brain dysfunction characterised by fluctuating mental state, inattention and altered behaviour.

INITIAL THOUGHTS

It is likely the patient is delirious due to the community-acquired pneumonia. His age, infection, pain and potential hypoxia are all precipitants of this disorder. You should also consider other factors such as polypharmacy or electrolyte abnormalities.

DIFFERENTIAL DIAGNOSIS

- Medical: delirium, sepsis, postoperative and post-traumatic states, or hallucinogenic medication.
- Neurological: cerebral vascular disease, stroke, tumour, contusion, subdural haematoma, meningitis and encephalitis, ophthalmic disorders, inner or middle ear disorders
- Psychiatric: alcohol withdrawal or intoxication, drug withdrawal or intoxication, schizophrenia, mood disorders, dementia, or mania
- Transient: sleep, food or sensory disturbances or deprivation, fatigue, prolonged isolation, chemical stimulation, or acute grief

INITIAL INSTRUCTIONS OVER PHONE

Ask the nurse to try to de-escalate the situation, if it is safe to do so, and if possible, repeat a full set of observations.

ASSESSMENT AND RESUSCITATION

- End of bed assessment: the patient seems to be distressed and agitated at the bedside.
- Airway: patent.
- Breathing: RR 21 breaths per minute, SpO_2 95% on room air, auscultation reveals crackles in the left upper zone.
- Circulation: BP 135/92 mmHg, HR 89 bpm, CRT < 2 s.
- Disability: temperature is 38.1°C, GCS 14/15, PEARL, CBG 6.8 mmol/L.
- Exposure: abdomen soft and non-tender, normal bowel sounds.

INITIAL INVESTIGATIONS

- Bedside: ECG (arrhythmias/myocardial infarction)
- Haematology: FBC (leukocytosis)
- Biochemistry: U&Es (urea part of CURB-65 score), CRP (inflammatory marker), LFTs
- Microbiology: sputum for MCS, blood cultures, urinary antigens (*Legionella*, pneumococcal antigens)
- Radiology: CXR (lobar or multilobar infiltrates)

 Clinical Tip

Note that any patient with a known cognitive impairment automatically receives 1 point for confusion on the CURB-65 score.

MAKING A DIAGNOSIS

The history and examination findings are suggestive of delirium secondary to severe pneumonia. Infection is a known precipitant of delirium. Remember there are many other causes of delirium, as demonstrated in Table 15.1.

MANAGEMENT

You should check previous cognitive assessments (Abbreviated Mental Test Score (AMTS), Mini-Mental State Examination (MMSE)) and use the confusion assessment method (CAM) tool to diagnose delirium. If uncertain of the diagnosis, you should treat it as delirium first. A multidisciplinary team approach is crucial to managing the condition. Patients will need one-to-one observation.

Conservative management is important. You should create a calming care environment with lighting appropriate to the time of day and accurate clocks in view of the patient. The patient should not be moved unless it is unavoidable, to help him to maintain a sense of familiarity. The team should interact with the patient regularly to keep him oriented in time and place, and allow visits from next of kin as well as doing stimulating activities. Triggers such as poor nutrition, poor sleep, sensory impairment, poor mobility, dehydration, constipation and pain should be addressed as much as possible.

Examination of the patient may reveal a precipitating factor and you should direct your management towards

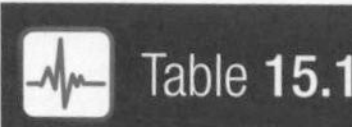

Table 15.1 DELIRIUMS mnemonic for treatable causes of delirium

Drugs
Emotional
Low PO_2 Anaemia Pulmonary embolism Myocardial infarction Stroke
Infection
Retention of urine and faeces
Ictal states
Undernutrition/dehydration
Metabolic disorders, including organ failure
Subdural

Source: Flaherty, J.H. and Morley, J.E. (2004) Delirium: a call to improve current standards of care. *The Journals of Gerontology: Series A*, *59*(4), pp. M341–M343.

addressing this. In this instance, you should give oxygen therapy and treat the patient's fever. You should also assess the patient's pain and give appropriate analgesia. The patient's infection may be resistant to the antibiotics, in which case you should check cultures and sensitivities to determine if you can offer a more specific treatment.

Sedation should be avoided unless the patient is a risk to himself and/or others and cannot be calmed down using more conservative approaches. If sedatives are used, it should be on a short term basis and reviewed at regular intervals.

Haloperidol is contraindicated for sedation under certain circumstances, including a history of Parkinson's disease, seizures or Lewy body dementia. It should also be avoided if the ECG reveals a QTc >470 ms or if the patient is too agitated to get a reliable ECG. Olanzapine at the lowest possible dose can be used (under specialist guidance) if haloperidol is contraindicated.

If there are no contraindications, prescribe the minimum dose required to sedate the patient. Dose required for sedation with oral haloperidol is age-dependent:

- >65 years: initially 0.5 mg (maximum 5 mg in 24 hours)
- 18–64 years: 1–10 mg in 1-3 divided doses , treatment should be started at the lowest possible dose and adjusted in increments at 2–4 hourly intervals if required

Delirium may take some time to resolve even once the acute trigger is addressed. Continue to monitor the patient and ensure there is a calm environment to help with the recovery process.

ESCALATION

If investigations reveal a complex organic cause you may need to bleep the on call specialist registrar to assist. For example, delirium may be the only manifestation of ischaemic heart disease in an older person. If the ECG reveals this, you should escalate.

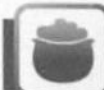

Clinical Tip

One third of delirium is preventable. Any patients presenting with any of the following risk factors require close supervision to prevent delirium and its sequelae: age >65, hip fracture, cognitive impairment, or deterioration of a severe illness. See Fig. 15.1 for an overview of risk factors.

STATION 15.5: SUICIDE RISK ASSESSMENT

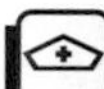

The Bleep Scenario

A 23 year old man who presented to A&E earlier is trying to leave the hospital. He had presented to the department after his partner found him with a self inflicted deep laceration on his right forearm and he is now attempting to leave before being formally assessed. His observations are: HR 92 bpm, BP 110/68 mmHg, RR 20 breaths per minute, SpO_2 96% on room air and temperature 37.5°C.

DEFINITION

Suicide is any act that deliberately brings about one's own death.

INITIAL THOUGHTS

You should be concerned about this patient's risk of suicide. Although this event was not intended to be fatal, there is an increased risk of committing suicide in the future. You should also consider what risk factors are present. In this case, the patient is male and in the 15–30 year age group.

INITIAL INSTRUCTIONS OVER PHONE

You should ask the nurse to do their best to comfort the patient until you arrive. In addition, ask for the patient to be moved to a private area for your consultation so he is more likely to engage.

ASSESSMENT AND RESUSCITATION

- End of bed assessment: the patient looks unkempt and there is a strong smell of alcohol.
- Airway: patent
- Breathing: RR 20 breaths per minute, SpO_2 96% on room air
- Circulation: CRT 3 s, BP 110/68 mmHg, HR 92 bpm
- Disability: PEARL, CBG 6.0 mmol/L, GCS 15. Temperature 37.5°C
- Exposure: exposure reveals the laceration has been sutured and dressed. You also notice scars from previous lacerations.

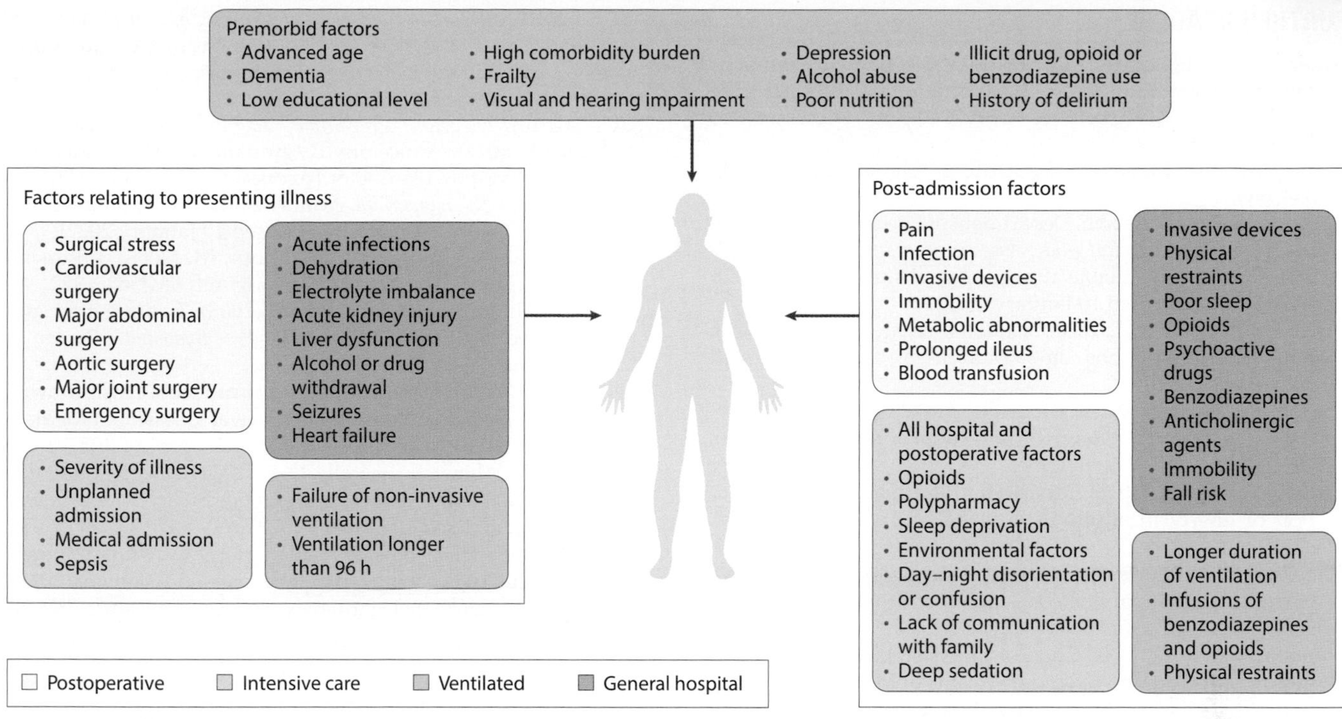

Fig. 15.1 Risk factors for delirum. (Source: Wilson, J.E. et al. [2020]. Delirium. *Nature Reviews Disease Primers, 6*, p. 90.)

MANAGEMENT

In order to manage this patient you will first have to conduct a thorough risk assessment, which involves four components:

1. Assess each of the components of suicide: ideation, intent, plan, access to lethal means, history of past suicide attempt
2. Evaluation of risk factors of suicide
3. Evaluation of the patient's current experience
4. Identification of potential targets for intervention

More than 700,000 people across the world die due to suicide every year. The greatest risk factor is a previous suicide attempt. Evidence suggests that men are three times more likely to commit suicide and tend to use more violent methods, such as firearms and hanging. In England and Wales, suicide is the leading cause of death in men aged 20–34 years in 2020 and suicide is most common amongst people aged 45–54 years old. Self-harm is associated with a 50–100 fold increased risk of future suicide. It is crucial to note that asking a patient about suicide or self-harm does not increase their risk.

Pathophysiology involves complex interactions between genetic and environmental factors. Evidence points towards a significant influence from serotonin system dysfunction. Neuroimaging studies indicate that suicidal behaviour is associated with structural and functional changes in parts of the prefrontal cortex involved with complex decision making and problem solving.

You should use your assessment to direct subsequent action. In the short term this may simply involve encouraging family and friend input or inpatient monitoring. If the risk assessment reveals psychiatric comorbidity (such as acute psychosis) or substance dependence, short term treatment with benzodiazepines may be indicated. The consequences of self harm and underlying physical illnesses should also be treated.

All patients who present in this way should be reviewed by the liaison psychiatry team, and may need admission under the Mental Health Act, or may be admitted voluntarily under the mental health team. They will also need follow up from the community mental health team or their general practitioner on discharge.

Management of these patients should include developing a safety plan for discharge, arranging ongoing psychosocial support and treatment for underlying psychiatric illness, if applicable. Safety plans should include reducing access to means of suicide, and increasing social support.

ESCALATION

It may be necessary to escalate to the on call mental health team if the patient is at serious risk and requires sectioning under the Mental Health Act. Indications include:

- The patient is still threatening to hurt or kill himself
- You become aware that he is looking for ways to kill himself
- The patient is seeking access to lethal means such as weapons or pills

FURTHER READING

Baker, C. (2021). *Suicide: summary of statistics*. House of Commons Library. Available at: https://researchbriefings.files.parliament.uk/documents/CBP-7749/CBP-7749.pdf. [Accessed 10 January 2022].

Byrne, P. (2007). Managing the acute psychotic episode. *BMJ, 334*, 686.

Centre for Suicide Research, Department of Psychiatry, University of Oxford (n.d.) *Clinical guide: Assessment of suicide risk in people with depression.* Available at: www.dpt.nhs.uk/download/2hn1ZTaUXY (accessed 10 January 2022).

Cole-King, A., & Oates, A. (2020). *Suicide risk management*. Available at: https://bestpractice.bmj.com/topics/en-gb/3000095. [Accessed 10 January 2022].

Curran, C., Byrappa, N., & McBride, A. (2004). Stimulant psychosis: systematic review. *British Journal of Psychiatry, 185*(3), 196–204.

Cutter, W. J., et al. (2011). Identifying and managing deprivation of liberty in adults in England and Wales. *BMJ, 342*, c7323.

Flaherty, J. H., & Morley, J. E. (2004). Delirium: A call to improve current standards of care. *The Journals of Gerontology: Series A, 59*(4), M341–M343.

Mental Capacity Act 2005 Code of practice. Available at: www.gov.uk/government/uploads/system/uploads/attachment_data/file/497253/Mental-capacity-act-code-of-practice.pdf (accessed 10 January 2022).

NICE. (2010). *Alcohol-use disorders: Diagnosis and management of physical complications*. Available at: www.nice.org.uk/guidance/cg100/chapter/Recommendations#acute-alcohol-withdrawal. [Accessed 10 January 2022].

NICE. (2010). *Delirium: Prevention, diagnosis and management*. Available at: www.nice.org.uk/guidance/cg103/evidence/full-guideline-pdf-134653069. [Accessed 10 January 2022].

NICE. (2021). *BNF haloperidol*. Available at: https://bnf.nice.org.uk/drug/haloperidol.html. [Accessed 10 January 2022].

Nicholson, T. R. J., Cutter, W., & Hotopf, M. (2008). Assessing mental capacity: The Mental Capacity Act. *BMJ, 336*, 322.

Shoptaw, S. J., Kao, U., & Ling, W. W. (2008). Treatment for amphetamine psychosis. *Cochrane Database Systematic Review, 4*, CD003026.

Sullivan, J. T., et al. (1989). Assessment of alcohol withdrawal: The revised clinical institute withdrawal assessment for alcohol scale (CIWA-Ar). *British Journal of Addiction, 84*, 1353–1357.

Warner, K. R., Weiner, E., & Kelly, D. L. (2021). *Brief psychotic disorder*. Available at: https://bestpractice.bmj.com/topics/en-gb/1118. [Accessed 10 January 2022].

WHO. (2021). *Fact sheet: Suicide*. Available at: www.who.int/news-room/fact-sheets/detail/suicide. [Accessed 10 January 2022].

Wilson, J. E., et al. (2020). Delirium. *Nature Reviews Disease Primers, 6*, 90.

Palliative Care

16

Content Outline

STATION 16.1: BREAKING BAD NEWS

The Bleep Scenario

An 85 year old female on the ward, Mrs Jones, has received results from a computed tomography (CT) scan, showing widespread metastatic cancer. You are on call and are contacted to review the scan and discuss the findings with the patient and her family.

DEFINITION

Breaking bad news can be one of the hardest as well as the most rewarding things you do as a doctor. Patients and relatives remember these conversations for the rest of their lives, so doing it well can make a big difference. There are some straightforward steps that can be adapted for each patient and family.

Clinical Tip

Shadow senior colleagues to gain confidence and tips. If you feel out of your depth, ask a senior member of staff to lead the discussion or ask them to observe you and give you feedback to improve your skills.

INITIAL THOUGHTS

Your response depends on your relationship with the patient. If this is an 'out-of-hours' request for a patient you are unfamiliar with, it may be more appropriate for her regular ward team in hours to deliver this news.

If the patient is under your care, and you feel comfortable explaining this, familiarise yourself with the patient's admission and check the CT report to ensure you are giving accurate information. If in any doubt, liaise with a senior colleague.

ASSESSMENT

GATHER INFORMATION

What was Mrs Jones' initial presentation to the hospital? What has she been told so far?

Mrs Jones is an 85 year old grandmother who lives at home with her husband of 50 years and a close family network. She attended hospital with weight loss, shortness of breath and difficulties mobilising. She is worried it might be cancer. The CT scan shows a large lung mass suspicious of cancer with multiple deposits within the liver and peritoneum, consistent with metastases.

WHAT ARE THE NEXT STEPS?

The oncologists will need contacting and the images discussed at a multidisciplinary team meeting. The notes suggest a poor performance status and, given the extent of disease, management options are likely to be palliative. You think it is unlikely she would tolerate further invasive investigations.

Clinical Tip

Tools such as SPICT (Supportive and Palliative Care Identifiers Tool) aid in identifying deteriorating patients who may benefit from palliative care. Timely use of this can help patients access appropriate support early.

GAIN CONSENT

Check before starting whether the patient, firstly, wants to hear about the scan results, and secondly, wants her next of kin to be involved. Ensure she has capacity for this decision.

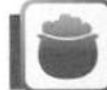

Clinical Tip

You may be asked by well-meaning relatives 'not' to disclose bad news to their loved ones. In a patient with capacity, this is illegal and unethical. However, phrasing it like that is not appropriate! Gently explain it is your duty to deliver information to any patient with capacity (providing the patient wishes to hear it) but reassure them you will offer the patient the opportunity for family to be present.

EFFECTIVE COMMUNICATION

There are different structures that can help to deliver bad news. A popular one is the SPIKES framework:

setting, perception, invitation, knowledge, empathy, strategy and summary.

SETTING

- A quiet, private room is preferable – with tissues available.
- Give your bleep to a colleague and ask staff to avoid disturbing you.

PERCEPTION

- Check understanding of the admission so far – does the patient know why the scan was requested?
- Use open questions and avoid jargon.

INVITATION

- Check how much the patient wants to know – do not force information on someone who does not wish to hear it.

KNOWLEDGE

- Offer a warning shot such as 'I'm afraid I have some bad news'.
- Gently explain in language appropriate to the patient and try to avoid euphemisms as these can be misinterpreted. Use clear language. Saying 'tumour' or 'mass' without 'cancer' can be ambiguous.
- Give Mrs Jones and her family time to digest this news. When she is ready, answer her questions and provide information about the next steps (including timescale).
- Ensure they know that support is available.

Clinical Tip

In patients whose first language is not English, a well-briefed professional interpreter should be used. Remember to look at the patient while you are speaking, rather than the interpreter. Preparing the interpreter in advance for the conversation, and debriefing with them afterwards, may help improve translation quality and interpreter well-being.

EMPATHY

- Acknowledge emotions – these can be wide-ranging and often unexpected.
- Use both verbal and non-verbal communication to demonstrate you care. Avoid closed body language and utilise eye contact appropriately.

STRATEGY AND SUMMARY

- Gently check understanding.
- Summarise the plan going forward.
- Offer a time to talk through any further questions.

Clinical Tip

A cup of tea can go a long way! It establishes connection and warmth between doctor and patient and is often greatly appreciated.

MANAGEMENT

Be prepared for grief. Amongst other feelings, it can manifest as anger, denial or depression. Provide space for release of emotions. Involvement of oncology/palliative care teams and referral for counselling may be helpful.

Acknowledging the emotional impact of these conversations on yourself will help maintain your well-being. Remember to debrief if you need to.

STATION 16.2: DEATH: THE LEGALITIES

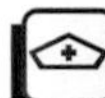

The Bleep Scenario

A patient on the acute medical unit ward has died. He has a do not attempt cardiopulmonary resuscitation (DNACPR) order in place and his death was expected. You are asked to verify the death.

DEFINITION

Death is the irreversible loss of capacity for consciousness and respiratory function. Confirmation can be made using either circulatory criteria following cardiorespiratory arrest, or neurological criteria in those who are brain-dead.

The latter requires two sets of brainstem function testing and includes patients who are mechanically ventilated. It is the former that you will be asked to do as a junior doctor.

Clinical Tip

Some patients may have expressed a wish for their body to be used for organ or tissue donation. Internal organs can only be retrieved in patients on life support machines who have been declared 'brain-dead'. However, tissues such as bone, tendons, corneas and heart valves, can be harvested up to 24 hours post-death in patients without contraindications. A transplant coordinator is available 24/7 to advise.

INITIAL THOUGHTS

Ensure this is an expected death and that a DNACPR order is in place.

ASSESSMENT

Before reviewing the patient, check the notes to confirm trajectory of illness and treatment limitations.

Try to ascertain: did the patient express any wishes regarding care after death or organ donation?

DEATH VERIFICATION

Often family and friends will be present, and it is important to express empathy and explain what you are

Table 16.1 An example of how a death certificate might be completed

SECTION	DISEASE/CONDITION
1a.	End-stage renal failure
1b.	Hypertensive nephropathy
1c.	Hypertension
2.	Insulin-dependent diabetes mellitus

about to do. Offer the opportunity for them to step outside if they would prefer. Exact guidelines for timing vary from trust to trust, so check local policy, but official guidelines suggest the patient must be observed for a minimum of 5 minutes:

- Feel for central pulse (carotid artery).
- Auscultate for heart sounds for 2 minutes.
- Auscultate for breath sounds for 3 minutes.
- Use a pen torch to check pupillary reaction – pupils will be fixed and dilated.
- Check response to voice and pain or pressure, e.g. by trapezius squeeze.
- Document the above in the notes, with the time and date you confirmed the death.

MANAGEMENT

DEATH CERTIFICATION

In the hospital setting, the cause of death should be discussed with the consultant in charge of the patient's care, before issuing a certificate.

Death certificates are legally required to be completed within 5 days (except in cases of coroner referrals and inquests).

Clinical Tip

It is important to record the cause of death accurately as the information is collected by the Office for National Statistics and used to target medical interventions based on frequency of underlying causes of death.

Filling out the death certificate can be complicated. Some death certificates will require information in all sections (1a–c, 2); others will only require a cause of death in section 1a (Table 16.1).

1a. Disease / condition leading directly to death
1b. Other disease / condition, if any, leading to 1a
1c. Other disease / condition, if any, leading to 1b
2. Other diseases / injuries / conditions contributing to the death but not related to the disease or causing it

Clinical Tip

Avoid 'modality of death' (e.g. respiratory arrest) or 'organ failure' (e.g. cardiac failure) alone, without comment on the condition leading to these. Also avoid abbreviations. Ask the bereavement office if unsure.

CORONER REFERRAL

Some deaths need referral to a coroner. The list below is not exhaustive and if unclear, discuss with your consultant or medical examiner. The following would warrant referral:

- Deaths due to:
  - Accident / suicide
  - Violence / neglect
  - Industrial disease
- Other:
  - Deaths during / secondary to an operation
  - Deaths in / shortly after release from police / prison custody
  - Cause of death unknown

FURTHER MANAGEMENT

Some patients will choose to have a burial or a cremation. An additional form is required for cremations, to be completed by a medical practitioner. These require additional details, including a summary of the patient's admission, any operations in the year before death, any concerns you have about the death and any implants (e.g. pacemaker) which may be hazardous to cremation staff if not removed.

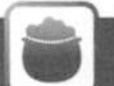

Clinical Tip

Many cultures and religions have certain rituals or beliefs that should be accommodated as far as practicable, if these happened to be important to the patient. For example, traditionally, in Islam, the dead should be buried within 24 h, and this may require the body to be released promptly.

STATION 16.3: PALLIATIVE CARE

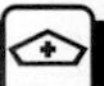

The Bleep Scenario

A 57 year old woman on the wards appears agitated. She has stage 4 breast cancer, with no more oncological interventions available. She has deteriorated over the last few days, and the ward team have documented that they feel she may be dying.

The consultant spoke to her family today to discuss treatment limitations. You are asked to review her.

DEFINITION

Palliative care is the targeted delivery of care to patients with non-curable conditions, with the aim of improving quality of life. This requires a holistic approach to address physical, psychological and spiritual needs to support those with advanced, incurable illness to 'live while they die'.

Palliative care is offered to patients with a broad range of diagnoses, with prognoses varying from days to years. Generalist palliative care can be provided by most healthcare professionals, with assistance from specialists for patients with complex needs.

Clinical Tip

The Department of Health's '5 priorities of care' for the dying patient support compassionate care for patients who are dying:

1. Recognise the possibility that a person may be dying.
2. Communicate effectively with the dying person and their loved ones.
3. Involve the dying person and their loved ones in decision making and care.
4. Support a patient's loved ones and listen to their needs.
5. Do create an individualised care plan.

INITIAL THOUGHTS

This woman may be reaching the end-of-life phase. She could be agitated for a variety of reasons, both related to and unrelated to her primary diagnosis. She will need a full assessment.

It is vital to review her notes to ascertain what investigations and conversations the ward team have had with her and her family. Her treatment limitations will need to be established.

DIFFERENTIAL DIAGNOSIS

- Cancer complications: pain, hypercalcaemia and cerebral metastases
- Medications: side effects and interactions, e.g. opioids, benzodiazepines and chemotherapy agents
- Medical: infection, constipation, urinary retention, acute renal / liver failure, hypoxia and electrolyte imbalance
- Environmental: unfamiliar surroundings and fear

INITIAL INSTRUCTIONS OVER PHONE

Ask the nurse if any pain and anxiolytic medications have been prescribed and whether the patient could receive one of these prior to your review. Establish whether a DNACPR order and/or a treatment escalation plan have been recorded. Clarify if there is an advance care plan or advance decision to refuse treatment.

Clinical Tip

- A DNACPR form aims to avoid circumstances of inappropriate CPR. It is a medical decision, made in discussion with the patient.
- An Advance Care Plan sets out a patient's wishes and priorities about their future care.
- An Advance Decision to Refuse Treatment (ADRT) is a legally binding document stating a patient's wishes to refuse certain treatments

ASSESSMENT AND RESUSCITATION

- End of the bed assessment: patient looks uncomfortable, grimacing, pointing to the site of her breast lesion.
- Airway: patent.
- Breathing: respiratory rate (RR) 25 breaths per minute, SpO_2 96% on room air, left-sided chest drain in situ for malignant pleural effusion (swinging). On auscultation, there are vesicular breath sounds.
- Circulation: heart rate (HR) 100 bpm, blood pressure (BP) 120/80 mmHg, heart sounds (HS) I + II + 0.
- Disability: Glasgow Coma Scale (GCS) 14/15, confused, temperature 36.8°C, capillary blood glucose (CBG) 6.0 mmol/L.
- Exposure: her abdomen is soft and non-tender with normal bowel sounds. Stool chart documents bowel last opened yesterday. Fluid chart documents 1l negative in the last 24 hours. No vomiting.

Clinical Tip

Observations may not be helpful if someone is actively dying, and it is important to assess whether these are appropriate before undertaking them. However, sometimes they may help exclude and correct reversible causes of symptoms, e.g. hypoxia causing delirium e.g. hypoxia causing delerium and should be tailored to the needs of the patient.

INITIAL INVESTIGATIONS

Consider whether the following investigations are appropriate or not.

- Bedside: bladder scan
- Haematology: full blood count (FBC: infection)
- Biochemistry: urea and electrolytes (U&Es), liver function tests (LFTs) for renal/liver failure Ca^{2+}. Mg^{2+}, PO_4, C-reactive protein (CRP: inflammation)
- Microbiology: blood and urine cultures (infection)
- Radiology: chest X-ray (consolidation), abdominal X-ray (obstruction), CT head (cerebral metastases)

MAKING A DIAGNOSIS

Consider if this is terminal agitation in a patient who is dying.

- Signs a patient may be dying include: changes in skin colour, cool extremities, Cheyne–Stokes breathing (irregular breathing characterised by pauses, followed by progressively deeper breathing), reduced or no oral intake, deteriorating swallow, change in continence and agitation unexplained by reversible causes

MANAGEMENT

Management should be targeted to the cause of symptoms and tailored to the need of the patient.

End-of-life injectable medications are generally prescribed in the last weeks or days of life, when it is anticipated that the oral route is not going to be available in the near future.

Remember that dosage of injectable opioids will vary depending on previous opioid doses.

Choice of end-of-life medication used varies between trusts. Table 16.2 is an example of a common selection of subcutaneous medications.

Table 16.2 A common anticipatory mediciation regime

SYMPTOM	EXAMPLE DRUG	PRN DOSE
Pain / breathlessness	Morphine sulfate N.B.: Caution: renal impairment	2.5 mg –5 mg SC hourly (or 1/6th of the 24-h SC opioid requirement)
Agitation	Midazolam* N.B.: Caution: renal impairment	2.5 mg–5 mg SC hourly
Nausea / vomiting	Levomepromazine	2.5 mg–6.25 mg SC 4-hourly
Chest secretions	Hyoscine butylbromide**	20 mg SC 2-hourly

PRN, as needed; SC, subcutaneously.
*Max dose of Midazolam in 24 hours = 30 mg (higher doses with specialist advice).
**Max dose of Hyoscine Butylbromide in 24 hours = 120 mg.

Table 16.3 Opioid conversions

MEDICATION	CODEINE	ORAL MORPHINE	SC MORPHINE	SC DIAMORPHINE
Equivalent dose	60 mg	6 mg	3 mg	2 mg
Conversion from oral morphine	× 10	–	÷ 2	÷ 3

SC, subcutaneous.

Table 16.4 Non-pharmacological management of breathlessness

Physiotherapy	Optimum positioning	• Drain secretions • Reduce work of breathing
	Breathing techniques, e.g. ABCT – active breathing cycle techniques	• ABCT is a three-phase technique to help clear secretions
	Non-invasive ventilation	• May assist in some cases, e.g. motor neurone disease
Occupational therapy	Energy conservation (5 Ps)	• Prioritising, planning, pacing, positioning, permission
	Adaptive equipment	• Such as perching stools
Relaxation/other techniques	'The calming hand'	• Five-stage method following the five fingers to help calm a breathless patient
	Fans/open windows	• Improve air circulation and may improve symptoms

Discuss these medications with the patient and her family, explaining their purpose and side effects, and work closely with the nursing team to ensure effectiveness is monitored.

If there are frequent medication requirements, a syringe driver may be used. Ask for assistance from your local specialist palliative care team if unsure how or when to prescribe.

Prescribing Tip

Check the most recent renal function tests as medications may need changing or the dose adjusting. Don't forget allergies and contraindications (Table 16.3).

Clinical Tip

Intravenous, subcutaneous fluids, or clinically assisted hydration towards the end of life is an emotive subject and there is a limited evidence base. It may improve delirium or myoclonus, but worsen oedema and effusions. There is little evidence to suggest it improves symptoms or survival. Seek senior support if requested by the family or patient. Wet sponges to moisten the lips can provide symptomatic relief of a dry mouth.

NON-PHARMACOLOGICAL MANAGEMENT OF BREATHLESSNESS

Dyspnoea can be secondary to a variety of different causes, and treatment will depend on aetiology. In addition to medications, consider non-pharmacological strategies (Table 16.4).

Other things to consider:

1. Is the patient about to die? Ensure her family are aware. Consider moving her to a side room and ensure her family and friends have open visiting access. A chaplain may be contacted to address any spiritual needs.
2. What is her preferred place of care? Fast-track discharge may be arranged to transfer a patient home or to a hospice. The multidisciplinary team will be crucial in facilitating this.
3. Does she need specialist palliative care input? Are there complex physical, psychological, social or spiritual needs that would benefit from specialist input?
4. Are there other treatment options that may be helpful? This may include palliative radiotherapy.

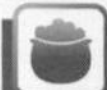

Clinical Tip

Spiritual care addresses a person's sense of meaning and purpose, their feeling of belonging and, ultimately, what is most important to them. Faith and religion may play a role, but spirituality encompasses a much broader definition of what makes someone who they are.

FURTHER READING

Academy of Medical Royal Colleges. (2008). *A code of practice for the diagnosis and confirmation of death*. Available at: www.aomrc.org.uk/wp-content/uploads/2016/04/Code_Practice_Confirmation_Diagnosis_Death_1008-4.pdf. [Accessed 9 January 2022].

Anonymous. (2009). *Medical certificate: Cremation 4*. Available at: https://assets.publishing.service.gov.uk/government/uploads/system/uploads/attachment_data/file/697078/cremation-form-4-medical-certificate.pdf. [Accessed 9 January 2022].

Baile, W. F., et al. (2000). SPIKES – a six-step protocol for delivering bad news: Application to the patient with cancer. *The Oncologist*, *5*(4), 302–311.

Mannix, K. (2017). *With the end in mind: Dying, death and wisdom in an age of denial*.

Marie Curie. (2019). *Providing spiritual care*. Available at: https://www.mariecurie.org.uk/professionals/palliative-care-knowledge-zone/individual-needs/spirituality-end-life. [Accessed 11 November 2022].

Medical Defence Union (MDU). (2019). *Breaking bad news*. Available at: www.themdu.com/guidance-and-advice/guides/breaking-bad-news. [Accessed 9 January 2022].

NHS Blood, & Transplant (n.d.). *Tissue donation*. Available at: www.organdonation.nhs.uk/helping-you-to-decide/about-organ-donation/tissue-donation/. [Accessed 9 January 2022].

NHS Scotland. (2019). *Supportive and Palliative Care Indicators Tool (SPICT)*. Available at: www.spict.org.uk/the-spict/. [Accessed 9 January 2022].

Office for National Statistics. (2008). *Guidance for doctors completing medical certificates of cause of death in England and Wales*. Available at: https://assets.publishing.service.gov.uk/government/uploads/system/uploads/attachment_data/file/757010/guidance-for-doctors-completing-medical-certificates-of-cause-of-death.pdf?_ga=2.71724819.1242743777.1566824500-1956202654.1565543358. [Accessed 9 January 2022].

Sadler, C., Watson, M., & Ganon, C. (2018–2019). *European certificate in essential palliative care: Handbook* (16th ed.). Esher: Princess Alice Hospice.

UK Donation Ethics Committee. (2016). *An ethical framework for donation after confirmation of death using neurological criteria (DBD)*. Academy of Medical Royal Colleges. Available at: https://bts.org.uk/wp-content/uploads/2018/01/Ethical_framework_donation_after_confirmation_death_using_neurological_criteria-2.pdf. [Accessed 9 January 2022].

West Midlands Palliative Care. (2019). *Physicians' guidelines for the use of drugs in symptom control*. Available at: westmidspallcare.co.uk. [Accessed 9 January 2022].

West Midlands Palliative Care Physicians. (2022). *Guidelines for the use of drugs in symptom control*. Available at: westmidspallcare.co.uk. [Accessed 9 January 2022].

General Surgery

17

Content Outline

STATION 17.1: ACUTE APPENDICITIS

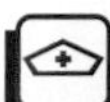

The Bleep Scenario

A 21 year old male has presented to the emergency department (ED) with right iliac fossa pain, nausea and vomiting. He has no past medical history.

His observations are: heart rate (HR) 115 bpm, blood pressure (BP) 125/60 mmHg, respiratory rate (RR) 15 breaths per minute, SpO_2 98% on room air and temperature 38.5°C. You are asked to review him.

DEFINITION

Acute appendicitis is acute inflammation of the appendix, secondary to obstruction of the appendix from hyperplasia of submucosal lymphoid follicles (60%), faecolith or faecal stasis (35%), foreign bodies (4%) or tumours (1%).

INITIAL THOUGHTS

A diagnosis of appendicitis is highly likely in this case given the location of the abdominal pain in the right iliac fossa. The classic history of appendicitis is migratory pain arising in the periumbilical area and moving to the right iliac fossa. As a part of the midgut, visceral pain from an inflamed appendix is perceived in the central abdomen, poorly localised initially. As the inflammation progresses, the parietal peritoneum is involved, and pain is sharper and better localised to the right iliac fossa (somatic pain). It is most commonly seen in adolescence or early adulthood. Other risk factors include low dietary fibre and smoking.

DIFFERENTIAL DIAGNOSIS

- Gastroenterology: viral gastroenteritis, inflammatory bowel disease and acute mesenteric adenitis
- Urology: urinary tract infection, renal colic, epididymo-orchitis and testicular torsion
- Gynaecology: pelvic inflammatory disease and ectopic pregnancy

INITIAL INSTRUCTIONS OVER PHONE

Ask the ED referrer to obtain intravenous (IV) access, take bloods and start IV fluids for resuscitation as required. Administer analgesia, antiemetics and arrange for a dipstick test of the urine. Ask the patient to remain nil by mouth.

ASSESSMENT AND RESUSCITATION

- End of the bed assessment: the patient is in obvious discomfort.
- Airway: patent.
- Breathing: RR 18 breaths per minute, SpO_2 98% on room air. On auscultation, there are vesicular breath sounds with good air entry bilaterally.
- Circulation: capillary refill time (CRT) <2 s. HR 95 bpm, regular. BP 125/60 mmHg, heart sounds (HS) I + II + 0.
- Disability: Glasgow Coma Scale (GCS) 15/15, pupils equal and reactive to light (PEARL), temperature 38.5°C, capillary blood glucose (CBG) 6.0 mmol/L.
- Exposure: his abdomen is tender with guarding in the right iliac fossa. There are no hernias. Genital examination and digital rectal exam are normal.

INITIAL INVESTIGATIONS

- Bedside: urine pregnancy test in women of childbearing age (in gynaecological causes of abdominal pain, to ensure it is safe to X-ray the patient) Electrocardiogram (ECG): preparation for surgery

- Haematology: full blood count (FBC: leukocytosis, anaemia, preparation for surgery)
- Biochemistry: urea and electrolytes (U&Es: acute kidney injury as a result of sepsis/dehydration, electrolyte imbalance), C-reactive protein (CRP: inflammation), venous or arterial lactate (if septic)
- Microbiology: blood cultures and urinalysis (infection)
- Radiology: erect chest X-ray (if signs of peritonitis [pneumoperitoneum]) and abdominal X-ray (if bowel obstruction suspected)

 **Clinical Tip**

In patients over the age of 50 (particularly if associated with a family history of colonic cancer, presence of associated colonic 'alarm' symptoms (abdominal pain, change in stool texture, change in stool frequency or blood in stool/rectal (PR) bleeding) or microcytic anaemia), consider a computed tomography (CT) scan to ensure there is no evidence of caecal mass suggesting malignancy prior to operation.

MAKING A DIAGNOSIS

Appendicitis is a clinical diagnosis. It is more common in adolescence or early adulthood.

- Symptoms: central abdominal pain migrating to the right iliac fossa, loss of appetite, nausea, vomiting and fever
- Signs: guarding and tenderness two-thirds along from the umbilicus to the right anterior superior iliac spine: this is McBurney's point (Fig. 17.1). Look for Rovsing's sign – tenderness in the right iliac fossa when palpating in the left iliac fossa

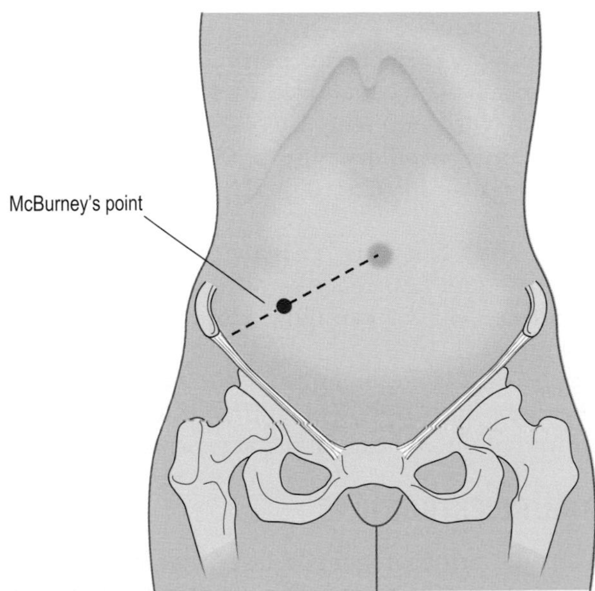

Fig. 17.1 McBurney's point. (Source: Dennis, M., Bowen, W.T. and Cho, L. [2020]. *Mechanisms of clinical signs*. Elsevier.)

 **Clinical Tip**

Although the base of the appendix is said to be roughly located around McBurney's point, its position may vary. Patients with atypical positioning of the appendix, such as retrocaecal or deep pelvic, may not elicit the typical exam findings.

MANAGEMENT

Keep the patient nil by mouth for theatre. Start a fluid balance chart and consider catheterisation, if unwell. Prescribe maintenance fluids once the patient is adequately resuscitated, along with analgesia and antiemetics.

The management of appendicitis is usually surgical, though conservative management with antibiotics is an alternative option. The decision of whether a conservative or surgical approach needs to be taken for this patient will be based on age, comorbidity, duration of the illness, history of previous surgical history and presence/absence of associated complications. The choice of surgical treatment between laparoscopic and open appendicectomy will depend on local policy, surgical preference and experience.

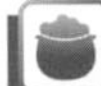 **Clinical Tip**

Upon the decision for laparoscopic or open appendicectomy, you will need to inform the emergency theatre coordinator, the ward nurses, the on call anaesthetist and the operating surgeon. You should be aware of relevant information when booking the case – the team will want to know when the patient will be fasted, any comorbidity, allergies and what tasks are outstanding (i.e. consent, informing next of kin).

ESCALATION

Contact the surgical registrar urgently if the patient becomes septic, perforates or if signs of peritonitis are noted on examination. The critical care team may need to be contacted if the patient is unwell and does not respond to initial resuscitative measures.

STATION 17.2: ACUTE CHOLECYSTITIS

 **The Bleep Scenario**

A 40 year old woman has presented to the ED with persistent right upper quadrant pain, nausea and fever. She has a known history of gallstones and biliary colic but reports her pain has not settled this time.

Her observations are: HR 115 bpm, BP 125/85 mmHg, RR 15 breaths per minute, SpO_2 98% on room air and temperature 38°C. You are asked to review the patient.

DEFINITION

Acute cholecystitis is an acute inflammatory disease of the gallbladder, often attributable to gallstones.

INITIAL THOUGHTS

This patient is likely to have a diagnosis of acute cholecystitis, given the history of right upper quadrant pain and the background of gallstones. In addition, the patient may be septic given the history of pyrexia. Ensure you follow your local sepsis protocol when assessing the patient. Other risk factors for the development of gallstones include increasing age, female gender and obesity.

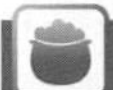 Clinical Tip

Intermittent obstruction of the gallbladder without inflammation causes intermittent pain and is known as biliary colic. Prolonged obstruction of the gallbladder outlet causes inflammation of the gallbladder and is known as cholecystitis.

DIFFERENTIAL DIAGNOSIS

- Gastroenterology: ascending cholangitis, perforated peptic ulcer, acute pancreatitis, gastro-oesophageal reflux disease and biliary colic
- Vascular: abdominal aortic aneurysm
- Cardiology: acute coronary syndrome
- Respiratory: right-sided pneumonia

INITIAL INSTRUCTIONS OVER PHONE

Ask the ED referrer to obtain IV access, take bloods and start IV fluids for resuscitation as required. Request that a pregnancy test is completed in this female patient of childbearing age.

ASSESSMENT AND RESUSCITATION

- End of bed assessment: the patient appears to be in obvious discomfort.
- Airway: patent.
- Breathing: RR 18 breaths per minute, SpO_2 98% on room air. On auscultation, there are vesicular breath sounds with good air entry bilaterally.
- Circulation: CRT <2 s, HR 90 bpm, regular, BP 110/60 mmHg, HS I + II + 0; jugular venous pressure (JVP) is normal.
- Disability: GCS 15/15, PEARL, temperature 38.2°C, CBG 5.5 mmol/L.
- Exposure: she is not jaundiced. Her abdomen is tender in the right hypochondrium with guarding. Normal bowel sounds. Calves unremarkable.

INITIAL INVESTIGATIONS

- Bedside: 12-lead ECG (rule out any cardiac causes for chest or upper abdominal pain), and urine hCG in women of childbearing age (gynaecological causes of abdominal pain, to ensure it is safe to X-ray the patient).
- Haematology: FBC (leukocytosis, anaemia, preparation for surgery).
- Biochemistry: CRP (inflammation), U&Es (acute kidney injury as a result of sepsis/dehydration, preparation for surgery), liver function tests (LFTs): cholestasis), amylase (pancreatitis), coagulation screen (preparation for surgery), venous or arterial lactate (sepsis screen).
- Microbiology: blood cultures and urinalysis (infection).
- Radiology: erect chest X-ray (if signs of peritonitis (pneumoperitoneum)), and an abdominal ultrasound scan (acute cholecystitis).

 Clinical Tip

Keep the patient nil by mouth for the abdominal ultrasound – having a meal may cause the gallbladder to contract, making it difficult to visualise on scanning. Features of acute cholecystitis on ultrasound are pericholecystic fluid, gallbladder wall thickening and radiological Murphy's sign (Fig. 17.2).

MAKING A DIAGNOSIS

According to the 2018 Tokyo guidelines, a suspected diagnosis of acute cholecystitis is given if there is one item in A and B. A definite diagnosis is given if there is one item in A, B and C:

A. Local signs of inflammation: Murphy's sign, right upper abdominal quadrant mass, pain or tenderness
B. Systemic signs of inflammation: fever, elevated white blood cell count, elevated CRP
C. Investigations: imaging findings characteristic of acute cholecystitis

 Clinical Tip

Murphy's sign is a specific, but not very sensitive, clinical sign for cholecystitis. Find the transpyloric plane (a horizontal plane about a hand's breath below the xiphisternum), where this crosses the right costal margin is the landmark for the fundus of the gallbladder. Palpate in the region just under the costal margin, and then ask the patient to inhale. If inspiration stops because of pain, and this is not reproduced when palpating the left upper quadrant, then Murphy's sign is positive.

MANAGEMENT

You should commence the patient on IV antibiotics. Co-amoxiclav is a typical choice but you should be guided

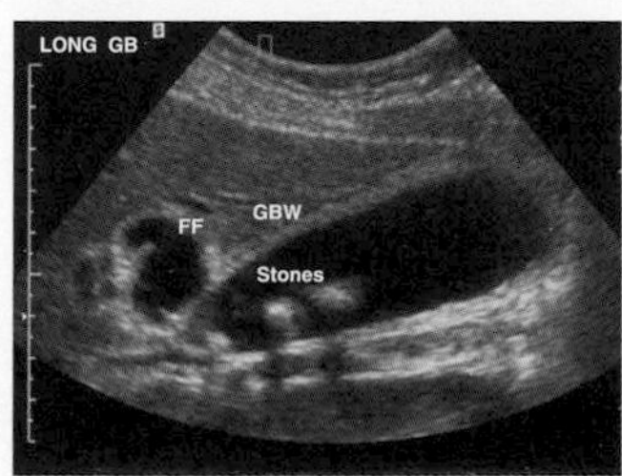

Fig. 17.2 Gallbladder with gallstones, thickened gallbladder wall (GBW) and pericholecystic fluid (FF). Together these findings constitute the sonographic signs of cholecystitis. (Source: Marx, J.A. et al. [2010]. *Rosen's emergency medicine*. 7th ed. Philadelphia, PA: Elsevier.)

by your trust's antimicrobial guidelines. Following resuscitation, the patient will require maintenance IV fluids. Start a fluid balance chart and consider catheterisation. Prescribe analgesia and antiemetics.

Ultimately, this patient will require a cholecystectomy. The timing of this will depend on local service provision and surgeon preference. Some centres manage acute cholecystitis conservatively with antibiotics. The patient will then be listed for an elective laparoscopic cholecystectomy in 6 weeks once the inflammation has settled. Other centres have pathways allowing for 'hot gallbladders', where laparoscopic cholecystectomy is performed on an acutely inflamed gallbladder in emergency theatre, following resuscitation and commencement of antibiotics.

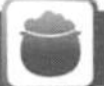

Clinical Tip

If an emergency laparoscopic cholecystectomy is decided upon by your seniors, inform the emergency theatre coordinator, the ward nurses, the on call anaesthetist and the operating surgeon. Know information relevant to booking the case – the team will want to know when the patient will be fasted, any comorbidity, allergies and what tasks are outstanding (i.e. consent, informing next of kin).

ESCALATION

Contact your surgical registrar to review the patient urgently if she becomes septic, perforates or if signs of peritonitis are noted on examination. The critical care team may need to be contacted if the patient is profoundly septic and not responding to resuscitation.

STATION 17.3: ACUTE CHOLANGITIS

The Bleep Scenario

A 43 year old man has presented to ED with right upper quadrant pain, jaundice and fever. He was recently listed for a cholecystectomy for gallstones.

His observations are: HR 110 bpm, BP 95/50 mmHg, RR 16 breaths per minute, SpO_2 95% on room air and temperature of 39°C. You are asked to review him.

DEFINITION

Acute cholangitis is an acute inflammation of the bile duct usually secondary to obstruction and infection in the bile duct.

INITIAL THOUGHTS

This patient reports fever, jaundice and right upper quadrant pain. Cholangitis should be suspected as there is evidence of systemic inflammation (fever/rigors or evidence of inflammation on bloods) and cholestasis (jaundice or obstructive LFTs). In addition, the patient may be septic. Ensure you follow your local sepsis protocol when assessing the patient. Risk factors for acute cholangitis include age over 50 years, history of gallstone or other biliary pathology, e.g. stricture of the biliary tree, or previous surgery to the bile ducts.

DIFFERENTIAL DIAGNOSIS

- Hepatobiliary: acute cholecystitis, acute pancreatitis, hepatic abscess and hepatitis
- Gastroenterology: peptic ulcer disease
- Urology: acute pyelonephritis
- Respiratory: right-sided pneumonia

INITIAL INSTRUCTIONS OVER PHONE

Ask the ED referrer to obtain IV access, take bloods and start IV fluids for resuscitation as required. Administer analgesia and antiemetics as required.

ASSESSMENT AND RESUSCITATION

- End of the bed assessment: the patient looks unwell and is visibly jaundiced.
- Airway: patent.
- Breathing: RR 20 breaths per minute, SpO_2 95% on room air. On auscultation, there are vesicular breath sounds with good air entry bilaterally.
- Circulation: CRT <2 s. HR 110 bpm, regular. BP 95/50 mmHg, HS I + II + 0. JVP is normal.
    - Administer 500 mL of crystalloid fluids stat to resuscitate the patient
- Disability: GCS 15/15, PEARL, temperature 39.0°C, CBG 8.8 mmol/L.
- Exposure: he is jaundiced. His abdomen is tender with guarding in the right hypochondrium. Normal bowel sounds. Calves unremarkable.

INITIAL INVESTIGATIONS

- Bedside: 12-lead ECG (rule out any cardiac causes for chest or upper abdominal pain), and urine hCG in women of childbearing age (gynaecological causes of abdominal pain, to ensure it is safe to X-ray the patient)
- Haematology: FBC (leukocytosis or anaemia)
- Biochemistry: U&Es (acute kidney injury as a result of sepsis/dehydration, electrolyte imbalance). LFTs (to check for obstructive pathology suggestive of gallstones). Amylase (acute pancreatitis), CRP (inflammation), arterial blood gas (ABG)/venous blood gas (to check lactate in cases of sepsis)
- Microbiology: blood cultures and urinalysis (infection)
- Radiology: erect chest X-ray (if signs of peritonitis [pneumoperitoneum]), abdominal ultrasound (gallstones if no known diagnosis and biliary duct dilatation suggestive of obstruction)

MAKING A DIAGNOSIS

According to the Tokyo 2018 guidelines, a suspected diagnosis of acute cholangitis is given if there is one item in A and one item in B or C. A definite diagnosis is given if there is one item in A, B and C:

A. Systemic inflammation: fever and/or shaking chills, evidence of inflammatory response on laboratory data (abnormal white cell count, increased CRP)
B. Cholestasis: jaundice, abnormal liver function tests (increased serum alkaline phosphatase, gamma-glutamyltransferase, aspartate aminotransferase and alanine transaminase levels)
C. Imaging: biliary dilatation, evidence of the aetiology on imaging (stricture, stone, stent, etc.)

Charcot's triad is also frequently used as diagnostic criteria for acute cholangitis. It compromises symptoms of: (1) fever with chills/rigor; (2) jaundice; and (3) right upper quadrant pain. It has high specificity but low sensitivity.

MANAGEMENT

The priority here is managing a septic patient. Commence antibiotics (after blood cultures) for suspected acute cholangitis. Follow local antimicrobial guidelines. Ensure the patient is adequately fluid-resuscitated and any electrolyte imbalance is corrected. Start a fluid balance chart and consider catheterisation. Prescribe analgesia and antiemetics.

The Tokyo guideline scores disease severity into three categories to aid management: grade I (mild), grade II (moderate) and grade III (severe). Grade I patients are usually managed conservatively, and biliary drainage is only considered if they do not respond to initial treatment measures within 24 hours. Grade II patients warrant early biliary drainage, within 48 hours. Grade III patients should receive aggressive medical management of sepsis, and emergent biliary drainage once the patient is haemodynamically stable.

An ultrasound scan of the abdomen and/or magnetic resonance cholangiopancreatogram (MRCP) (Fig. 17.3) needs to be considered to confirm biliary obstruction. However, if the patient is in extremis, your senior may well proceed to biliary drainage. You will have to correct the patient's clotting. Recall that vitamin K is a fat-soluble vitamin and with biliary obstruction, absorption may be impaired; therefore, vitamin K needs to be administered intravenously.

This patient will require a cholecystectomy, for longer term management, if the obstruction is due to gallstones.

ESCALATION

Contact the surgical registrar urgently if the patient is in extremis to consider biliary drainage, usually via endoscopic retrograde cholangiopancreatography (ERCP). If the patient is not suitable for endoscopy (e.g. as a result of previous bowel surgery such as gastric bypass with secondary altered anatomy making it unsuitable), radiological drainage (percutaneous transhepatic cholangiopancreatography) may be considered. Choice of drainage will also depend on local services. The critical care team may need to be contacted if the patient is profoundly septic and not responding to resuscitation.

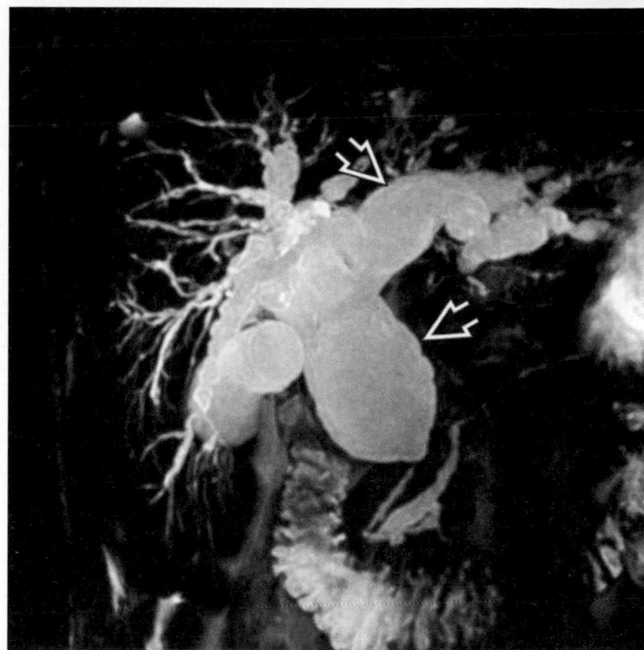

Fig. 17.3 Coronal magnetic resonance cholangiopancreatogram (MRCP) reveals massive dilation of the intrahepatic and proximal extrahepatic bile ducts, a type 4 choledochal cyst, responsible for the ascending cholangitis and abscess. (Source: Zaheer, A. and Raman, S.P. [2022]. *Diagnostic imaging: Gastrointestinal*. Elsevier.)

The endoscopy team needs to be contacted to perform ERCP, though some general surgeons can perform this procedure. If radiological drainage is considered, you will need to speak to the interventional radiology team. You should discuss the results of the clotting screen with the haematologist on call if there are derangements to be corrected.

STATION 17.4: ACUTE PANCREATITIS

The Bleep Scenario

A 60 year old man has presented to the ED with vomiting and severe epigastric pain radiating to the back. He reports a history of gallstones.

His observations are: HR 105 bpm, BP 110/65 mmHg, RR 15 breaths per minute, SpO_2 93% on room air and temperature 37.7°C. You are asked to review the patient.

DEFINITION

Acute pancreatitis is an acute inflammation of the pancreas, with variable involvement of other regional or remote organ systems. It is commonly related to gallstones and/or alcohol use.

INITIAL THOUGHTS

Severe epigastric pain radiating to the back is a classical presentation of acute pancreatitis. Your assessment should look for potential underlying causes for acute pancreatitis. The most common aetiologies in the UK are gallstones and alcohol. Gallstones are thought to cause a back pressure in the pancreatic duct stimulating enzymes and autodigestion of the pancreas. The mechanism for alcohol is unclear. Other causes include hypercalcaemia, ERCP, viral infections, medications, hereditary causes, ampullary or pancreatic tumours, steroids or autoimmune pancreatitis.

DIFFERENTIAL DIAGNOSIS

- Cardiac: acute coronary syndrome
- Gastrointestinal: peptic ulcer disease, peptic ulcer perforation, intestinal obstruction, viral gastroenteritis, acute mesenteric ischaemia, Boerhaave's syndrome
- Hepatobiliary: cholecystitis, acute cholangitis
- Vascular: abdominal aortic aneurysm

INITIAL INSTRUCTIONS OVER PHONE

Ask the ED referrer to consider supplementary oxygen, aiming for oxygen saturations > 94%, obtain IV access, take bloods and start IV fluids for resuscitation as required.

ASSESSMENT AND RESUSCITATION

- End of the bed assessment: the patient is visibly distressed and in pain.
- Airway: patent.
- Breathing: RR 22 breaths per minute, SpO_2 96% on 2 L via nasal cannula. On auscultation, there are vesicular breath sounds with good air entry bilaterally.
- Circulation: CRT 3 s. HR 115 bpm, regular. BP 110/65mmHg, HS I + II + 0. JVP is normal.
  - Administer 500 mL of crystalloid fluids stat to resuscitate the patient
- Disability: GCS 15/15, PEARL, temperature 38.5°C, CBG 7.0 mmol/L.
- Exposure: he is not jaundiced. His abdomen is tender in the epigastrium with guarding but no pulsatile/expansile mass is palpable. No radiofemoral delay. Normal bowel sounds. Calves unremarkable.

Clinical Tip

There are many severity 'prediction' scoring systems. The modified Glasgow score is commonly used to predict the severity of pancreatitis and should be calculated on admission and after 48 hours. Scores ≥3 predict severe pancreatitis. This score is only 70% sensitive and sole reliance on this score can miss 30% of patients with severe pancreatitis.

The mnemonic PANCREAS aids in recalling the parameters involved. One point is given for each of the following:
P: PO_2 <7.9kPa
A: age >55
N: (neutrophils) white cell count > 15 x 10^9/L
C: calcium <2 mmol/L
R: renal function – urea > 16 mmol/L
E: enzymes – lactate dehydrogenase > 600 IU/L, or AST >200 IU/L
A: albumin <3 × 2 g/L
S: sugar – blood glucose >10 mmol/L.

INITIAL INVESTIGATIONS

- Bedside: 12-lead ECG (rule out any cardiac causes for chest or upper abdominal pain), and urine hCG in women of childbearing age (gynaecological causes of abdominal pain, to ensure it is safe to X-ray the patient)
- Haematology: FBC (leukocytosis, anaemia, to calculate Glasgow score)
- Biochemistry: U&Es, LFTs, ABG and bone profile (to calculate Glasgow score, LFTs also to rule out differentials of upper abdominal pain). CRP (inflammation), amylase (to aid diagnosis of acute pancreatitis)
- Microbiology: urinalysis (infection)
- Radiology: erect chest X-ray (pneumoperitoneum, may show a sentinel bowel loop). Abdominal ultrasound (gallstones or biliary dilatation; this should be completed even if there is a history of alcohol excess)

Clinical Tip

A CT pancreas may be considered on admission if there is diagnostic uncertainty (i.e. normal amylase) (Fig. 17.4). However, with a clear diagnosis, CT is reserved for severe cases after 4 days or if a complication develops.

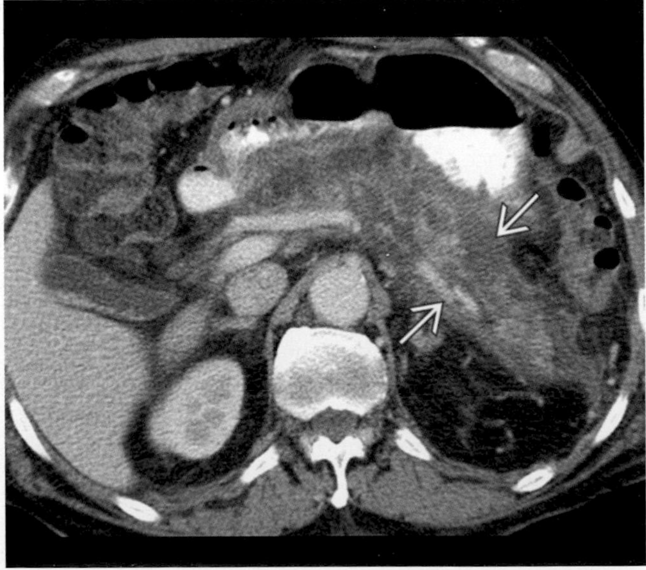

Fig. 17.4 Acute pancreatitis on computed tomography (CT). This CT shows severe acute necrotising pancreatitis with heterogeneous and diminished enhancement of the pancreas. (Source: Lamps, L.W. and Kakar, S. [2022]. *Diagnostic pathology: Hepatobiliary and pancreas*. Elsevier.)

MAKING A DIAGNOSIS

- Symptoms: severe epigastric pain radiating to the back, nausea, vomiting and anorexia
- Signs: abdominal tenderness and guarding may be noted. Cullen and Grey Turner signs are evidence of retroperitoneal haemorrhage at the periumbilical skin and both flanks respectively; these are late signs
- Investigations: raised serum lipase or amylase three times above normal, radiological evidence of pancreatitis

The revised Atlanta classification defines acute pancreatitis as having two of three criteria:

1. Abdominal pain consistent with pancreatitis (severe epigastric pain radiating to the back)
2. Raised serum lipase or amylase three times above normal
3. Radiological evidence of pancreatitis

MANAGEMENT

Continue fluid resuscitation, paying attention to correcting potential electrolyte derangements, and monitoring blood sugars. Start a fluid balance chart and consider catheterisation. Prescribe analgesia and antiemetics. Insulin may be required if the patient is hyperglycaemic. Start a proton pump inhibitor for gastro-protection.

In the context of alcoholic pancreatitis, start an alcohol withdrawal regime in line with local protocols.

If gallstones are confirmed, and there is evidence of biliary obstruction with a stone or associated cholangitis, ERCP may be considered. ERCP and definitive sphincterotomy may be considered in unfit patients to reduce the risk of recurrent pancreatitis. In milder cases, the patient should have a cholecystectomy on the same admission or within 2 weeks once recovered. In severe cases, cholecystectomy needs to be considered at a later date once all complications have resolved.

ESCALATION

Contact the critical care outreach team, especially if the patient has a high severity score or has developed organ failure. The gastroenterology team may need to be contacted if ERCP is required, though some general surgeons can perform this procedure. There may need to be discussion with the regional hepatopancreatic biliary team if there are complications such as pancreatic necrosis, particularly associated with infection and multiorgan failure in early stages, infected peripancreatic fluid collection or development of pseudocysts at later stages.

STATION 17.5: BOWEL OBSTRUCTION

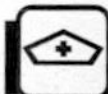

The Bleep Scenario

A 65 year old woman has presented to the ED with abdominal pain and distension. She is vomiting and has not opened her bowels for 5 days. She reports a history of previous abdominal surgery.

Her observations are: HR 110 bpm, BP 105/60 mmHg, RR 15 breaths per minute, SpO_2 98% on room air and temperature 37.8°C. You are asked to review her.

DEFINITION

Bowel obstruction is a mechanical obstruction of the small and/or large bowel.

INITIAL THOUGHTS

This woman presents with a history of suspected bowel obstruction, most likely small-bowel obstruction given the failure to open bowels, abdominal pain, distension and vomiting. Common aetiologies for bowel obstruction are adhesions and hernias in the case of the small bowel and malignancy for the large bowel. Other causes include strictures (associated with Crohn's disease, diverticular disease or postoperative), volvulus, foreign bodies and gallstone ileus.

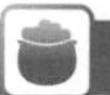

Clinical Tip

Vomiting is an earlier feature than constipation in small-bowel obstruction, while the reverse is true for large-bowel obstruction, where vomiting can even be absent.

DIFFERENTIAL DIAGNOSIS

- Gastroenterology: bowel obstruction, acute colonic pseudo-obstruction, toxic megacolon, pseudomembranous colitis, ileus, infectious gastroenteritis, diverticulitis and appendicitis
- Hepatobiliary: ascites
- Vascular: abdominal aortic aneurysm and mesenteric artery ischaemia
- Urology: urinary tract infection
- Other: trauma and gastrointestinal foreign body

INITIAL INSTRUCTIONS OVER PHONE

Ask the ED referrer to obtain IV access, take bloods and start IV fluids for resuscitation. Advise analgesia as required.

Clinical Tip

Assessment should look for red-flag signs of malignancy – weight loss, change in bowel habit or PR bleeding.

ASSESSMENT AND RESUSCITATION

- End of the bed assessment: the patient looks dehydrated and has bilious vomit in a bowl.
- Airway: patent.
- Breathing: RR 15 breaths per minute, SpO_2 98% on room air. On auscultation, there are vesicular breath sounds with good air entry bilaterally.
- Circulation: CRT 2 s, HR 110 bpm, regular. BP 100/60 mmHg, HS I + II + 0. JVP is normal.
  - Administer 500 mL of crystalloid fluids stat to resuscitate the patient.
- Disability: GCS 15/15, PEARL, temperature 37.8°C, CBG 6.0 mmol/L.
- Exposure: her abdomen is distended and generally tender, but with no guarding or signs of peritonism. No masses palpable in the abdomen. She has a midline laparotomy scar. There are no hernias, and bowel sounds are tinkling. Digital rectal examination showed an empty rectum.

INITIAL INVESTIGATIONS

- Bedside: 12-lead ECG (rule out any cardiac causes for chest or upper abdominal pain), and urine hCG in women of childbearing age (in gynaecological causes of abdominal pain, to ensure it is safe to X-ray the patient)
- Haematology: FBC (leukocytosis or anaemia)
- Biochemistry: U&Es (acute kidney injury as a result of dehydration, electrolyte imbalance), CRP (inflammation) and ABG (acid–base imbalance)
- Microbiology: urinalysis (infection)
- Radiology: erect chest X-ray (if signs of peritonitis [pneumoperitoneum]), and abdominal X-ray (bowel obstruction) (Fig. 17.5)

MAKING A DIAGNOSIS

- Symptoms: vomiting, failure to pass flatus or stool, abdominal distension and pain
- Investigations: abdominal X-ray demonstrating distended loops of small/large bowel or appearances of caecal/sigmoid volvulus. As a guide, the 3, 6, 9 rule suggests the upper limits of normal: 3 cm for small bowel, 6 cm for large bowel and 9 cm for caecum.

Clinical Tip

It is important to ascertain whether the constipation is complete or partial, as it will influence further management. If there is partial obstruction, the patient will still be able to pass flatus and stool, but these may be reduced in quantity. Complete obstruction describes no passage of stool or flatus.

MANAGEMENT

This scenario is most likely adhesional small-bowel obstruction. In addition to fluid resuscitation followed by maintenance fluids, insert a wide-bore nasogastric tube to decompress the stomach – so-called 'drip and suck'. Once aspirated to dryness, ask for 4-hourly nasogastric aspiration. Keep the patient nil by mouth until reviewed by your senior colleagues. Start a fluid balance

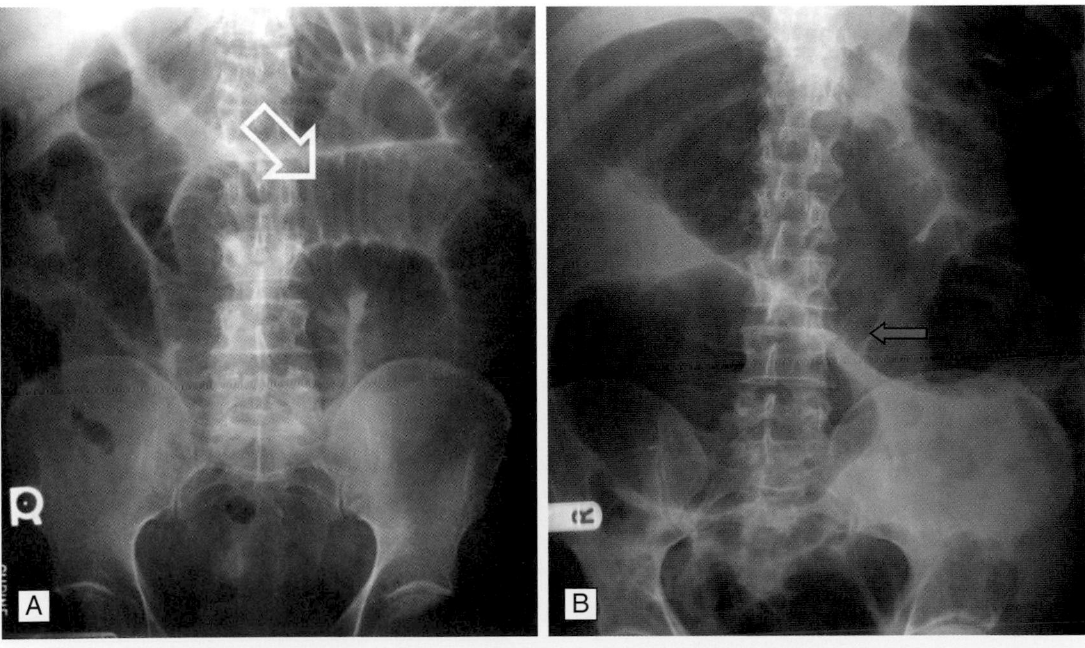

Fig. 17.5 Plain abdominal X-rays showing obstruction. (A) Supine film in a patient with small-bowel obstruction showing valvulae conniventes (arrow). (B) X-ray demonstrating large-bowel obstruction with arrow at a haustration. (Source: Garden, O.J., Parks, R.W. and Wigmore, S.J. (Eds.) [2022]. *Principles and practice of surgery*. Elsevier.)

chart, catheterise the patient and measure hourly urine output. Correct any electrolyte abnormalities. Prescribe analgesia and antiemetic.

Adhesional small-bowel obstruction may resolve with conservative (drip-and-suck) management. If initial conservative management fails, or generally in the case of complete small-bowel obstruction, the patient will require surgery. Correction of the underlying cause is also necessary, e.g. tumour resection, hernia repair. Perforation or impending perforation requires immediate surgical intervention. Sigmoid volvulus may be decompressed via a colonoscopy. Once hydrated well, a CT abdomen and pelvis with contrast is required to identify the aetiology and completeness of the obstruction, to look for complications such as ischaemia or perforation or if the diagnosis is inconclusive on X-ray. Your senior can advise you if further imaging is indicated.

Be aware of closed-loop obstruction, where there is a blockage at two points. The segment of bowel between the two points continues to distend and is at risk of necrosis and perforation. The same is true of large-bowel obstruction where there is a competent ileocaecal valve. Since the colon does not decompress into the ileum, the caecum may be at risk of perforation.

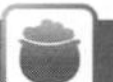

Clinical Tip

If surgery is decided upon by your seniors, inform the emergency theatre coordinator, the ward nurses, the on call anaesthetist and the operating surgeon. Know information relevant to booking the case – the team will want to know when the patient will be fasted, any comorbidity, allergies and what tasks are outstanding (i.e. consent, informing next of kin). Most patients undergoing emergency laparotomy will require a high dependency unit (HDU) or intensive therapy unit (ITU) bed, so you may need to coordinate this with the intensivists.

Prescribing Tip

In cases of complete small-bowel obstruction, antiemetics may not provide symptomatic relief. The nasogastric decompression is more effective in relieving nausea. There may be some benefit in partial small-bowel obstruction. It is important to note that metoclopramide is contraindicated in bowel obstruction as it is a prokinetic agent.

ESCALATION

Contact your surgical registrar to review the patient urgently if she becomes septic, perforates or if signs of peritonitis are noted on examination. The critical care team should be contacted, particularly if the patient has significant renal failure. You may need to discuss any further scans such as CT with radiology if indicated.

In cases of sigmoid volvulus, you may be asked to contact endoscopy and gastroenterology for a colonoscopy to decompress the volvulus. However, this can also be performed by the surgical team.

STATION 17.6: ACUTE DIVERTICULITIS

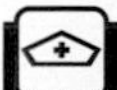

The Bleep Scenario

A 60 year old woman has presented to the ED with left iliac fossa pain and malaise. She reports a history of constipation.

Her observations are: HR 105 bpm, BP 136/74 mmHg, RR 18 breaths per minute, SpO_2 98% on room air and a temperature of 38.0°C. You are asked to review the patient.

DEFINITION

Acute diverticulitis is acute inflammation of colonic diverticulum or diverticula.

INITIAL THOUGHTS

This patient is likely to have a diagnosis of acute diverticulitis, given the location of the pain, history of constipation and her age. A large proportion of the population will have diverticulosis; that is, the presence of diverticula. These are outpouchings of the colonic mucosa through natural weaknesses in the colonic wall where vasa recta pierce the wall; this happens as the pressure within the colon is increased. Diverticulitis can present when a diverticulum becomes inflamed, secondary to blockage from hard faeces (Fig. 17.6).

Risk factors include age >50 years, low dietary fibre, western diet and obesity (body mass index > 30).

DIFFERENTIAL DIAGNOSIS

- Gastrointestinal: bowel obstruction, stercoral perforation, appendicitis, inflammatory bowel disease and ischaemic colitis
- Urology: renal colic and urinary tract infection
- Gynaecological: pelvic inflammatory disease and salpingitis

INITIAL INSTRUCTIONS OVER PHONE

Ask the ED referrer to obtain IV access, take bloods and start IV fluids for resuscitation as required. Advise analgesia as required.

ASSESSMENT AND RESUSCITATION

- End of the bed assessment: the patient is in obvious discomfort.
- Airway: patent.
- Breathing: RR 18 breaths per minute, SpO_2 98% on room air. On auscultation, there are vesicular breath sounds with good air entry bilaterally.
- Circulation: CRT <2 s, HR 80 bpm, regular. BP 135/70 mmHg, HS I + II + 0.
- Disability: GCS 15/15, PEARL, temperature 38.2°C, CBG 6.5 mmol/L.

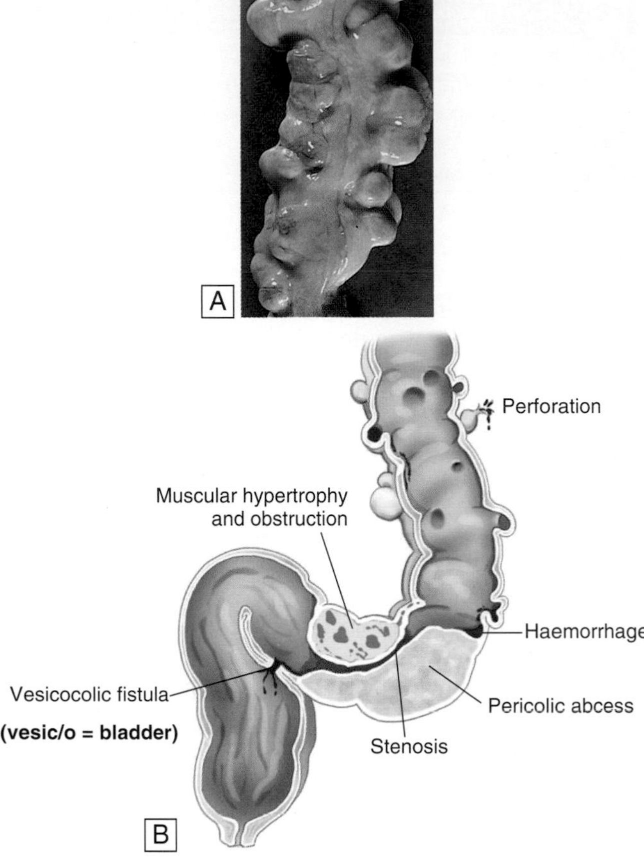

Fig. 17.6 (A) Diverticulosis (outpouchings of colonic mucosa). Diverticulosis can lead to diverticulitis (B) and its subsequent complications. (Source: Damjanov, I., & Linder, J. (1996). *Pathology: a color atlas.* Mosby Inc.)

- Exposure: she is tender in the left iliac fossa with guarding and percussion tenderness locally. Normal bowel sounds. There are no hernias. Digital rectal exam is normal.

INITIAL INVESTIGATIONS

- Haematology: FBC (leukocytosis or anaemia)
- Biochemistry: CRP (inflammation), U&Es (acute kidney injury as a result of sepsis/dehydration, electrolyte imbalance), venous or arterial lactate (septic screen). Cross-match (if there is anaemia secondary to PR bleeding)
- Microbiology: blood cultures and urinalysis (infection)
- Radiology: erect chest X-ray (if there are signs of peritonitis [pneumoperitoneum]) and abdominal X-ray (if bowel obstruction is suspected)

MAKING A DIAGNOSIS

- Symptoms: left iliac fossa pain, history of constipation, PR bleeding, fever
- Signs: guarding and tenderness in the left iliac fossa, palpable masses, peritonitis
- Investigations: leukocytosis and/or raised CRP

MANAGEMENT

Commence the patient on antibiotics if she is pyrexial with raised inflammatory markers. Follow the trust's local antimicrobial guidelines. Prescribe analgesia and antiemetics. Keep the patient nil by mouth until your senior reviews her. Following resuscitation, the patient will require maintenance IV fluids. Start a fluid balance chart and consider catheterisation. Prescribe analgesia and antiemetics. Management is often conservative, but CT may be considered if the patient does not improve, or there are concerns regarding diagnosis or complications of diverticulitis. Colonoscopy or CT colon will need to be organised as an outpatient to rule out underlying colonic malignancy.

Acute diverticulitis may also result in abscess formation. This may again be treated with a course of antibiotics or may necessitate drainage as well. With more severe cases (i.e. patients with generalised peritonitis) the patient will require surgery. A Hartmann's procedure is commonly used to manage perforated diverticulitis with faecal peritonitis. It involves laparotomy, resection of diseased bowel, with the formation of an end-colostomy and leaving a rectal stump. A fistula may also develop with nearby structures – bladder or vagina.

 Clinical Tip

If surgery is decided upon by your seniors, inform the theatre coordinator, the ward nurses, the on call anaesthetist and the operating surgeon. Know information relevant to booking the case – the team will want to know when the patient will be fasted, any comorbidity, allergies and what tasks are outstanding (i.e. consent, informing next of kin). Most patients undergoing emergency laparotomy will require an HDU or ITU bed, so you may need to coordinate this with the intensivists.

 Clinical Tip

The Hinchey classification is useful in describing complicated diverticulitis. Hinchey stage I is diverticulitis with pericolic abscess. Hinchey stage II is diverticulitis with distant abscess (retroperitoneal or pelvic). Stage III involves purulent peritonitis and stage IV is faecal peritonitis.

ESCALATION

Contact your surgical registrar to review the patient if she does not respond to initial resuscitation and antibiotic therapy, to plan further management. If the patient is unwell with generalised peritonitis and/or septic, contact the critical care outreach team. You may need to speak to the on call radiologist if a CT scan is indicated. They will also be involved if there are abscesses or collections to drain percutaneously.

STATION 17.7: LOWER GASTROINTESTINAL BLEEDING

The Bleep Scenario

A 70 year old woman has presented to the ED with PR bleeding. She does not report any pain. She has a past medical history of breast cancer and hypertension.

Her observations are: HR 100 bpm, BP 100/70 mmHg, RR 16 breaths per minute, SpO_2 96% on room air and a temperature 37.8°C. You are asked to review the patient.

DEFINITION

Lower gastrointestinal bleeding is defined as having a source of bleeding distal to the ligament of Treitz. Be aware, however, that 15% of PR bleeds have an upper gastrointestinal source.

INITIAL THOUGHTS

There are several aetiologies that can cause PR bleeding. Diverticulosis is a common cause, as a result of bleeding from the vessels within the diverticula. Colorectal malignancy can present with lower gastrointestinal bleeding and should always be considered. Haemorrhoids are also a common cause of PR bleed. These are enlargements of vascular cushions in the anus. Also consider inflammatory bowel disease in a young patient. In this case, haemorrhoids are a likely diagnosis given the absence of abdominal pain, but it is crucial to rule out an underlying malignancy (Fig. 17.7).

Clinical Tip

Remember to consider other sources of bleeding such as haematuria or vaginal bleeding, as they can sometimes be mistaken for PR bleeding.

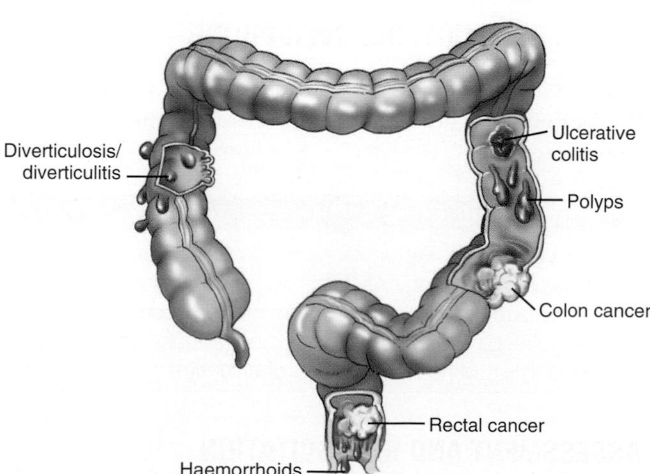

Fig. 17.7 Common causes of lower gastrointestinal bleeding. (Source: Leonard, P. [2022]. *Building a medical vocabulary with Spanish translations*. Elsevier Saunders.)

DIFFERENTIAL DIAGNOSIS

- Lower gastrointestinal: diverticular disease, colorectal cancer, haemorrhoids, inflammatory bowel disease, colonic angiodysplasia, ischaemic or infective colitis and mesenteric ischaemia
- Upper gastrointestinal (rapid transport): peptic ulcer disease, oesophageal varices and oesophagitis
- Haematological: coagulopathy and thrombocytopenia
- Other: vasculitides and trauma

INITIAL INSTRUCTION OVER PHONE

Ask the ED referrer to obtain IV access, take bloods and start IV fluids for resuscitation as required.

ASSESSMENT AND RESUSCITATION

- End of the bed assessment: the patient appears pale.
- Airway: patent.
- Breathing: RR 18 breaths per minute, SpO_2 98% on room air. On auscultation, there are vesicular breath sounds with good air entry bilaterally.
- Circulation: CRT 3 s, HR 100 bpm, regular. BP 105/70 mmHg, HS I + II + 0. JVP is normal.
  - Administer 500 mL of crystalloid fluids stat to resuscitate the patient.
  - 12-lead ECG: No signs of ischaemia noted.
- Disability: GCS 15/15, PEARL, temperature 36.5°C, CBG 5.5 mmol/L.
- Exposure: abdomen soft and non-tender. No masses felt. Digital rectal examination did not reveal haemorrhoids or masses. There is fresh blood on the glove.

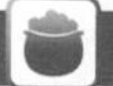

Clinical Tip

Melaena is a black, tarry stool and is strongly suggestive of an upper gastrointestinal source of bleeding. Haematochezia is the passage of fresh blood per anus and is suggestive of a colonic source of bleeding. It is useful to clarify if the fresh blood is mixed in the stool, suggesting a colonic source, or just covering the stool or on the toilet paper, suggesting haemorrhoids or a rectal lesion.

INITIAL INVESTIGATIONS

- Haematology: FBC (anaemia or leukocytosis). Group and save and cross-match 4 units of blood in preparation for transfusion if there are signs of ongoing severe bleeding. ABG (to obtain haemoglobin (Hb) level)
- Biochemistry: U&Es (acute kidney injury, electrolyte imbalance). CRP (inflammation)
- Microbiology: urinalysis (infection)

MANAGEMENT

Determine the volume and rate of bleeding. Identify the likely aetiology and any comorbidities that may adversely affect the outcome, as this will affect management. Continue fluid resuscitation, start a fluid balance chart and consider catheterisation. You should be aware of the major haemorrhage protocol.

Stop antihypertensive medication and withhold antiplatelets or anticoagulants. Look to reverse any clotting abnormalities. You can also give the patient 1 g tranexamic acid, an antifibrinolytic, although the evidence is limited.

An ABG will give you a quick Hb level and may direct you to transfuse the patient prior to the formal lab results. Transfuse if Hb is <8.0 g/dL. You may transfuse at a higher threshold if the patient has a history of cardiac ischaemia.

80–85% of patients with PR bleeding settle spontaneously. However, if bleeding is brisk and ongoing, consider a CT angiogram to identify the source. Bleeding will need to be at a certain rate to identify a bleeding point (0.5 mL/hour), so this may not be useful if bleeding is intermittent. However, if a bleeding point is identified it may allow an interventional radiologist to embolise the source. Both lower and upper gastrointestinal endoscopy can also be considered either acutely or at intervals to investigate the source of bleeding. A small proportion of patients may require surgery to identify and arrest the bleed.

ESCALATION

Put out a major haemorrhage call if the patient is in extremis. Inform your surgical registrar of the patient urgently if the patient is haemodynamically unstable; they will plan further management. Contact the critical care outreach team to review the patient if she is not responding to initial resuscitative measures. Discuss reversal of anticoagulation or correction of clotting with a haematologist. If a CT angiogram is indicated, speak to the interventional radiologists.

You may need to organise an endoscopy with the endoscopy suite or gastroenterology team, or mobilise emergency theatres by speaking to the theatre coordinator and on call anaesthetist.

STATION 17.8: HERNIAS

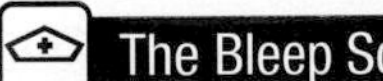

The Bleep Scenario

A 45 year old man has presented to the ED with pain and swelling in his right groin. He was previously fit and well.

His observations are: HR 90 bpm, BP 126/84 mmHg, RR 15 breaths per ute, SpO_2 97% on room air and temperature of 37.4°C. You are asked to review him.

DEFINITION

A hernia is a protrusion of a viscus or part of a viscus through its normal containing structures.

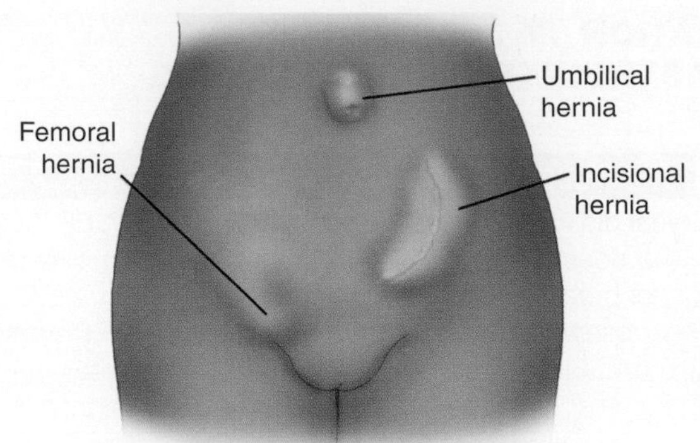

Fig. 17.8 Abdominal wall hernias. (Source: Leonard, P. [2022]. *Building a medical vocabulary with Spanish translations*. Elsevier Saunders.)

INITIAL THOUGHTS

The history given is suggestive of a hernia. There are several factors that can influence the development of a hernia. Indirect inguinal hernias are related a patent processus vaginalis. Direct inguinal hernias are related to a weakness in the abdominal wall, sometimes secondary to previous surgery or collagen disorders. There are several different types of hernias which you may come across on a surgical placement. This may include epigastric, umbilical, Spigelian, incisional, inguinal and femoral hernias (Fig. 17.8). The approach to assessment will be similar.

Risk factors for inguinal hernias include male gender, old age, smoking, family history, abdominal aortic aneurysm, defective transversalis fascia and connective tissue disorders.

DIFFERENTIAL DIAGNOSIS

- Lower gastrointestinal: inguinal or femoral hernia, abscess, lymphadenopathy
- Urology: renal colic, testicular pain, hydrocele
- Vascular: femoral aneurysm, saphena varix

INITIAL INSTRUCTIONS OVER PHONE

Ask the nurse to provide analgesia as required. As the patient is otherwise well, further action can await review.

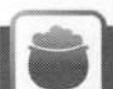

Clinical Tip

Hernia can contain fat or, more seriously, bowel, thus causing bowel obstruction. As a hernia becomes incarcerated, the blood supply to its contents can be compromised. This is a strangulated hernia. Your assessment should look for signs of a strangulated hernia or bowel obstruction.

ASSESSMENT AND RESUSCITATION

- End of the bed assessment: the patient looks well but shows discomfort in his groin.

- Airway: patent.
- Breathing: RR 18 breaths per minute, SpO_2 99% on room air. On auscultation, there are vesicular breath sounds with good air entry bilaterally.
- Circulation: CRT <2 s. HR 80 bpm, regular. BP 130/80 mmHg, HS I + II + 0.
- Disability: GCS 15/15, PEARL, temperature 37°C, CBG 5.5 mmol/L.
- Exposure: abdomen soft and non-tender. Bowel sounds are normal, and no bowel sounds are audible over the lump. There is a tender lump in the right groin, with a cough impulse. Scrotal examination is normal.

Clinical Tip

A cough impulse is indicative of the presence of a hernia and is elicited by palpating the lump and asking the patient to cough. The test is positive if you see or feel the lump increase in size on coughing. It can also be completed if the lump is not visible, by palpating the external ring and asking the patient to cough.

INITIAL INVESTIGATIONS

- Haematology: FBC (leukocytosis or anaemia)
- Biochemistry: U&Es (electrolyte imbalance), CRP (inflammation)
- Microbiology: urinalysis (infection)
- Radiology: abdominal X-ray (bowel obstruction). Ultrasound scan of groin (if the diagnosis is unclear)

MAKING A DIAGNOSIS

- Symptoms: pain and swelling in the groin
- Signs: cough impulse on examination of the lump

MANAGEMENT

Differentiate between an inguinal and a femoral hernia,which is more likely to strangulate. Inguinal hernias are more likely in males. Locate the pubic tubercle, an inguinal hernia will be above and medial to this. A femoral hernia will be below and lateral to the pubic tubercle (Fig. 17.9).

Is the hernia reducible? For an inguinal hernia, recall your anatomy before attempting reduction. The deep inguinal ring is 1 cm above the halfway point between the anterior superior iliac spine and pubic tubercle (midpoint of the inguinal ligament). The superficial ring is about 1 cm above and lateral to the pubic tubercle. Give the patient analgesia. Apply gentle but constant pressure to see if the swelling can be reduced back past the deep ring.

If reducible, then the patient does not need emergency admission, and can be seen in clinic or booked for elective repair. If irreducible then urgent repair should be considered. If there is bowel obstruction, the patient will need a nasogastric tube, IV fluids and emergency hernia repair with possible bowel resection.

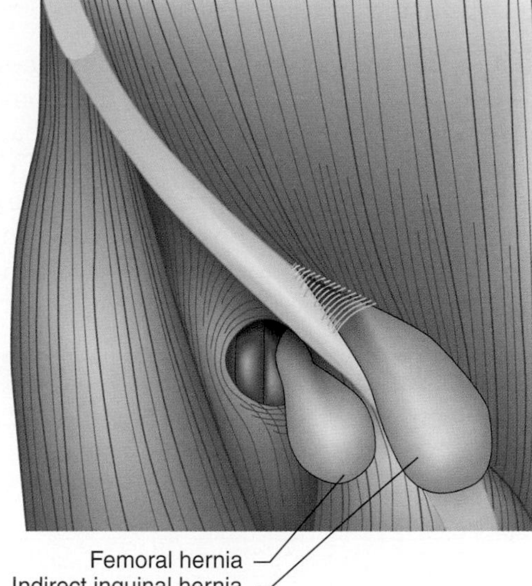

Fig. 17.9 Exit of inguinal and femoral hernias. (Source: Garden, O.J., Parks, R.W. and Wigmore, S.J. (Eds.) [2022]. *Principles and practice of surgery*. Elsevier.)

Clinical Tip

If the patient requires emergency surgery, inform the emergency theatre coordinator, the ward nurses, the on call anaesthetist and the operating surgeon. Know information relevant to booking the case – the team will want to know when the patient will be fasted, any comorbidity, allergies and what tasks are outstanding (i.e. consent, informing next of kin).

ESCALATION

Contact your surgical registrar to review the patient urgently if the hernia is irreducible or associated with suspected bowel obstruction; they will plan further management.

STATION 17.9: HIGH ILIOSTOMY OUTPUT

The Bleep Scenario

A 30 year old male is admitted to the surgical ward. He has recently had a laparotomy, with resultant formation of a stoma. He has now returned with high stoma output.

His observations are: HR 110 bpm, BP 110/75 mmHg, RR 18 breaths per minute, SpO_2 98% on room air and temperature 37.5°C. You are asked to review him.

DEFINITION

A stoma is an opening on the surface of the abdominal wall, either naturally or surgically created, connecting a hollow viscus (bowel or bladder) to the outside environment. Normal distal ileostomy output is 500–700 mL/day. There are different values given for a high-output stoma, usually greater than 1000–2000 mL in 24 hours.

INITIAL THOUGHTS

With high stoma output, you will want to know the type of stoma (Fig. 17.10), how often the stoma bag needs changing and the contents of the stoma bag. You are concerned about dehydration, electrolyte disturbance and impaired renal function. Consider the cause of the high-output stoma; possible causes include short-bowel syndrome, abdominal sepsis, incomplete bowel obstruction and medication.

Clinical Tip

Most water reabsorption occurs in the large bowel, so an ileostomy will have more watery effluent. The more proximal the stoma, the more watery. Therefore, a colostomy will have more formed stool produced.

INITIAL INSTRUCTIONS OVER PHONE

Ask a nurse to obtain IV access, take initial bloods and start IV fluids for resuscitation as required.

ASSESSMENT AND RESUSCITATION

- End of the bed assessment: the patient looks dehydrated.
- Airway: patent.
- Breathing: RR 18 breaths per minute, SpO_2 98% on room air. On auscultation, there are vesicular breath sounds with good air entry bilaterally.
- Circulation: CRT 3 s. HR 110 bpm, regular. BP 110/75 mmHg, HS I + II + 0.
  - Administer 500 mL of crystalloid fluids stat to resuscitate the patient.
- Disability: GCS 15/15, PEARL, temperature 36.7°C, CBG 6.0 mmol/L.
- Exposure: his abdomen is soft, non-tender with a well-healing midline laparotomy wound. He has a stoma located in the right iliac fossa that looks pink and healthy. Normal bowel sounds. Calves unremarkable.

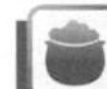

Clinical Tip

Review the patient's drug chart to check if any medications are contributing to the high-output stoma, e.g. prokinetics, metformin or rapid withdrawal of some drugs (e.g. steroids or opiates).

INITIAL INVESTIGATION

- Bedside: ABG (acid–base imbalance)
- Haematology: FBC (leukocytosis or anaemia)
- Biochemistry: CRP (inflammation). Electrolytes, such as magnesium, phosphate and U&Es (acute kidney injury, electrolyte imbalance)
- Microbiology: effluent sample (pathogenic organisms)
- Radiology: abdominal X-ray (subacute obstruction or evidence of colitis)

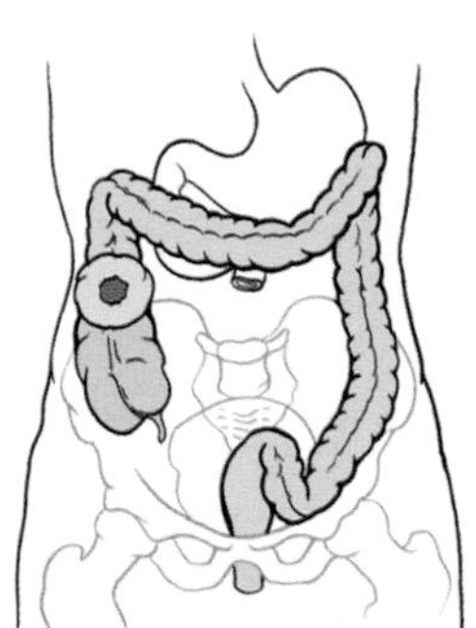

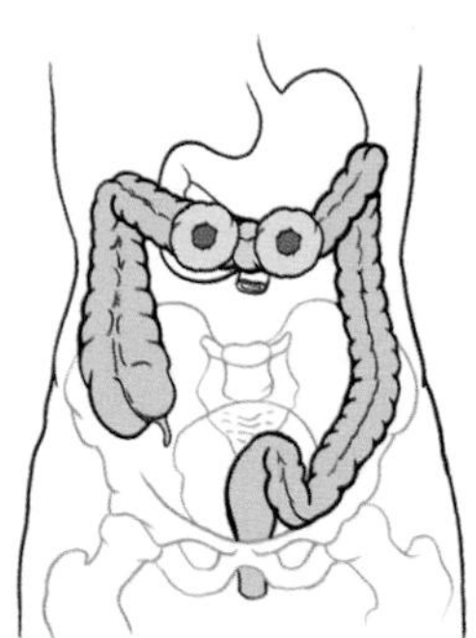

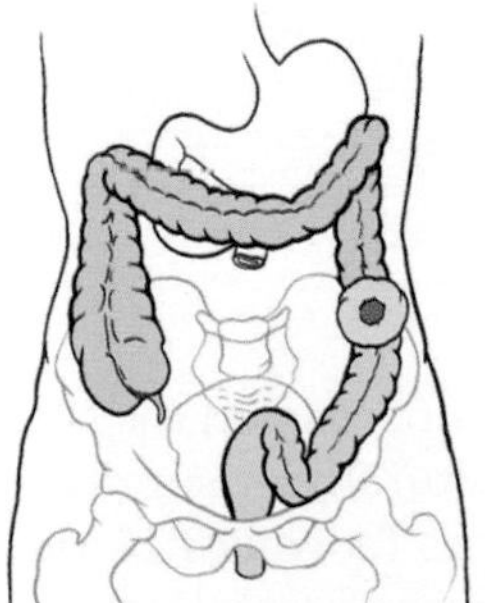

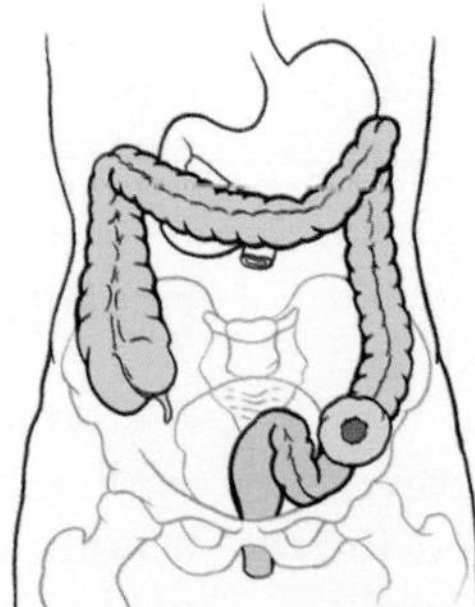

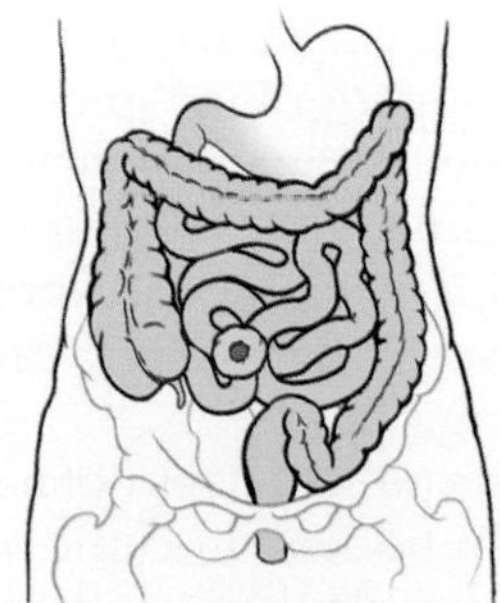

Fig. 17.10 Types of ostomies and intestinal diversions. (Source: Stromberg, H.K. [2022]. *Study guide for medical-surgical nursing: Concepts and practice.* Elsevier.)

MAKING A DIAGNOSIS

Assess the stoma type; colostomies are more likely in the left side of the abdomen, and ileostomies on the right. Ileostomies are spouted, while colostomies are flush with the skin. Examine the bag contents. Watery, green effluent is in keeping with ileostomy while a colostomy produces more formed brown stool. If the contents are urine, then the patient has a urostomy (i.e. ileal conduit). Both ileostomy and colostomy can be end-stomas (one lumen) or a loop (two lumens).

Examine the stoma with the bag off. Have a replacement stoma bag ready. The patient may have the relevant equipment to aid in removing the bag, as well as having a replacement. Protect nearby wounds. Look for a parastomal hernia, protrusion or retraction of the stoma. Assess the quality of the skin around the stoma and the mucosa of the stoma.

MANAGEMENT

Prescribe maintenance fluids once the patient has been adequately resuscitated. Start a fluid balance chart and consider catheterisation. Correct any electrolyte derangement. Nephrotoxic medications will need to be stopped if there are signs of renal compromise.

This patient's stoma is an ileostomy. His high-output ileostomy can be managed by starting loperamide 4 mg four times daily and Dioralyte, if bowel infection is not suspected. Rehydrate with IV fluids.

You should also inform the consultant who has operated on the patient. The specialist stoma nurse may need to get involved if there is concern about stoma care.

ESCALATION

Inform your surgical registrar urgently if there are signs of sepsis, electrolyte imbalance, acute kidney injury or no response to initial resuscitative measures.

FURTHER READING

BMJ Best Practice. *Acute appendicitis.* Available at: https://bestpractice.bmj.com/topics/en-gb/290/history-exam. [Accessed 20 April 2020].

BMJ Best Practice. *Acute cholecystitis.* Available at: https://bestpractice.bmj.com/topics/en-gb/3000084?q=Acute%20cholecystitis&c=suggested. [Accessed 20 April 2020].

BMJ Best Practice. *Large bowel obstruction.* Available at: https://bestpractice.bmj.com/topics/en-gb/877?q=Large%20bowel%20obstruction&c=suggested . [Accessed 20 April 2020].

BMJ Best Practice. *Small bowel obstruction.* Available at: https://bestpractice.bmj.com/topics/en-gb/993. [Accessed 20 April 2020].

Fozard, J. B., et al. (2011). ACPGBI position statement on elective resection for diverticulitis. *Colorectal Disease, 13*(3), 1–11.

Kiriyama, S., et al. (2018). Tokyo guidelines 2018: Diagnostic criteria and severity grading of acute cholangitis. *Journal of Hepato-Biliary-Pancreatic Sciences*, *25*(1), 17–30.

Longmore, M., et al. (2014). *Oxford handbook of clinical medicine* (9th ed.). New York: Oxford University Press.

Masamichi, Y., et al. (2018). Tokyo guidelines 2018: Diagnostic criteria and severity grading of acute cholecystitis. *Journal of Hepato-Biliary-Pancreatic Sciences*, *25*(1), 41–54.

Mountford, C. G., Manas, D. M., & Thompson, N. P. (2014). A practical approach to the management of high output stoma. *Gastroenterology*, *5*, 203–207.

NICE. (2014). *Gallstone disease: Diagnosis and management*, CG188. Available at: www.nice.org.uk/guidance/cg188/chapter/1-Recommendations#managing-gallbladder-stones. [Accessed 20 April 2020].

NICE. (2018). *Acute pancreatitis*. NICE guideline NG104. Available at: www.nice.org.uk/guidance/ng104/chapter/Recommendations#identifying-the-cause. [Accessed 20 April 2020].

Royal College of Surgeons of England. (2013). *Commissioning guide: Rectal bleeding*. Available at: www.rcseng.ac.uk/library-and-publications/rcs-publications/docs/rectal-bleeding-guide/. [Accessed June 2017].

Wilson, D. (1990). Hematemesis, melena, and hematochezia. In H. K. Walker, W. D. Hall, & J. W. Hurst (Eds.), *Clinical methods: The history, physical, and laboratory examinations* (3rd ed.) (pp. 439–442). Boston, MA: Butterworths.

18 Renal and Urology

Content Outline

STATION 18.1: URINARY RETENTION

The Bleep Scenario

A 75 year old male was admitted 3 days ago with a neck-of-femur fracture after falling at home. He is now complaining of abdominal pain, constipation and inability to urinate since last night.

His observations are: heart rate (HR) 92 bpm, blood pressure (BP) 155/60 mmHg, respiratory rate (RR) 18 breaths per minute, SpO_2 96% on room air and temperature of 37.4°C. You are asked to review him.

DEFINITION

Urinary retention is the inability to urinate voluntarily. The presentation may be acute or acute on chronic.

Acute urinary retention is a medical emergency characterised by the inability to pass urine over a period of hours.

Chronic urinary retention is a gradual (over months or years) development of the inability to empty the bladder completely. It is characterised by a residual bladder volume greater than 1 litre or associated with the presence of a distended or palpable bladder.

INITIAL THOUGHTS

The patient is demonstrating symptoms of acute urinary retention – inability to urinate, pain and bloating of the lower abdomen.

It is likely that he has been commenced on strong analgesia following his neck of femur fracture, which could be causing constipation and subsequent urinary retention.

Other causes to consider include urinary tract infection (UTI), prostatic enlargement, stones or blood clots in urethra, urethral stricture, malignancy and Iatrogenic causes.

DIFFERENTIAL DIAGNOSIS

- Gastroenterology: constipation, bowel obstruction, appendicitis
- Vascular: abdominal aortic aneurysm
- Urology: UTI
- Urological: gynaecological surgery
- Latrogenic: catheters, medication and neurological disorders

INITIAL INSTRUCTIONS

Request a bladder scan is completed if the nursing staff have been trained to perform this procedure.

ASSESSMENT AND RESUSCITATION

- End of the bed assessment: the patient looks agitated by the abdominal discomfort.
- Airway: patent.
- Breathing: RR 18 breaths per minute, SpO_2 96% on room air. On auscultation, there are vesicular breath sounds with good air entry bilaterally.
- Circulation: capillary refill time (CRT) <2 s, HR 92 bpm, regular. BP 155/60 mmHg, heart sounds (HS) I + II + 0. Jugular venous pressure (JVP) is normal.
- Disability: Glasgow Coma Scale (GCS) 15/15, pupils equal and reactive to light (PEARL), temperature 37.4°C, capillary blood glucose (CBG) 11.2 mmol/L.
- Exposure: lower abdominal tenderness reported and dullness to percussion. Palpable, distended bladder. Calves are unremarkable. On digital rectal exam, smooth, enlarged prostate is palpable.

Clinical Tip

Complete a digital rectal examination in male patients to assess the size of the prostate and a pelvic exam in female patients to look for pelvic masses.

Prescribing Tip

Review the patient's drug chart, paying attention to precipitants such as opioid analgesia, antimuscarinics, sympathomimetics and anaesthetics.

INITIAL INVESTIGATIONS

- Haematology: full blood count (FBC: anaemia or leukocytosis)
- Biochemistry: urea & electrolytes (U&Es), C-reactive protein (CRP: inflammation)
- Microbiology: urine dip and microscopy, culture and sensitivity (MC&S: infection)
- Radiology: bladder ultrasound (urinary retention). Renal ultrasound and computed tomography (CT) kidneys, ureters and bladders (CTKUB: if obstructive pathology suspected, hydronephrosis). Magnetic resonance imaging (MRI) spine (if signs suggestive of cauda equina syndrome are present, e.g. loss of power or sensation, bladder or bowel incontinence, saddle anaesthesia)

MAKING A DIAGNOSIS

- Symptoms: acute inability to pass urine, painful lower abdomen. In cases of chronic retention, the patient may report urinary frequency, hesitancy, urgency and the feeling of incomplete emptying.
- Signs: palpable bladder, dull to percuss over lower abdomen
- Investigations: bladder ultrasound showing post-void residual volume ≥100 mL

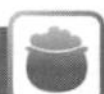 **Clinical Tip**

Postvoid residual volume measures the amount of urine in the bladder after urination. A post-void residual volume of ≥100 mL implies the bladder is not empty.

MANAGEMENT

The most likely diagnosis in this case is acute urinary retention secondary to constipation. Urgent catheterisation is indicated. Record the residual volume (normal bladder size 400–500 mL). Catheterisation may be avoided if the residual volume is less than 200 mL.

Ensure to treat the underlying cause, e.g. antibiotics for UTI.

In males over the age of 65 with recurrent acute retention or acute on chronic urinary retention, guidance currently recommends starting an alpha-1 blocker (modified-release alfusozin or tamsulosin) at least 24 hours before removing the catheter. It is licensed for use for 2–3 days during catheterisation and for 1 day after removal. However, some experts recommend that it is continued until a cause has been identified. In cases where surgical correction may be required, e.g. malignancy or if a urethral stricture is suspected, refer to the urology team for assessment and subsequent management. They may advise to keep the catheter in situ until surgical correction is completed.

Monitor the kidney function to look for any complications of retention, such as acute kidney injury (AKI) or hydronephrosis. If any complications are present, then a trial without catheter (TWOC) is not appropriate and the patient should be discussed with urology.

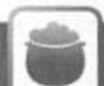 **Clinical Tip**

It is important to consider high-pressure chronic retention in cases where renal impairment and/or hydronephrosis are noted. Patients often report a history of nocturnal enuresis, alongside other lower urinary tract symptoms including hesitancy, slow stream, incomplete emptying and urgency. If suspected, a prompt referral to urology is required for diagnosis with urodynamic testing, and management to minimise the risk of complications.

In cases where there are no complications and the retention is relieved, a TWOC is completed. If the patient is unable to pass urine after a TWOC, generally the patient can be discharged with a catheter and referred to the urology team for follow-up.

ESCALATION

Providing you can insert the catheter and the retention is relieved without any complications, the situation may not need escalating to a senior acutely.

If the patient develops AKI and/or hydronephrosis secondary to the retention or bladder outlet obstruction is suspected, the case should be escalated to your senior and referred to urology.

STATION 18.2: PYELONEPHRITIS

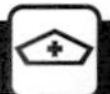 **The Bleep Scenario**

A 25 year old female has been admitted into the emergency department (ED) with flank pain, rigors and pyrexia. She has no significant past medical history.

Her observations are: HR 110 bpm, BP 95/53 mmHg, RR 22 breaths per minute, SpO_2 96% on room air and temperature 38.5°C. You are asked to review her.

DEFINITION

Pyelonephritis, sometimes referred to as an upper UTI, is an infection of the renal parenchyma of one or both kidneys. It is commonly caused by ascending bacterial infection from the bladder, but can also occur secondary to blood-borne organisms.

INITIAL THOUGHTS

Any patient with a high temperature and rigors should be assessed for sepsis.

Pyelonephritis is likely to be the diagnosis given the history of fever in association with flank pain. Risk factors for pyelonephritis include: female gender, immunocompromise, pregnancy, catheter in situ, history of renal/ureteric stones and sexually transmitted infections.

Clinical Tip

Remember to rule out an ectopic pregnancy in females of childbearing age presenting with severe abdominal pain. Pregnancy also warrants more aggressive treatment, often with intravenous (IV) antibiotics in the case of pyelonephritis.

DIFFERENTIAL DIAGNOSIS

- Gastrointestinal: appendicitis, cholecystitis, gastroenteritis, pancreatitis
- Renal: UTI, renal colic
- Gynaecological: ectopic pregnancy, pelvic inflammatory disease, ruptured ovarian cyst
- Musculoskeletal: psoas abscess

INITIAL INSTRUCTIONS OVER PHONE

Ask the nurse to consider supplementary oxygen, aiming for oxygen saturations of more than 94%. Obtain IV access, take initial bloods and start IV fluids as per the sepsis protocol. Request that a urine dipstick and pregnancy test are completed. Advise analgesia cautiously, starting with step 1 of the analgesic ladder and avoiding nephrotoxic medication in large doses.

ASSESSMENT AND RESUSCITATION

- End of the bed assessment: the patient appears drowsy but is rousable. She has an empty vomit bowl next to the bedside.
- Airway: patent.
- Breathing: RR 22 breaths per minute, SpO_2 96% on room air. On auscultation, there are vesicular breath sounds with good air entry bilaterally.
- Circulation: CRT 3 s and clammy to touch, HR 110 bpm, regular. BP 95/53 mmHg, HS I + II + 0. JVP is normal. Dry mucous membranes, reduced skin turgor.
  - Administer 500 mL of crystalloid fluids to resuscitate the patient.
- Disability: GCS 15/15, PEARL, temperature 38.5°C, CBG 5.6 mmol/L.
- Exposure: abdominal tenderness reported on palpation of left renal angle. Bowel sounds present. Calves unremarkable. Pregnancy test negative.

INITIAL INVESTIGATIONS

- Bedside: urine pregnancy test in females of childbearing age (gynaecological causes of abdominal pain, to ensure it is safe to X-ray the patient)
- Haematology: FBC (anaemia or leukocytosis)
- Biochemistry: U&Es (AKI, electrolyte imbalance), liver function tests (rule out biliary causes of abdominal pain), CRP (inflammation), amylase (pancreatitis), venous blood gas (lactate as per sepsis protocol)
- Microbiology: blood cultures and urine MC&S (infection)
- Radiology: a renal ultrasound scan (USS: structural abnormalities), renal CT (pyelonephritis and features of renal stones)

Prescribing Tip

Try to obtain a urine sample for culture before starting empirical antibiotics, if possible, although do not delay treatment.

Clinical Tip

Haematuria and proteinuria can occur with UTIs. Urine dipstick should not be used in patients: (1) with an indwelling catheter or (2) aged over 65 years as dipstick testing becomes more unreliable. Nitrite is produced by a bacterial enzyme that converts nitrates into nitrites. However, this enzyme is not present in all bacteria and a negative result does not exclude a UTI. The presence of leukocytes is also a good indicator of UTI.

MAKING A DIAGNOSIS

- Symptoms: symptoms of UTI (dysuria, increased frequency, increased urgency) plus systemic symptoms of pyelonephritis (fever, malaise, nausea, vomiting, flank pain, acute inability to pass urine, painful lower abdomen). The presence of UTI symptoms, in the absence of significant systemic symptoms, is suggestive of a lower UTI (Fig. 18.1)

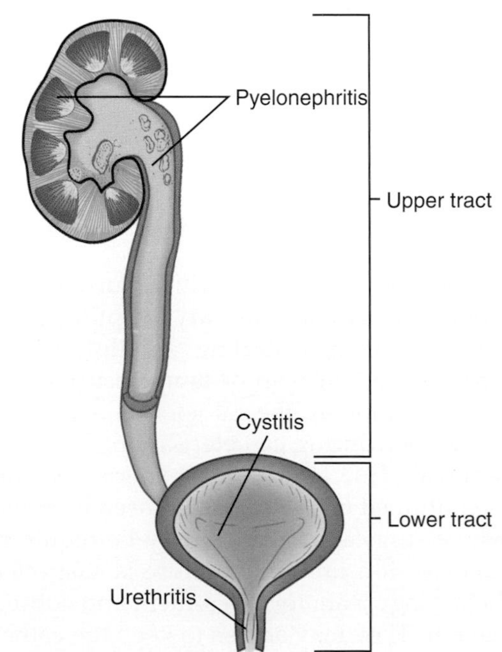

Fig. 18.1 Urinary tract infections. (Source: Harding, M. et al. [2020]. *Lewis's medical-surgical nursing: assessment and management of clinical problems.* 11th ed. Elsevier Mosby.)

- Signs: temperature ≥ 38.5°C, renal angle tenderness – typically unilateral
- Investigations: midstream urine or catheter specimen of urine and culture showing bacteraemia

MANAGEMENT

This patient demonstrates signs of sepsis and should be managed using your local sepsis protocol. Start IV antibiotics within the hour, with guidance from your hospital antimicrobial guidelines. The most common causative bacterium in cases of pyelonephritis is *Escherichia coli*. Other causative pathogens include *Klebsiella*, *Proteus*, *Pseudomonas* and *Enterobacter* species. If the patient does not respond to antibiotics you may have to contact microbiology to discuss sensitivities based on the growth of blood and urine cultures.

Some patients will need a referral for further investigation of an underlying risk factor. These include men following the first episode of pyelonephritis with no obvious cause, women with recurrent pyelonephritis and those where *Proteus* species is identified as the causative organism.

ESCALATION

A senior doctor should review patients who meet the sepsis criteria. If the patient is in septic shock, it may be necessary to escalate to the critical care team.

STATION 18.3: ACUTE KIDNEY INJURY

The Bleep Scenario

A 62 year old male is admitted to a medical ward with pneumonia. He is responding well to his antibiotics. His bloods from today have shown an acute rise in urea and creatinine, and he is scoring on the AKI scale.

His observations are: HR 115 bpm, BP 110/75 mmHg, RR 24 breaths per minute, SpO_2 92% on 2 L of oxygen and temperature 37.8°C. You are asked to review him.

DEFINITION

AKI is a reversible decline in renal excretory function over hours to days due to a number of causes. It results in a failure to maintain fluid, electrolyte and acid–base homeostasis

INITIAL THOUGHTS

You have been informed that the patient has developed AKI. AKIs present with an array of potential symptoms; they are commonly picked up during a routine blood test and in this case the patient may not be symptomatic.

AKI can also present with patients becoming acutely unwell.

AKI can either be classified as acute or acute on chronic. Those with acute on chronic AKI will have a background of chronic kidney disease with a rise in serum creatinine compared to their baseline. Risk factors include increased age, chronic kidney disease, heart failure, diabetes, peripheral vascular disease and previous episodes of AKI.

DIFFERENTIAL DIAGNOSIS (Fig. 18.2)

- Prerenal (most common) is due to hypoperfusion of the kidneys leading to reduced glomerular filtration
- Intrinsic renal is secondary to structural damage of the kidney. It can also be due to damage to renal cells from persistent prerenal or postrenal causes
- Postrenal (least common) is due to acute obstruction of the flow of urine resulting in increased intratubular pressure and decreased glomerular filtration rate

INITIAL INSTRUCTIONS OVER PHONE

Advise the ED referrer to consider supplementary oxygen, aiming for oxygen saturations > 94%. Obtain IV access, take bloods and start IV fluids for resuscitation as required. Request a urine dipstick.

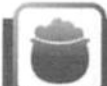

Clinical Tip

Assessment should identify any concerning features, including metabolic acidosis, hyperkalaemia, fluid overload, uraemia and bleeding.

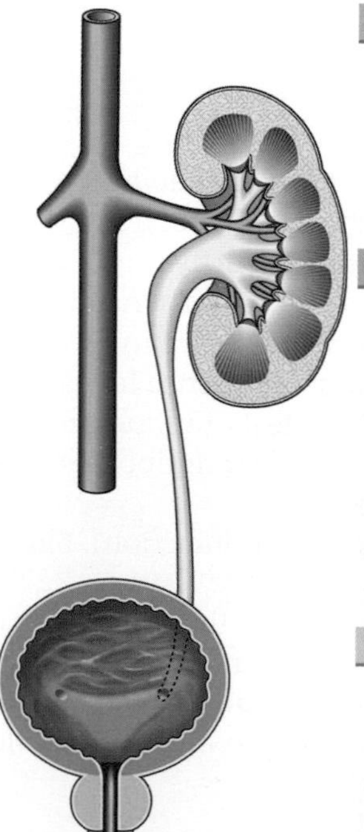

PRERENAL

Impaired perfusion:
- Cardiac failure
- Sepsis
- Blood loss
- Dehydration
- Vascular occlusion

RENAL

Glomerulonephritis
Small-vessel vasculitis
Acute tubular necrosis
- Drugs
- Toxins
- Prolonged hypotension

Interstitial nephritis
- Drugs
- Toxins
- Inflammatory disease
- Infection, including COVID-19

POSTRENAL

Urinary calculi (bilateral)
Retroperitoneal fibrosis
Benign prostatic hypertrophy
Bladder cancer
Prostate cancer
Cervical cancer
Urethral stricture/valves
Meatal stenosis/phimosis

Fig. 18.2 Causes of acute kidney injury. (Source: Walker, B.R. and Colledge, N.R. [2023]. *Davidson's principles and practice of medicine*. Elsevier Health Sciences.)

ASSESSMENT AND RESUSCITATION

- End of the bed assessment: the patient is agitated and is vomiting into a bowl.
- Airway: patent.
- Breathing: RR 24 breaths per minute, SpO_2 92% on 2 L oxygen. On auscultation, there are vesicular breath sounds with good air entry bilaterally.
- Circulation: CRT <2 s, HR 115 bpm, regular. BP 110/75 mmHg, HS I + II + 0. JVP is normal.
  - Administer crystalloid fluids. Generally, this is in a stepwise regimen of 2, 4, 6, 8, 12-hourly but should be tailored to the patient's requirements (e.g. if the patient has congestive cardiac failure, administration will need to be slower).
  - 12-lead electrocardiogram (ECG): normal ECG, no signs of hyperkalaemia.
  - Catheter in situ: urine output 200 mL over the past 8 hours.
- Disability: GCS 15/15, PEARL, CBG 13.1 mmol/L, temperature 37.8°C.
- Exposure: abdomen soft and non-tender. Lower-limb exam shows no signs of deep-vein thrombosis but there is mild bilateral pitting oedema. No rash noted.

Prescribing Tip

Review the patient's drug chart; stop or adjust any nephrotoxic medications. Common nephrotoxic medications (using the mnemonic CANDAM): contrast media, angiotensin-converting enzyme (ACE) inhibitors/angiotensin receptor blockers, non-steroidal anti-inflammatory drugs (NSAIDs), diuretics, antibiotics (e.g. vancomycin, aminoglycosides) and metformin.

INITIAL INVESTIGATIONS

- Haematology: FBC (leukocytosis or anaemia)
- Biochemistry: U&Es (electrolyte imbalance, stage the AKI), CRP (inflammation). Further investigations to consider: creatinine kinease (rhabdomyolysis), urine for albumin:creatinine ratio (chronic kidney disease), urine sodium and Bence Jones protein (myeloma), immunology tests (antineutrophil cytoplasmic antibodies, antinuclear antibodies, immunoglobulins, complement)
- Microbiology: urine MC&S (urine infection), blood cultures (infection)
- Radiology: chest X-ray (signs of fluid overload). Consider renal USS within 12 hours (renal obstruction) or within 24 hours (if AKI fails to respond to treatment, small, scarred kidneys may be visible on USS)

MAKING A DIAGNOSIS

Detect an AKI using the following criteria:

- A rise in serum creatinine of ≥26 µmol/L within 48 hours
- Be aware that in the absence of a baseline creatinine value, a high serum creatinine level may indicate AKI, even if the rise in creatinine over 48 hours is less than 26 µmol/L (particularly if the patient has been unwell)
- A ≥50% rise in serum creatinine (more than 1.5 times baseline) known or presumed to have occurred within the past 7 days
- A fall in urine output to <0.5 mL/kg/hour for more than 6 hours (if it is possible to measure this, for example, if the person has a catheter)
- AKI can be classified into three stages:

ACUTE KIDNEY INJURY STAGES

STAGE	CREATININE	URINE OUTPUT
1	Creatinine rise of ≥26 µmol/L within 48 hours or Creatinine rise of 1.50–1.99 × from baseline within 7 days	<0.5 mL/kg/hour for >6 hours
2	Creatinine rise of 2.00–2.99 × from baseline within 7 days	<0.5 mL/kg/hour for >12 hours
3	Creatinine rise of ≥3.00 × from baseline within 7 days. For acute injury with pre-existing chronic kidney disease: Current creatinine ≥354 µmol/L with either • Rise of ≥26 µmol/L within 48 hours or • Rise of ≥50% from baseline within 7 days. Any requirement for renal replacement therapy	<0.3 mL/kg/hour for 24 hours or Anuria for 12 hours

MANAGEMENT

Treat the AKI by reversing any potential causes, e.g. if the patient is hypotensive secondary to septic shock, treat the sepsis appropriately.

Stop all nephrotoxic medications. Monitor fluid balance by inserting a catheter if appropriate and record daily weights. Optimise fluid balance, treat hypovolaemia and avoid dehydration by administering IV fluids. Patients with AKI may require aggressive IV hydration. Monitor kidney function daily for signs of improvement. While patients are in AKI, medications must be reviewed regularly and dose adjustments made.

ESCALATION

Not all patients with AKI need a referral to the renal team. Early referral is recommended in patients with severe AKI (AKI stage 3) and with complications refractory to medical treatment. Complex fluid regimens in patients with concurrent renal and cardiac failure can be discussed with the renal team. Also, consult the renal team in the event of any complex drug dosing queries for these patients. In the event of deterioration despite treatment, patients should be discussed with the medical registrar, renal team or intensive care team if unstable for consideration of renal replacement therapy (RRT).

RRT is indicated for patients not responding to medical management with the following conditions:

- Refractory hyperkalaemia
- Fluid overload
- Pulmonary oedema
- Metabolic acidosis
- Uraemia

STATION 18.4: HAEMATURIA

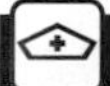

The Bleep Scenario

A 75 year old male with dementia, admitted on the medical ward, has pulled out his catheter. He is confused and there appears to be some bleeding from his urethra.

His observations are: HR 90 bpm, BP 145/75 mmHg, RR 24 breaths per minute, SpO_2 93% on room air and temperature 37.8°C. You are asked to review him.

DEFINITION

Haematuria is the presence of blood in the urine, which can be macroscopic (visible haematuria (VH)/gross haematuria) or microscopic (non-visible/dipstick-positive haematuria). Non-visible haematuria can be further subdivided into symptomatic non-visible haematuria (s-NVH) and asymptomatic non-visible haematuria (a-NVH).

INITIAL THOUGHTS

First consider the acute management of the catheter being removed, as frank bleeding would need assessment urgently. You should consider why the patient is catheterised and if this is clinically necessary. In the above case there is an obvious cause of the haematuria; however, you must consider other differentials. If the confusion is acute you should also look for potential causes of acute delirium, such as sepsis, stroke and myocardial infarction.

DIFFERENTIAL DIAGNOSIS

- Infection: UTI, cystitis, urethritis
- Tumour: renal carcinoma, carcinoma of the bladder, prostate cancer, urethral cancer
- Trauma: renal tract trauma due to accidents, catheter or foreign body, rapid emptying of an overdistended bladder (e.g. after catheterisation for acute retention), prolonged severe exercise
- Inflammation: glomerulonephritis, Henoch–Schönlein purpura, IgA nephropathy
- Structural: calculi (renal, bladder, ureteric), simple cysts, polycystic renal disease, congenital
- Haematological: sickle cell disease, coagulation disorders, anticoagulation therapy
- Surgery: invasive procedures to the prostate or bladder
- Toxins: sulfonamides, cyclophosphamide
- Other: genital bleeding, menstruation, Munchausen's syndrome

Clinical Tip

Consider other causes of red or dark urine:

- Haemoglobinuria: dipstick positive but no red cells on microscopy
- Myoglobinuria
- Food: beetroot
- Drugs: rifampicin, nitrofurantoin, senna
- Porphyria: urine darkens on standing
- Bilirubinuria: obstructive biliary disease

INITIAL INSTRUCTIONS OVER PHONE

Ask the ED referrer to obtain IV access and take bloods. Establish volume of blood loss and administer fluid resuscitation as required. Request a urine dipstick.

ASSESSMENT AND RESUSCITATION

- End of the bed assessment: the patient appears very agitated and confused. There is minimal blood on the patient's sheets.
- Airway: patent.
- Breathing: RR 24 breaths per minute, SpO_2 93% on room air. On auscultation, there are vesicular breath sounds with good air entry bilaterally.
- Circulation: CRT <2 s, HR 90 bpm, regular. BP 145/75 mmHg, HS I + II + 0. JVP is normal. No clinical signs of dehydration.
- Disability: GCS 15/15, PEARL, temperature 37.8°C, CBG 5.3 mmol/L.
- Exposure: abdomen soft and non-tender. Minimal bleeding from the urethral meatus. Macroscopic haematuria noted in the urine, no clots evident. Calves are unremarkable.

INITIAL INVESTIGATIONS

- Haematology: FBC (anaemia or leukocytosis)
- Biochemistry: U&Es (electrolyte disturbance), clotting screen (coagulopathy), CRP (inflammation), group and save and cross-match (in cases of severe bleeding, when transfusion may be considered)
- Microbiology: urine dip and MC&S (infection). Albumin:creatinine ratio (renal disease)
- Radiology: CT urogram (CTU) or ultrasound (malignancy, stones). CT is the imaging modality of choice

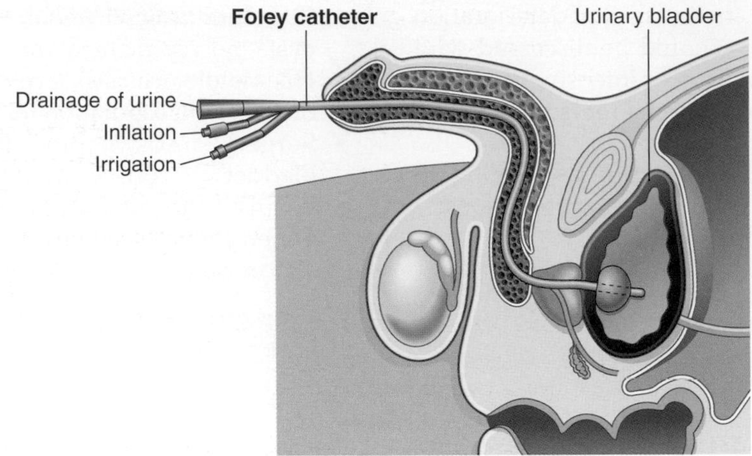

Fig. 18.3 Foley catheter in place in the urinary bladder. The three-way catheter has three separate lumens: for drainage of urine, for inflation of balloons in the bladder and for introduction of irrigating solutions into the bladder. (Source: Chabner, D.E. [2021]. *The language of medicine*. Elsevier.)

 **Clinical Tip**

Urine dipstick of fresh voided urine sample is a sensitive means of detecting haematuria. Significant haematuria is considered 1+ or greater. Trace haematuria should be considered negative. Routine microscopy for confirmation of dipstick haematuria is not necessary.

 **Clinical Tip**

A fifth of macroscopic haematuria is associated with urological malignancy. If malignancy is suspected, the patient will require imaging such as CTU and cystoscopy. Cystoscopy will usually be organised after haematuria settles; however, in cases of ongoing haematuria it will be requested on a more urgent basis.

 **Clinical Tip**

Measuring the blood pressure, U&Es and the albumin: creatinine ratio will exclude haematuria secondary to renal disease.

MAKING A DIAGNOSIS

Significant haematuria is defined as:

- Any single episode of VH
- Any single episode of s-NVH (in the absence of UTI or other transient causes)
- Persistent a-NVH (in the absence of UTI or other transient causes). Persistence is defined as two out of three dipsticks positive for NVH

MANAGEMENT

If there is massive blood loss and haemodynamic instability, an urgent referral to urology is needed as well as consent for blood transfusion. Monitor closely for signs of active bleeding. Reinsert a catheter to avoid urethral obstruction from clots. If the patient is passing clots, insert a three-way catheter (Fig. 18.3), which also allows irrigation of the bladder. If urethral trauma is suspected, catheterisation may be difficult, requiring experience and early discussion with urology.

With confused patients it is important to rationalise why they need interventions. If the patient is likely to pull tubes out, you should weigh the clinical need and risk of patient removal. If catheterisation is necessary in confused patients you can bandage the catheter around the patient's leg or use dummy catheters. In cases where these interventions have failed it may be appropriate to use hand control mittens. However, before using hand mittens, deprivations of liberty safeguards documentation should be completed.

Although there appears to be a justification for the haematuria in this case (i.e. catheter-related), it may be appropriate to consider further investigations and referral.

INDICATIONS FOR UROLOGICAL REFERRAL FOR FURTHER INVESTIGATION

- All patients with VH
- All patients with s-NVH
- All patients with a-NVH aged ≥ 40 years

INDICATIONS FOR UROLOGICAL REFERRAL FOR SUSPECTED BLADDER AND RENAL CANCER

- Aged ≥ 45 with the following:
  - Unexplained visible haematuria without UTI
  - Visible haematuria that persists or recurs after successful treatment of UTI
- Aged ≥ 60 with unexplained non-visible haematuria and either dysuria or a raised white cell count on a blood test

INDICATIONS FOR RENAL REFERRAL

- For patients who have had a urological cause excluded or have not met the referral criteria for a urological assessment

- Evidence of declining estimated glomerular filtration rate (eGFR) >10 mL/minute at any stage within the previous 5 years or by >5 mL/minute within the previous year
- Stage 4 or 5 chronic kidney disease (eGFR ≤30 mL/minute)
- Significant proteinuria (albumin:creatinine ratio ≥30 mg/mmol)
- Isolated haematuria (in the absence of significant proteinuria) with hypertension in those aged younger than 40 years
- Visible haematuria coinciding with intercurrent (usually upper respiratory tract) infection

ESCALATION

There is any evidence of hypotension or a low haemoglobin secondary to acute blood loss, refer urgently to urology for advice. If you struggle to pass the catheter during reinsertion, seek help from a senior. If this fails then contact the urology team.

STATION 18.5: RENAL COLIC

 **The Bleep Scenario**

A 45 year old male has presented with severe abdominal pain, radiating from his loin to groin, and nausea. He appears to be clinically dehydrated on assessment. He has no significant past medical history to report.

His observations are: HR 115 bpm, BP 130/85 mmHg, RR 20 breaths per minute, SpO_2 94% on room air and temperature 37.4°C. You are asked to review him.

DEFINITION

Renal colic is an acute and severe abdominal pain, radiating from the loin to the groin, secondary to obstruction of flow of urine in the ureter by a urinary stone.

INITIAL THOUGHTS

The location of the pain is highly suggestive of renal colic. Dehydration is a well-known risk factor for renal stones.

Other risk factors for stone formation include: being male, age 40–60 years, excessive dietary intake of oxalate, urate, sodium and animal protein, obesity, positive family history of renal stone formation, anatomical abnormalities of the urinary tract, certain gastrointestinal (e.g. Crohn's disease, malabsorptive conditions) and genetic (e.g. cystinuria, renal tubular acidosis, cystic fibrosis) conditions.

DIFFERENTIAL DIAGNOSIS

- Renal: pyelonephritis, obstruction of the ureter (e.g. blood clot, stricture, urothelial tumour), acute renal infarction, renal rupture, renal abscess
- Gastrointestinal: gastro-oesophageal reflux disease (GORD), acute cholecystitis, biliary colic, appendicitis, peritonitis, gastroenteritis, inflammatory bowel disease, bowel obstruction or ischaemia
- Gynaecological: ectopic pregnancy, endometriosis, ovarian torsion or cyst rupture, pelvic inflammatory disease, salpingitis
- Vascular: aortic or iliac aneurysms
- Other: musculoskeletal pain, pneumonia or pleurisy, shingles, testicular torsion, factitious renal colic

 **Clinical Tip**

Make sure you rule out a leaking abdominal aortic aneurysm as it can closely mimic renal colic, and if missed can be fatal.

INITIAL INSTRUCTIONS OVER THE PHONE

Advise the nurse to give analgesia and complete a urine dipstick test.

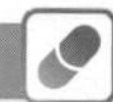 **Prescribing Tip**

Provide adequate analgesia – NSAIDs are generally used first-line. For rapid relief of severe pain, a rectal suppository of diclofenac can be used. If NSAIDs are contraindicated, prescribe paracetamol ± weak opioids. Manage nausea and active vomiting with antiemetics; IV administration is often preferred as oral antiemetics are not practical.

 **Clinical Tip**

Make sure you exclude the main complications of urinary stones on assessment – obstruction of urinary flow and infection.

ASSESSMENT AND RESUSCITATION

- End of the bed assessment: the patient is alert, but is in obvious pain. He is clutching the right side of his abdomen.
- Airway: patent.
- Breathing: RR 20 breaths per minute, SpO_2 94% on room air. On auscultation, there are vesicular breath sounds with good air entry bilaterally.
- Circulation: CRT <2 s, HR 115 bpm, regular. BP 130/85 mmHg, HS I + II + 0. JVP is normal. Dry mucous membranes, reduced skin turgor.
  - Administer crystalloid fluids to resuscitate the patient.
- Disability: GCS 15/15, PEARL, temperature 37.4°C, CBG 7.2 mmol/L.
- Exposure: abdominal tenderness on palpation of right renal angle. Bowel sounds present.

INITIAL INVESTIGATIONS

- Bedside: urine pregnancy test in females of childbearing age (gynaecological causes of abdominal pain, to ensure it is safe to X-ray the patient)
- Haematology: FBC (leukocytosis)

- Biochemistry: U&Es (assess renal function), CRP (inflammation), calcium, phosphate and urate levels (assess for potential electrolyte imbalances that may cause renal stones)
- Microbiology: urine dip and MC&S (infection, haematuria)
- Radiology: CT KUB (diagnose renal stones, look for complications, e.g. hydronephrosis), US KUB (diagnose renal stones), abdominal X-ray (some renal calculi are visible on plain film) (Fig. 18.4).

Clinical Tip

Urgent imaging should be offered to all patients to confirm diagnosis and assess the likelihood of spontaneous stone passage, by assessing the size and location of the stone (within 24 hours). Most adults will be offered a low dose non-contrast CT. Children, young people and females of child-bearing age should be offered ultrasound first-line.

MAKING A DIAGNOSIS

- Symptoms: acute, severe (mostly unilateral) flank pain radiating from loin to groin, which occurs in spasms. Associated symptoms may include nausea, vomiting, haematuria, increased urinary frequency or dysuria
- Signs: renal angle tenderness on the affected side, ipsilateral flank tenderness
- Investigations: CT KUB or US KUB to diagnose renal stones

MANAGEMENT

The primary diagnosis in this case is renal colic secondary to renal or ureteric stones. Arrange immediate hospital admission if the patient is septic, at risk of AKI, has a solitary or transplanted kidney, bilateral obstruction is suspected, the patient is dehydrated and cannot take fluids orally due to nausea and vomiting or if the diagnosis is unclear.

Encourage oral intake of fluids; adult patients should aim to have 2.5–3 L/day. If there is concern about dehydration or patients are unable to drink orally due to nausea or vomiting, consider prescribing IV fluids.

Further management depends on the size and location of the stone, and whether there are signs of infection. Patients with urinary stones and signs of infection need urgent urology referral for rapid renal decompression, via nephrostomy or stent insertion, and IV antibiotics.

If the stone is <5 mm, it is very likely to pass spontaneously and 'watchful waiting' can be considered. It can also be considered if the stone is > 5 mm with safety netting and adequate counselling of the risks and benefits.

Active surgical management to remove the stone is indicated if the stone fails to pass or there is readmission with ongoing/increasing pain. Surgical options include: ureteroscopy, percutaneous nephrolithotomy and open surgery. The choice of surgical procedure depends on factors such as the size of the stone, the age of the patient, any obvious contraindications, if previous procedures have failed and upon anatomical considerations.

Extracorporeal shock wave lithotripsy (ESWL) is a non-invasive outpatient treatment that focuses shock waves on the stone to break it up. The smaller stone particles can then pass spontaneously. Ureteroscopy involves the use of various energy sources (e.g. lasers) to again break up the stone. Percutaneous nephrolithotomy is considered for renal stones when ESWL and ureteroscopy fail. This is a procedure in which a nephroscope is passed percutaneously into the collecting system and the stone is fragmented and extracted through the nephroscope. Open surgery is rarely indicated but it is required in cases where all the above have failed, are unlikely to be successful or where complications have occurred.

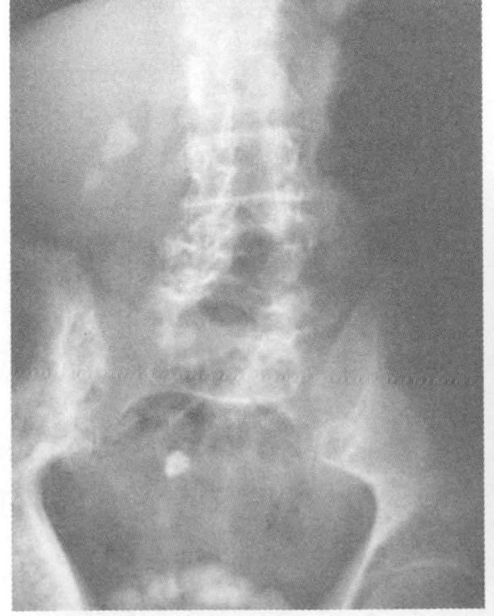

A radiolucent kidney stone can be seen on the KUB at the ureterovesical junction.

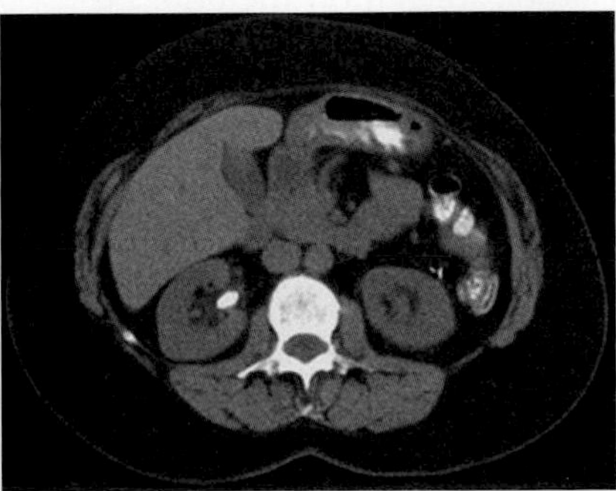

A large stone is seen in the renal pelvis of the right kidney.

Fig. 18.4 Renal stones on abdominal X-ray and computed tomography scan. A radiolucent kidney stone can be seen on the kidneys, ureters and bladder (KUB) at the ureterovesical junction. A large stone is seen in the renal pelvis of the right kidney. (Source: Used with permission of GE Healthcare.)

ESCALATION

Refer to urology on an urgent basis if the patient has signs of infection, recurring severe pain or there is evidence of hydronephrosis on CT scan.

If the stone is >5 mm, complications are present or the stone does not pass spontaneously, you should discuss with urology for further management.

FURTHER READING

Carlo, N., & Muir, G. (2012). Chronic urinary retention in men: How we define it, and how does it affect treatment outcome? *British Journal of Urology International*, *110*, 1590–1594.

NICE. (2013). *Acute kidney injury: Prevention, detection and management*. NG148. Available at: www.nice.org.uk/guidance/ng148. [Accessed 25 July 2022].

NICE. (2015). *Urological cancers – recognition and referral*. Available at: https://cks.nice.org.uk/urological-cancers-recognition-and-referral#!scenario. [Accessed 16 January 2022].

NICE. (2019). *LUTS in men*. Available at: https://cks.nice.org.uk/topics/luts-in-men/management/urinary-retention/. [Accessed 16 January 2022].

NICE. (2020). *Renal or ureteric colic – acute*. Available at: https://cks.nice.org.uk/topics/renal-or-ureteric-colic-acute/. [Accessed 16 January 2022].

NICE. (2021). *Management of acute pyelonephritis*. Available at: https://cks.nice.org.uk/topics/pyelonephritis-acute/management/management/. [Accessed 16 January 2022].

Pickard, R., et al. (2015). Medical expulsive therapy in adult with ureteric colic: A multicentre, randomised, placebo-controlled trial. *The Lancet*, *386*(9991), 341–349.

Renal Association and British Association of Urological Surgeons. (2008). Joint consensus statement on the initial assessment of haematuria. Available at: www.baus.org.uk/_userfiles/pages/files/News/haematuria_consensus_guidelines_July_2008.pdf. [Accessed 16 January 2022].

19 Vascular

Content Outline

STATION 19.1: AORTIC DISSECTION

 The Bleep Scenario

A 70 year old male has presented to the emergency department (ED) with a 2-hour history of severe, tearing chest pain radiating to the back. He has a past medical history of hypertension and diabetes.

His observations are: heart rate (HR) 140 bpm, blood pressure (BP) 155/80 mmHg, respiratory rate (RR) 24 breaths per minute, SpO_2 94% on room air and temperature 37.1°C. You are asked to review him.

DEFINITION

Aortic dissection results from a tear in the aortic intima. The subsequent blood flow between the intima and the media results in the formation of a false lumen. The tear may extend through the adventitia, leading to rupture, or through the intima at a secondary location, leading to re-entry into the aorta.

INITIAL THOUGHTS

Consider the common causes of chest pain. The history is strongly suggestive of an aortic dissection – severe, tearing chest pain radiating to the back. Any condition that increases intimal shear stress or decreases arterial wall strength is considered to be a risk factor for aortic dissection. Hypertension, connective tissue diseases (e.g. Marfan's or Ehlers–Danlos syndrome), increasing age, family history, atherosclerosis, aortic valve disease (bicuspid valve), previous aneurysms, pregnancy and cocaine abuse are important risk factors to consider.

DIFFERENTIAL DIAGNOSIS

- Cardiac: acute coronary syndrome, cardiac tamponade, pericarditis, aortic aneurysm
- Chest: pulmonary embolism, pneumothorax, mediastinitis
- Gastrointestinal: pancreatitis, oesophageal perforation
- Locomotor: musculoskeletal pain

INITIAL INSTRUCTIONS OVER PHONE

Ask the ED referrer to consider supplementary oxygen, aiming for oxygen saturations > 94%. Obtain intravenous (IV) access with two large-bore cannulae, take initial bloods and start IV fluids for resuscitation as required. Advise analgesia, and it is crucial to reduce BP.

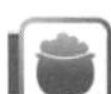 Clinical Tip

Look for signs of end-organ ischaemia as you are assessing the patient. Renal ischaemia may present with deranged creatinine levels and refractory hypertension. Acute limb ischaemia with limb pain and paralysis. Patients with mesenteric ischaemia may present with abdominal pain. Spinal cord ischaemia is a rare complication, presenting with paraplegia. Patients are also at risk of stroke if the carotid artery is involved.

ASSESSMENT AND RESUSCITATION

- End of the bed assessment: the patient is sweaty, confused and appears short of breath.
- Airway: patent.
- Breathing: RR 30 breaths per minute, SpO_2 94% on room air. On auscultation, there are vesicular breath sounds with good air entry bilaterally.
- Circulation: capillary refill time (CRT) >2 s. HR 130 bpm, regular. BP 160/80 mmHg in both arms. Heart sounds are dual, with an early diastolic murmur suggestive of aortic regurgitation. Jugular venous pressure (JVP) is normal.
  - 12-lead electrocardiogram (ECG): may show evidence of myocardial ischaemia or may be normal, depending on the degree of coronary vessel involvement.
- Disability: Glasgow Coma Scale (GCS) 14/15, E4V4M6. Pupils equal and reactive to light (PEARL), temperature 37.5°C, capillary blood glucose (CBG) 8.4 mmol/L.
- Exposure: no focal neurological deficits.

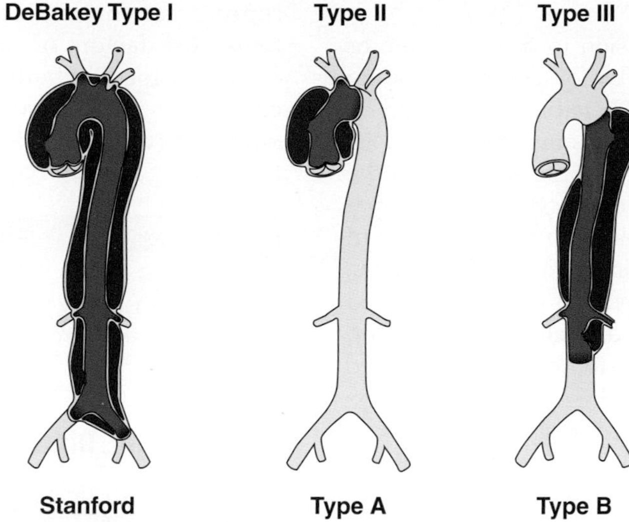

DeBakey

Type I	Originates in the ascending aorta, propagates at least to the aortic arch and often beyond it distally
Type II	Originates in and is confined to the ascending aorta
Type III	Originates in the descending aorta and extends distally down the aorta or, rarely, retrograde into the aortic arch and ascending aorta

Stanford

Type A	All dissections involving the ascending aorta, regardless of the site of origin
Type B	All dissections not involving the ascending aorta

Fig. 19.1 Common classifications of thoracic aortic dissection. (Source: Hartjes, T. (Ed.) [2022]. *AACN core curriculum for progressive and critical care nursing.* Elsevier.)

INITIAL INVESTIGATIONS

- Haematology: full blood count (FBC: anaemia or infection), group and save and cross-match (if transfusion necessary, in preparation for theatre)
- Biochemistry: troponin (myocardial infarction), D-dimer (pulmonary embolism, to risk stratify the likelihood of aortic dissection), urea and electrolytes (U&Es) and liver function tests (LFTs: to assess for organ hypoperfusion)
- Radiology: chest X-ray (CXR: pulmonary causes of chest pain, to look for signs of aortic dissection), computed tomography (CT) angiography (in stable patients for a definitive diagnosis of aortic dissection) or bedside ultrasound echocardiogram (to aid diagnosis in unstable patients)

 **Clinical Tip**

Features suggestive of aortic dissection on a chest X-ray include widening of the aortic silhouette or mediastinum, pleural effusion and enlargement of the aortic knuckle. The absence of these features does not rule out dissection.

MAKING A DIAGNOSIS

- Symptoms: acute, severe tearing chest pain radiating to the back
- Signs: discrepancy in BP between both arms is a hallmark feature
- Investigation: imaging will determine the type of aortic dissection. Type A dissection involves the ascending aorta. Type B dissection involves the rest of the aorta, usually beyond the origin of the left subclavian artery (Fig. 19.1)

MANAGEMENT

Initial management is determined by the type of aortic dissection, as seen on cardiac imaging. Type A aortic dissection requires immediate surgical intervention, whilst type B dissections are initially managed medically.

It is important to ensure the patient has been given adequate pain relief; any persisting pain may indicate progression of the dissection or impending rupture.

TYPE A

The patient will need a blue-lighted transfer to the nearest cardiothoracic surgery centre. Surgical repair, involving excision of the intimal tear and placement of a graft, should be performed immediately in type A aortic dissection unless the patient has any contraindications to surgery. The surgical team will make this decision. Mortality in type A aortic dissection remains high, even with immediate surgical intervention.

TYPE B

The patient will require admission to coronary care or the high dependency unit (HDU) for closer monitoring and control of BP and pain. IV beta-blockers should be given if the patient is hypertensive, aiming for a systolic BP of 100–120 mmHg, to minimise shear stress on the aorta. If beta-blockers are contraindicated or if the patient is not responding to beta-blockers, consider calcium channel antagonists and/or renin–angiotensin inhibitors. Surgical or endovascular interventions can be considered in patients with type B aortic dissection who develop complications, such as end-organ ischaemia secondary to occlusion of a major aortic branch, aortic rupture or extension of the dissection. Updated analysis of data from the International Registry of Aortic Dissection (IRAD) suggests that there may also be some benefit to endovascular intervention in patients with uncomplicated type B aortic dissection with refractory pain and hypertension.

 **Clinical Tip**

The IRAD shows that hypotension, absence of chest/back pain and branch vessel involvement are predictors of in-hospital mortality.

ESCALATION

All suspected cases of aortic dissection should be immediately referred to the cardiothoracic or vascular team, as immediate surgical repair will be required in some cases. Untreated type A aortic dissection has a 50% mortality rate within the first 48 hours.

STATION 19.2: ABDOMINAL AORTIC ANEURYSM

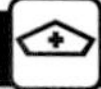 **The Bleep Scenario**

A 74 year old man presents to ED via an ambulance, with a painful and distended abdomen. He is known to have a past medical history of hypertension and hypercholesterolaemia.

His observations are: HR 140 bpm, BP 70/60 mmHg, RR 30 breaths per minute, SpO_2 94% on room air and temperature 37.0°C. You are asked to review him.

DEFINITION

Abdominal aortic aneurysm (AAA) is a pathological, full-thickness dilatation of the abdominal aorta, at least 1.5 times larger than the expected normal diameter.

INITIAL THOUGHTS

The primary differential until proven otherwise is a ruptured AAA, which is classically associated with a triad of abdominal pain, abdominal distension/swelling and haemodynamic instability. However, note that this triad is only present in 50% of cases and often AAA rupture presents with non-specific abdominal symptoms. Risk factors of AAA include age, male gender, family history, hypertension, hypercholesterolaemia, connective tissue disorders and smoking. However, note that ruptured AAA is more common in women than men.

 **Clinical Tip**

You should rule out aortic dissection, which may present similarly but typically involves sharp chest pain, and is likewise a surgical emergency.

DIFFERENTIAL DIAGNOSIS

- Vascular: aortic dissection, ulcerated aortic plaque, inferior wall myocardial infarction
- Gastrointestinal: ischaemic bowel, bowel obstruction, diverticulitis, appendicitis, pancreatitis, gastroenteritis, gastrointestinal bleed, peritonitis

INITIAL INSTRUCTIONS OVER PHONE

Advise the ED referrer to obtain IV access with two large-bore cannulae, take bloods, start oxygen, aiming for oxygen saturations > 94%, and commence hypotensive fluid resuscitation.

ASSESSMENT AND RESUSCITATION

- End of the bed assessment: the patient is sweaty, confused, and appears short of breath.
- Airway: patent.
- Breathing: RR 30 breaths per minute, SpO_2 94% on room air. On auscultation, there are vesicular breath sounds with good air entry bilaterally.
- Circulation: CRT > 2 s. HR 140 bpm, regular. BP 70/60 mmHg in both arms. HS I + II + 0. Peripheral pulses are absent.
  - Administer 500 mL of crystalloid fluids stat to resuscitate the patient
  - 12-lead ECG: assess cardiac comorbidities and rule out myocardial ischaemia.
- Disability: the patient is confused. GCS 13/15, E3V6M4. PEARL. Temperature 37.5°C. CBG 8.6 mmol/L.
- Exposure: an expansile, pulsatile, tender abdominal mass is palpated.

INITIAL INVESTIGATIONS

- Haematology: FBC (anaemia, leukocytosis)
- Biochemistry: C-reactive protein (CRP: inflammation). U&Es (to assess for organ hypoperfusion, electrolyte imbalance). Group and save and cross-match (in preparation for transfusion and surgery)
- Microbiology: blood cultures (infectious AAA)

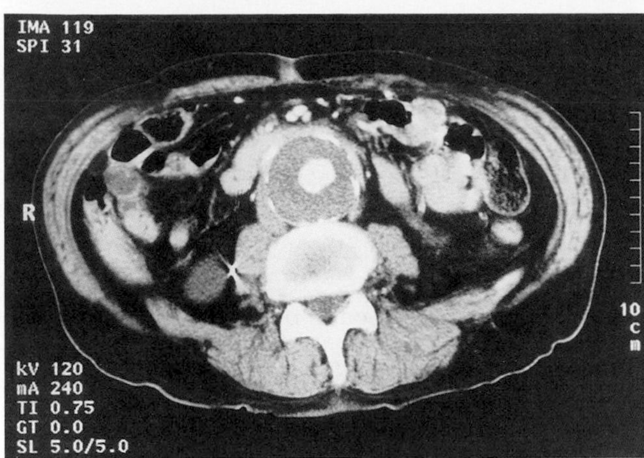

Fig. 19.2 Computed tomography scan of an abdominal aortic aneurysm. Contrast in the lumen of the vessel, a thick layer of mural thrombus and calcification in the aneurysm wall are shown. (Source: Crawford, M.H., DiMarco, J.P. and Paulus, W.J. (Eds.) [2004]. *Cardiology*. 2nd ed. St Louis, MO: Mosby.)

- Radiology: CT aorta is the imaging modality of choice in suspected or confirmed cases as long as the patient is stable (Fig. 19.2). Bedside aortic ultrasound (if there is a delay in CT aorta/instability of patient)

 **Clinical Tip**

Signs suggestive of a contained ruptured AAA on CT include large aneurysm sac, increase in aneurysm size, a thrombus and high-attenuation crescent sign, focal discontinuity in circumferential wall calcification and the 'draped aorta sign'.

 **Clinical Tip**

Patients who have a documented history of AAA and present symptomatically do not require further investigation. They can be immediately transferred to the operating theatre. However, if the patient is stable, a CT is desirable, as it will aid in planning for cases that are suitable for endovascular repair.

MAKING A DIAGNOSIS

- Symptoms: painful and distended abdomen. Symptoms of cerebral hypoperfusion may be present, such as lightheadedness, dizziness, headache, fatigue or confusion.
- Signs: an expansile, pulsatile, tender abdominal mass is classically associated with AAA, but is not a sensitive sign due to the retroperitoneal position of the abdominal aorta. Other signs that may be present are hypotension and the absence of peripheral pulses.

MANAGEMENT

RUPTURED AAA

You should commence fluids in cases of haemodynamic instability, targeting a systolic BP around 70 mmHg to maintain cerebral and cardiac perfusion. Aggressive fluid resuscitation may worsen bleeding.

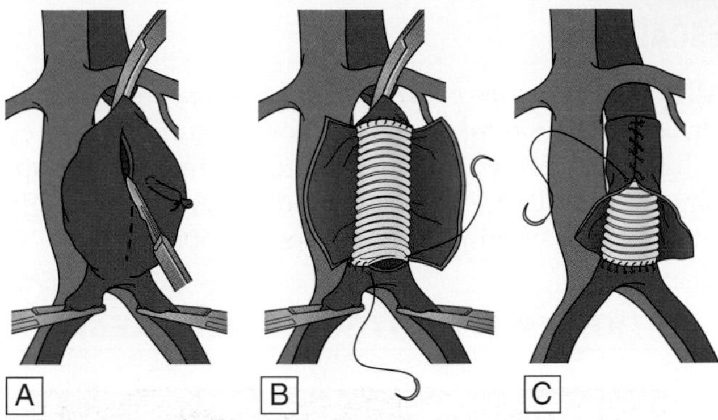

Fig. 19.3 Surgical repair of an abdominal aortic aneurysm. (A) Incising the aneurysmal sac. (B) Insertion of synthetic graft. (C) Suturing native aortic wall over synthetic graft. (Source: Cooper, K. and Gosnell, K. [2022]. *Foundations and adult health nursing*. Elsevier.)

You should prepare packed red blood cells, clotting factors and platelets, in anticipation of the need for transfusion during surgical repair.

Surgical repair, either endovascular repair or open surgery (Fig. 19.3), is necessary for all patients with a ruptured AAA. Open surgery involves replacement of the affected aortic segment with a graft. Endovascular repair involves the placement of a graft via the femoral arteries.

Endovascular repair is more beneficial than open surgical repair for the majority of people, especially in males over the age of 70 and females of any age. CT imaging will assist in determining the patient's anatomical suitability for an endovascular repair. Open surgical repair provides a better balance of risk and benefit in males under 70.

 **Clinical Tip**

If the team is going to operate, inform the theatre coordinator, ward nurses, on call anaesthetist and the operating surgeon. The team will want to know when the patient will be fasted, if there are any comorbidities, allergies and what tasks are outstanding (i.e. consent, informing next of kin). Most patients undergoing emergency laparotomy will require a HDU or intensive therapy unit bed, so you may need to coordinate this with the intensive care team.

NON-RUPTURED SYMPTOMATIC AAA

Patients who have non-ruptured, symptomatic AAAs are at increased risk of AAA rupture, and urgent surgical (open or endovascular) repair is indicated.

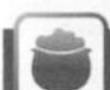 **Clinical Tip**

Most AAAs present asymptomatically and are found incidentally or on routine screening of patients with risk factors. Asymptomatic AAA should be monitored in the outpatient setting, as the risk of rupture is low (<1% per year) if the AAA is under 5.5 cm in diameter. Elective surgery may be undertaken for AAAs > 5.5 cm diameter or > 4 cm diameter with growth > 1 cm in 1 year to minimise the risk of AAA rupture.

ESCALATION

All suspected cases of AAA should be immediately referred to the vascular registrar or consultant, as they will require immediate surgical repair in cases of ruptured AAA. Untreated ruptured AAA is invariably fatal, usually within hours of presentation.

STATION 19.3: ACUTE LIMB ISCHAEMIA

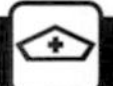 The Bleep Scenario

A 64 year old male has presented to the ED with acute onset of pain, numbness and weakness in his left leg. He has a history of hypertension and myocardial infarction.

His observations are: HR 90 bpm, BP 145/90 mmHg, RR 16 breaths per minute, SpO_2 94% on room air and temperature 37.0°C. You are asked to review him.

DEFINITION

Acute limb ischaemia is defined as a sudden decrease in limb perfusion, threatening limb viability.

INITIAL THOUGHTS

Acute limb ischaemia is a surgical emergency and should be urgently excluded in this case. This man reports key symptoms (pain, numbness and weakness) and has strong risk factors of limb ischaemia (history of hypertension and coronary artery disease). You should consider the causes of reduced limb perfusion. Causes of acute limb ischaemia include thrombosis, emboli and arterial dissection or trauma.

DIFFERENTIAL DIAGNOSIS

- Vascular: deep-vein thrombosis (DVT), vasospasm, arterial dissection
- Orthopaedics: compartment syndrome, soft-tissue trauma
- Neurological: neuropathy, cord compression/ischaemia

INITIAL INSTRUCTIONS OVER PHONE

Ask the ED referrer to obtain IV access, take initial bloods and give analgesia as required.

 Clinical Tip

The severity of acute limb ischaemia is classified as viable, threatened and non-viable depending on the degree of sensory loss, muscle weakness and Doppler signal. Your assessment should ascertain the severity and aetiology of limb ischaemia as this will guide further management.

Pain, pallor, paraesthesia, paralysis, pulselessness and perishing cold/poikilothermia (6 Ps) are classical features of an acute bloodless leg, requiring urgent revascularisation within 6 hours.

ASSESSMENT AND RESUSCITATION

- End of the bed assessment: the patient is distressed; his left leg is pale.
- Airway: patent.
- Breathing: RR 16 breaths per minute, SpO_2 98% on room air. On auscultation, there are vesicular breath sounds with good air entry bilaterally.
- Circulation: CRT >2 s, HR 80 bpm, regular, BP 140/90 mmHg assessed in both arms. HS I + II + 0. Cold and pale left lower limb with absent popliteal, dorsalis pedis and posterior tibial pulses. Upper-limb and right-lower-limb pulses are present.
  - Assess lower limb pulses with a Doppler instrument – audible flow indicates a better prognosis.
  - Ankle–brachial index can be taken if there is audible Doppler flow – ankle–brachial index in acute limb ischaemia is a predictor of outcome.
  - 12-lead ECG: to assess cardiac comorbidities and suitability for revascularisation.
- Disability: GCS 15/15, PEARL, temperature 37.5°C, CBG 8.4 mmol/L.
- Exposure: abdomen soft and non-tender, with normal bowel sounds. Left lower limb tender, pale in appearance, with associated paraesthesia, sensory loss and reduced power (4/5).

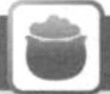 Clinical Tip

Calf muscle tenderness is a worrying sign as it may be late and can indicate the development of compartment syndrome.

INITIAL INVESTIGATIONS

- Haematology: FBC (anaemia or leukocytosis), thrombophilia screen (in selected cases – clotting disorder)
- Biochemistry: U&Es (biochemical baseline) and coagulation profile (coagulopathy)
- Radiology: arteriography, CT angiography or magnetic resonance (MR) angiography (localise obstruction)

 Clinical Tip

Patients should have an on-table angiogram; imaging should not delay management if immediate revascularisation is required.

MAKING A DIAGNOSIS

Limb ischaemia can be separated into acute or chronic, depending on the duration of symptoms. Acute limb ischaemia is the presence of symptoms of limb ischaemia (6 Ps) for 2 weeks or less, typically presenting within hours in patients without underlying vascular disease. Onset in patients with vascular disease is variable. Chronic limb ischaemia is the presence of symptoms for greater than 2 weeks.

- Symptoms and signs: 6 Ps – paraesthesia, pain, pallor, pulselessness, poikilothermia and paralysis
- Aetiology: thrombosis (60% of causes; commonly associated with atherosclerotic plaques, bypass grafts and aneurysms), emboli (30%; cardiac or paradoxical), arterial dissection or trauma

MANAGEMENT

All patients with acute limb ischaemia should receive heparin as a bolus, followed by continuous heparin infusion to prevent further propagation of thromboemboli.

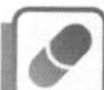 **Prescribing Tip**

Heparin is contraindicated in cases where there is a history of heparin-induced thrombocytopenia.

Acute limb ischaemia with no sensory or motor deficits and an audible Doppler signal indicates a viable limb. Mild sensory deficits (involvement of toes) with no motor deficit and an inaudible arterial Doppler signal indicate a marginally threatened limb. Moderate sensory deficits (more than toe involvement), rest pain, motor deficit and an inaudible arterial Doppler signal indicate an immediately threatened limb. Viable, marginally threatened and immediately threatened limbs are all indications for immediate revascularisation. Profound sensory and motor deficits and inaudible arterial and venous Doppler signals indicate an irreversibly damaged limb (Fig. 19.4). This is an indication for amputation.

Revascularisation can be achieved through endovascular catheterisation or open surgery, and sometimes by thrombolysis, especially for occluded bypasses. This decision will be made by the vascular team. In general, endovascular catheterisation is preferred in viable or marginal cases, and open surgery is preferred in patients with an immediately threatened limb.

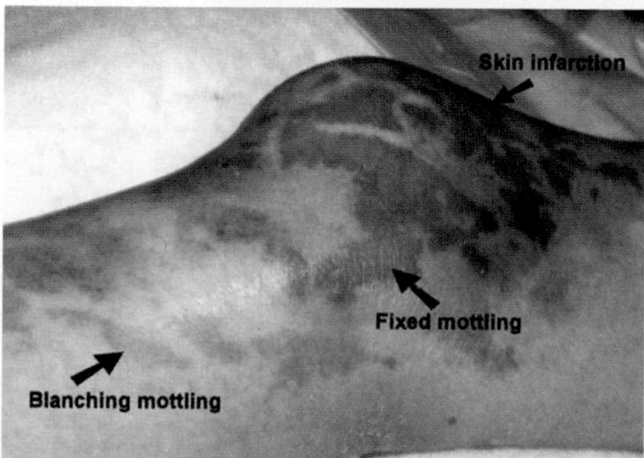

Fig. 19.4 Skin changes resulting from severe acute limb ischaemia. Fixed mottling of the skin is indicative of non-viability. (Source: Watson, P. and O'Brien, J. [2016]. *The junior doctor survival guide*. Elsevier.)

 **Clinical Tip**

If surgery is decided upon by your seniors, inform the theatre coordinator, ward nurses, on call anaesthetist and the operating surgeon. Know information relevant to booking the case. The team will want to know when the patient will be fasted, if there are any comorbidities, allergies and what tasks are outstanding (i.e. consent, informing next of kin).

ESCALATION

Irreversible nerve and muscle damage can occur within hours of presentation. All suspected cases of acute limb ischaemia should be immediately referred to the vascular registrar or consultant, as urgent revascularisation may be required.

STATION 19.4: DEEP-VEIN THROMBOSIS

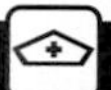 **The Bleep Scenario**

A 67 year old female has presented to the ED with a 1 day history of painful, swollen and erythematous left calf. She had a left-sided total hip arthroplasty last week.

Her observations are: HR 80 bpm and regular, BP 130/90 mmHg, RR 16 breaths per minute, SpO_2 97% on room air and temperature 37.5°C. You are asked to review her.

DEFINITION

Deep vein thrombosis (DVT) is a blood clot in the distal venous system.

INITIAL THOUGHTS

DVT is your primary differential, taking into account the unilateral presentation of symptoms and the background of recent surgery. Risk factors for DVT relate to Virchow's triad (endothelial damage, venous stasis and hypercoagulability). These include immobility, recent surgery, travel, thrombophilia, pregnancy, contraceptive use, malignancy and age.

DIFFERENTIAL DIAGNOSIS

- Unilateral: DVT, cellulitis, thrombophlebitis, lymphoedema, Baker's cyst or trauma, e.g. calf muscle tear or haematoma
- Bilateral: drug-induced (e.g. vasodilators such as amlodipine, nifedipine), hypoalbuminaemia, cardiac failure, renal failure, venous insufficiency, pregnancy or pelvic mass

INITIAL INSTRUCTIONS OVER PHONE

Advise the ED referrer to obtain IV access and take bloods.

Clinical Tip

Assessment must rule out the potentially fatal complication of pulmonary embolus. Any presence of chest pain, breathlessness or haemoptysis should raise your suspicion. In addition, an examination of the peripheral vascular system must be completed, as a massive DVT in the lower extremity (phlegmasia cerulea dolens) can compromise vascular supply and lead to acute limb ischaemia.

ASSESSMENT AND RESUSCITATION

- End of the bed assessment: the patient looks comfortable. You note that her left calf is swollen and erythematous.
- Airway: patent.
- Breathing: RR 16 breaths per minute, SpO_2 98% on room air. On auscultation, good air entry both sides with no added breath sounds.
- Circulation: CRT <2 s, HR 80 bpm, regular. BP 130/90 mmHg assessed in both arms, HS I + II + 0. Peripheral pulses are present.
  - 12-lead ECG: to assess cardiac function and look for signs of pulmonary embolus.
- Disability: GCS 15/15, PEARL, temperature 37.5°C, CBG 7.5 mmol/L.
- Exposure: left-calf oedema, erythema and tenderness. No other significant findings.

INITIAL INVESTIGATIONS

- Haematology: FBC (anaemia, bleeding risk, underlying predispositions such as malignancy)
- Biochemistry: D-dimer (diagnostic aid). U&Es and LFTs (therapeutic drug dose adjustment, impairment). Coagulation profile (coagulopathies, prerequisite prior to anticoagulants)
- Radiology: duplex ultrasound (evidence of thrombus in deep veins) (Fig. 19.5). CXR, CT abdomen and pelvis and/or mammogram (malignancy in cases of unprovoked thrombus)

MAKING A DIAGNOSIS

Initial evaluation and management are dependent on the pretest probability of DVT, as determined by the two-step Wells score (Table 19.1).

LOW PRETEST PROBABILITY

Patients in whom DVT is suspected but with a low pretest probability should receive a D-dimer test within 4 hours. If this is not possible, offer interim therapeutic anticoagulation whilst awaiting the result. A negative D-dimer in these patients usually excludes a DVT. If this is the case, consider an alternative diagnosis and discuss the signs and symptoms of DVT and where to seek further medical help if required. A positive result is an indication for investigation with ultrasound.

HIGH PRETEST PROBABILITY

Patients with a high pretest probability require urgent venous duplex ultrasound (DUS) within 4 hours, to rule out DVT (Fig. 19.6). If a venous DUS cannot be completed within 4 hours, a D-dimer test and interim therapeutic anticoagulation should be given. Findings on ultrasound consistent with DVT in patients with a high pretest probability are diagnostic. Patients with a high pretest probability with negative ultrasound findings should receive a D-dimer test if not previously done. Repeat the venous DUS

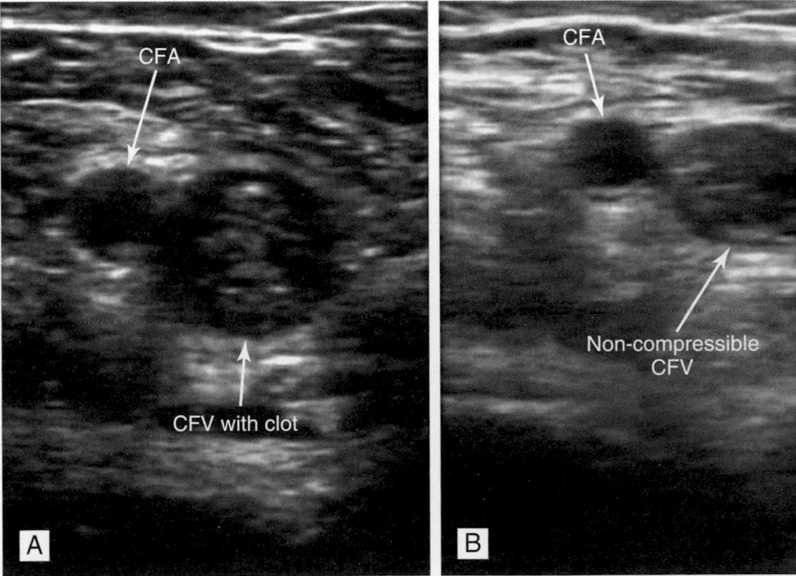

Fig. 19.5 Two-dimensional duplex ultrasound of a common femoral vein (CFV) with deep-vein thrombosis (DVT). (A) Without compression. (B) With compression (minimally compressible due to DVT). CFA, common femoral artery. (Source: Zaidi, G. and Tsegaya, A. [2015]. Ultrasonography for deep venous thrombosis. *Critical Care in Ultrasound*, pp. 60–65.)

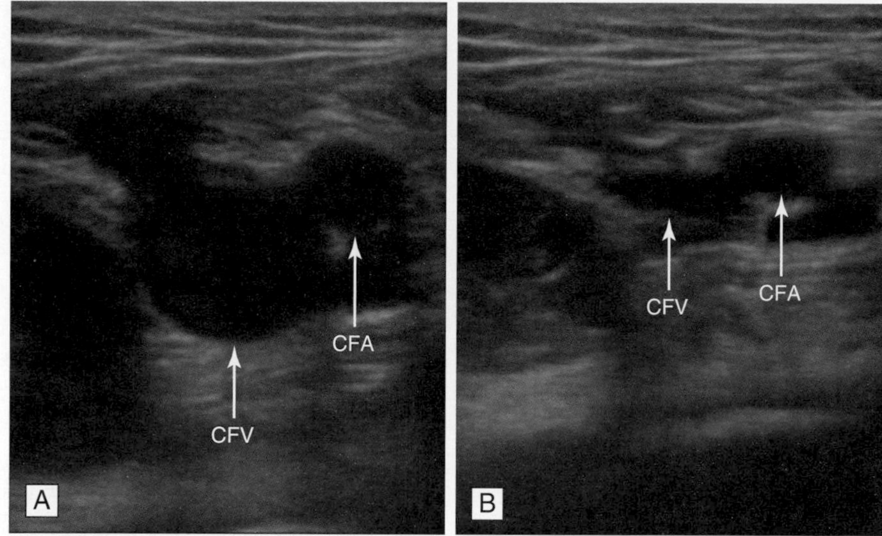

Fig. 19.6 Two-dimensional duplex ultrasound of a common femoral vein (CFV) without deep-vein thrombosis (DVT). (A) Without compression. (B) With compression, showing complete apposition of the anterior and posterior walls of the vein. CFA, common femoral artery. (Source: Zaidi, G. and Tsegaya, A. [2015]. Ultrasonography for deep venous thrombosis. *Critical Care in Ultrasound*, pp. 60–65.)

Table 19.1 Two-step Wells score[a]

CLINICAL FEATURE	POINTS
Active cancer (treatment ongoing, within 6 months, or palliative)	1
Paralysis, paresis or recent plaster immobilisation of the lower extremities	1
Recently bedridden for 3 days or more or major surgery within 12 weeks requiring general or regional anaesthesia	1
Localised tenderness along with the distribution of the deep venous system	1
Entire leg swollen	1
Calf swelling at least 3 cm larger than asymptomatic side	1
Pitting oedema confined to the symptomatic leg	1
Collateral superficial veins (non-varicose)	1
Previously documented DVT	1
An alternative diagnosis is at least as likely as DVT	−2

[a]1 point or less indicates a low pretest probability of deep-vein thrombosis (DVT).
2 points or more indicate a high pretest probability of DVT.

6–8 days later for all patients with a positive D-dimer test and a negative ultrasound scan, and no anticoagulation cover.

DUS should note the location of the DVT, as this influences management.

MANAGEMENT

ANTICOAGULATION

A proximal DVT is of greater clinical significance, as it confers a 50% risk of developing a pulmonary embolism. Distal venous thrombi are often smaller and capable of spontaneous thrombolysis, conferring a lower risk of pulmonary embolism.

Direct oral anticoagulants, such as apixaban or rivaroxaban, should be considered the first line. The choice of agent will depend on patient factors such as hepatic/renal function, pregnancy, cancer, obesity and bleeding risk. Trust guidelines and professional preferences will also influence it. Direct oral anticoagulants, unlike warfarin, do not require monitoring.

If neither apixaban or rivaroxaban is suitable, offer low-molecular-weight heparin (LMWH) for at least 5 days, followed by dabigatran or edoxaban. Alternatively, LMWH in conjunction with warfarin can be given for at least 5 days until the international normalised ratio is at least 2.0 in two consecutive readings, followed by warfarin alone.

Symptomatic distal DVT and asymptomatic distal DVT with evidence of extension towards the proximal veins follow the same treatment algorithm: anticoagulation for at least 3 months.

After 3 months of anticoagulation, the risks and benefits of continuing anticoagulation should be considered. Consider extending the treatment period for patients with unprovoked proximal DVT if their risk of venous thromboembolism recurrence is high, and there is no risk of major bleeding. Patients with active cancer should receive anticoagulant therapy for at least 6 months.

OTHER TREATMENT OPTIONS

Thrombolysis can be considered in patients who have symptomatic iliofemoral DVTs with symptoms less than 14 days' duration, good functional status, a life expectancy of 1 year or more and a low risk of bleeding.

Inferior vena cava filters are considered in patients when anticoagulation is contraindicated and should be removed once anticoagulation can be commenced.

Prescribing Tip

All patients should have their bleeding risk assessed before commencing anticoagulation. Patient factors that confer a bleeding risk include active bleeding, acquired bleeding disorders (e.g. acute liver failure), acute stroke, thrombocytopenia, uncontrolled systolic hypertension and uncontrolled inherited bleeding disorders.

ESCALATION

Pulmonary embolism secondary to a DVT can lead to significant illness. The patient should be reviewed by the medical registrar or consultant who will direct further management.

FURTHER READING

Bates, S. M., & Ginsberg, J. S. (2004). Treatment of deep-vein thrombosis. *New England Journal of Medicine*, *351*(3), 268–277.

Bjork, M., et al. (2020). Editor's choice: European Society for Vascular Surgery (ESVS) 2020 clinical practice guideline on the management of acute limb ischaemia. *European Journal of Vascular and Endovascular Surgery*, *59*(2), 173–218.

Braverman, A. C. (2010). Acute aortic dissection. *Circulation*, *122*(2), 184–188.

Callum, K., & Bradbury, A. (2000). Acute limb ischaemia. *BMJ*, *320*(7237), 764–767.

Creager, M. A., Kaufman, J. A., & Conte, M. S. (2012). Acute limb ischemia. *New England Journal of Medicine*, *366*(23), 2198–2206.

Erbel, R., et al. (2014). ESC guidelines on the diagnosis and treatment of aortic diseases: Document covering acute and chronic aortic diseases of the thoracic and abdominal aorta of the adult. The Task Force for the Diagnosis and Treatment of Aortic Diseases of the European Society of Cardiology (ESC). *European Heart Journal*, *35*(41), 2873–2926.

Gerhard-Herman, M. D., et al. (2016). AHA/ACC guideline on the management of patients with lower extremity peripheral artery disease. A report of the American College of Cardiology/ American Heart Association Task Force on Clinical Practice Guidelines, *69*(11), e71–e126.

Hagan, P. G., et al. (2000). The International Registry of Acute aortic Dissection (IRAD): New insights into an old disease. *JAMA*, *283*(7), 897–903.

Kearon, C., et al. (2016). Antithrombotic therapy for VTE disease: Chest guideline and expert panel report. *Chest*, *149*(2), 315–352.

Kent, K. C. (2014). Abdominal aortic aneurysms. *New England Journal of Medicine*, *371*(22), 2101–2108.

Layden, J., et al. (2012). Diagnosis and management of lower limb peripheral arterial disease: Summary of NICE guidance. *BMJ*, *345*.

Lederle, F. A., et al. (2002). Immediate repair compared with surveillance of small abdominal aortic aneurysms. *New England Journal of Medicine*, *346*(19), 1437–1444.

Lee, T. H., & Goldman, L. (2000). Evaluation of the patient with acute chest pain. *New England Journal of Medicine*, *342*(16), 1187–1195.

Metcalfe, D., Holt, P. J. E., & Thompson, M. M. (2011). The management of abdominal aortic aneurysms. *BMJ*, *342*.

Moll, F. L., et al. (2011). Management of abdominal aortic aneurysms. Clinical practice guidelines of the European Society for Vascular Surgery. *European Journal of Vascular and Endovascular Surgery*, *41*(1), S1–S58.

NICE. (2020a). *Abdominal aortic aneurysm: Diagnosis and management*. NG156. Available at: www.nice.org.uk/guidance/ng156/chapter/Recommendations#diagnosis. [Accessed 7 January 2022].

NICE. (2020b). *Venous thromboembolic diseases: Diagnosis, management and thrombophilia testing*. NG158. Available at: www.nice.org.uk/guidance/ng158. [Accessed 7 August 2020].

Nienaber, C. A., & Eagle, K. A. (2003). Aortic dissection: New frontiers in diagnosis and management part 1: From etiology to diagnostic strategies. *Circulation*, *108*(5), 628.

Nienaber, C. A., & Eagle, K. A. (2003). Aortic dissection: new frontiers in diagnosis and management part 2: therapeutic management and follow-up. *Circulation*, *108*(6), 772.

Norgren, L. et al. Inter-Society Consensus for the Management of Peripheral Arterial Disease (TASC II). *European Journal of Vascular and Endovascular Surgery*, *33*(1, Supplement), S1–S75.

Riambau, V., et al. (2017). Management of descending thoracic aorta disease. *European Journal of Vascular and Endovascular Surgery*, *53*(1), 4–52.

Rutherford, R. B., et al. (1997). Recommended standards for reports dealing with lower extremity ischemia: Revised version. *Journal of Vascular Surgery*, *26*(3), 517–538.

Tendera, M., et al. (2011). ESC guidelines on the diagnosis and treatment of peripheral artery diseases: Document covering atherosclerotic disease of extracranial carotid and vertebral, mesenteric, renal, upper and lower extremity arteries: The Task Force on the Diagnosis and Treatment of Peripheral Artery Diseases of the European Society of Cardiology (ESC). *European Heart Journal*, *32*(22), 2851–2906.

Trimarchi, S., et al. (2010). Importance of refractory pain and hypertension in acute type B aortic dissection: Insights from the International Registry of Acute Aortic Dissection (IRAD). *Circulation*, *122*(13), 1283–1289.

Wells, P. S., et al. (2003). Evaluation of D-dimer in the diagnosis of suspected deep-vein thrombosis. *New England Journal of Medicine*, *349*(13), 1227–1235.

Orthopaedics

20

Content Outline

STATION 20.1: ACUTE OSTEOMYELITIS

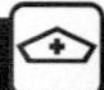 The Bleep Scenario

Your are bleeped by the ED nurse. A 59 year old diabetic woman has presented with painful foot ulcers, associated with foot swelling and fever. She has a past medical history of asthma, poorly controlled type 2 diabetes mellitus with neuropathy, diabetic foot ulcers and chronic kidney disease.

Her observations are: heart rate (HR) 104 bpm, blood pressure (BP) 112/87 mmHg, respiratory rate (RR) 18 breaths per minutes, SpO_2 94% on room air and temperature 38.8°C. You are asked to review her.

DEFINITION

Osteomyelitis is an inflammatory condition of the bone caused by an infecting organism, most commonly *Staphylococcus aureus*. It usually involves a single bone but rarely can affect multiple sites.

INITIAL THOUGHTS

This woman has signs of sepsis. Osteomyelitis is rare in healthy adults. It is more common in children (especially the long bones of boys), diabetics, immunocompromised, in those with sickle cell disease, tuberculosis, following orthopaedic surgery or trauma, intravenous (IV) drug users or in those with indwelling lines. Bacteria can reach the bone directly or indirectly. Direct inoculation can occur through open wounds, or during open orthopaedic surgery. Indirect infections can come from the blood stream or from adjacent tissue or prosthetics.

DIFFERENTIAL DIAGNOSIS

- Rheumatology: gout
- Trauma and orthopaedics: trauma (soft-tissue injury or fracture)
- Other: cellulitis
- Haematology: acute sickle cell crisis

 Clinical Tip

The key to distinguishing between trauma and osteomyelitis is the duration of symptoms. Symptoms should rapidly settle following minor trauma. Persistent pain and swelling in response to the initial injury, as well as increased inflammatory markers, raise the clinical suspicion of osteomyelitis. It is therefore important to tell patients being discharged with a history of minor trauma to return if their symptoms do not settle or if they become systemically unwell.

INITIAL INSTRUCTIONS OVER PHONE

Ask the nurse to give supplementary oxygen, aiming for oxygen saturations > 94%. Also, ask them to obtain IV access, take bloods and start IV fluids for resuscitation as per the sepsis protocol.

ASSESSMENT AND RESUSCITATION

- End of the bed assessment: the patient appears distressed and in pain.
- Airway: patent.
- Breathing: RR 18 breaths per minute, SpO_2 94% on room air. On auscultation, there are vesicular breath sounds with good air entry bilaterally.
- Circulation: capillary refill time (CRT) 3 s, HR 110 bpm, regular. BP 112/87 mmHg, heart sounds (HS) I + II + 0, jugular venous pressure (JVP) normal.
    - Administer 500 mL of crystalloid fluids stat to resuscitate the patient.
- Disability: Glasgow Coma Scale (GCS) 15/15, pupils equal and reactive to light (PEARL), temperature 38.8°C, capillary blood glucose (CBG) 7.1 mmol/L.
- Exposure: abdomen soft and non-tender. Bowel sounds are normal. Ulceration noted around the feet and ankles bilaterally. A deep ulcer is noted on the left foot dorsum, with associated tenderness, swelling, erythema and warmth. The patient

has palpable pulses and reduced sensation up to the ankle bilaterally.

INITIAL INVESTIGATIONS

- Haematology: full blood count (FBC: leukocytosis).
- Biochemistry: C-reactive protein (CRP) and erythrocyte sedimentation rate (ESR): inflammation. Venous blood gas (VBG: lactate as per sepsis protocol). Urea and electrolytes (U&Es: electrolyte imbalance). Blood glucose and HbA_{1c} in patients with diabetes; blood sugar control.
- Microbiology: blood cultures, urine microscopy, culture and sensitivity (MC&S), joint aspiration (infection) and bone culture (gold standard for diagnosis)
- Radiology: magnetic resonance imaging (MRI: acute osteomyelitis) (Fig. 20.1), X-ray (osteomyelitis, other bone pathology: fractures, bone tumours), computed tomography (CT: to visualise the extent of bone destruction and identify complications, e.g. sequestrum, reservoirs of infection forming in areas of bone necrosis).

Clinical Tip

Osteopenia is the first sign that is seen on plain radiographs; it appears around 6 to 7 days following the onset of infection. Evidence of bone destruction, cortical breaches, involucrum and periosteal reaction are seen shortly after. Sequestra, a complication of diabetic foot, can be seen as early as 10 days.

MAKING A DIAGNOSIS

- Symptoms: redness, swelling and reduced mobility at the site of infection. History of systemic symptoms, e.g. malaise, lethargy, pain or fever
- Signs: a focus for infection, pyrexia, localised signs of inflammation such as swelling, erythema and decreased sensation in cases of diabetic foot
- Investigations: raised inflammatory markers, positive blood cultures, positive culture from bone or joint aspiration and image findings consistent with a bone or joint infection

MANAGEMENT

Treatment of osteomyelitis is typically twofold: appropriate antibiotic therapy and surgical removal of infected or necrotic tissue. You must ensure the patient is haemodynamically stable. Start a fluid balance chart and consider catheterisation. The affected limb should be immobilised and analgesia should be given.

CHOICE OF ANTIBIOTIC THERAPY

Bone biopsy can help targeted antibiotic therapy, which is usually prolonged and requires a peripherally inserted central catheter (PICC) line. *Staphylococcus aureus*, as a skin commensal, is the commonest cause. The probability of more atypical infections is increased in IV drug users (*Pseudomonas, Escherichia* and *Klebsiella*), those with sickle cell disease (*Salmonella*) and neonates (*Haemophilus* and *Streptococcus*). Cultures and sensitivities will aid antibiotic choice. In the absence of this information,

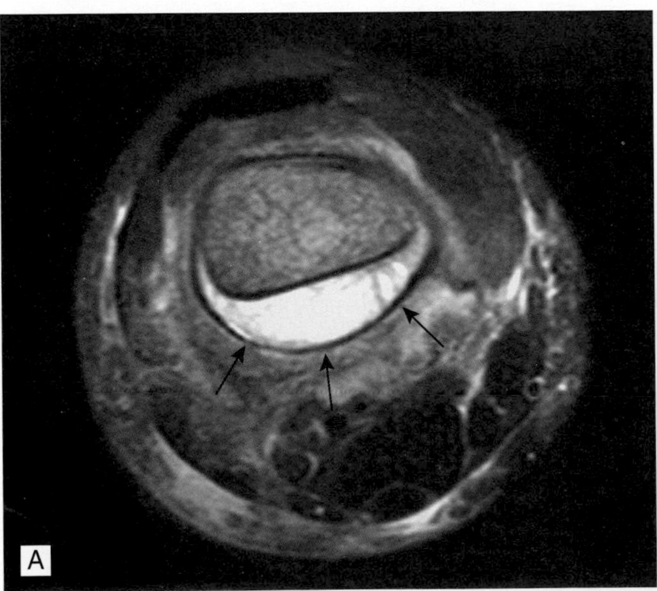

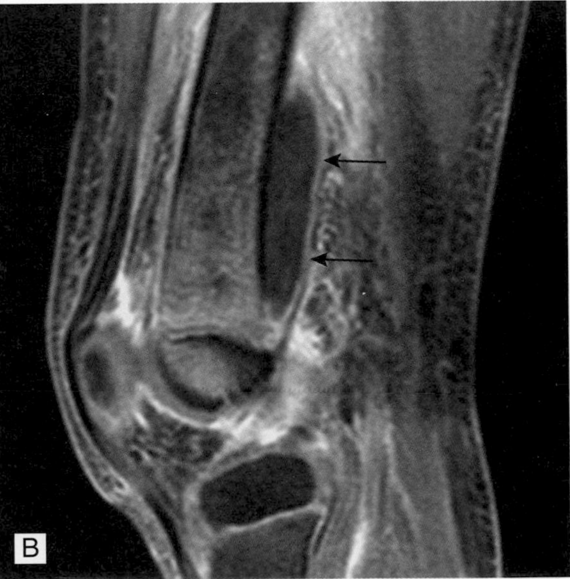

Fig. 20.1 Acute osteomyelitis of a distal femur. (A) T2-weighted fat-saturated axial magnetic resonance imaging (MRI) shows a large subperiosteal abscess (arrows) at the posterior aspect of the femur. Increased signal is seen within the bone, and there is adjacent soft-tissue oedema. (B) T1-weighted fat-saturated postgadolinium sagittal MRI shows the longitudinal extent of the subperiosteal abscess with an enhancing wall (arrows). (Source: Coley, B.D. [2013]. *Caffey's pediatric diagnostic imaging*. Elsevier.)

broad-spectrum, empirical antibiotics should be given. Culture-specific treatment should be in accordance with local trust policy or microbiology advice.

False-negative blood or biopsy cultures are common in patients who have already been initiated on antibiotic therapy. If possible obtain cultures before commencing antibiotics; however, this should not delay treatment.

The duration of treatment for acute infection is usually 4–6 weeks, transitioning to oral antibiotics once clinical symptoms stabilise and inflammatory markers are decreasing.

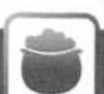

Clinical Tip

Although treatment is guided by clinical response and level of inflammatory markers, an early drop in CRP should not be an indication to discontinue antibiotics. Patients typically require at least 4 weeks of antimicrobial therapy. Changes on the X-ray lag at least 2 weeks behind a normal CRP.

SURGERY

Indications for surgery are failure to respond to antibiotics, infected surgical wounds or chronic osteomyelitis with necrotic bone and soft tissue. The purpose is to preserve viable tissue and prevent recurrent systemic infection. Orthopaedics will drain the area and debride the infected tissue. Specialist advice should be sought regarding the management of diabetic feet; this may involve the vascular team or the endocrinology team or both. Tissue viability nursing input may also be needed.

It is important to be aware of the complications. Patients are at risk of chronic infection, osteonecrosis (which can require amputation), septic arthritis, Marjolin ulcers (squamous cell carcinoma occurring over traumatised skin) and pathological fractures. Surgical amputation may be advised by the vascular team if the affected part of the limb is not salvageable.

ESCALATION

If the patient is haemodynamically unstable, escalate to your seniors urgently. It is important to refer to orthopaedics early as investigations can be complex, and delayed treatment increases the potential for complications.

STATION 20.2: COLLES' FRACTURE

The Bleep Scenario

You are called by the ED nurse about a 74 year old woman who has presented with a painful right wrist following a fall. She tripped over the kerb whilst rushing to catch the bus, landing on her outstretched hand. She denies any loss of consciousness or trauma to the head or neck. She is known to have hypertension, osteoporosis and iron-deficiency anaemia.

Her observations are: HR 85 bpm, BP 135/84 mmHg, RR 12 breaths per minute, SpO_2 98% on room air and temperature 36.5°C. You are asked to review her.

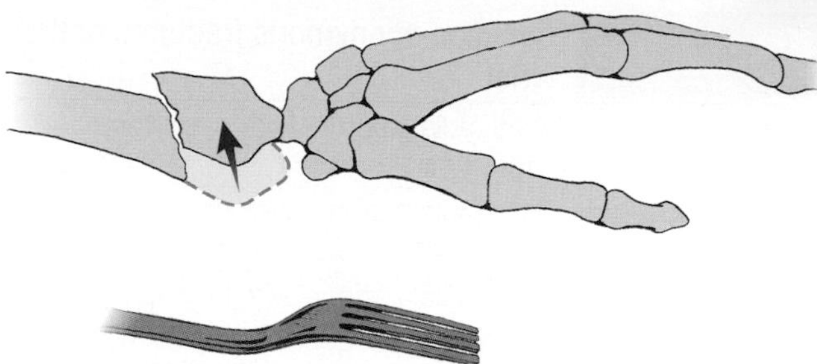

Fig. 20.2 Colles' fracture with resultant dinner-fork deformity. (Source: Manske, R.C. [2022]. *Fundamental orthopedic management for the physical therapist assistant e-book.* Elsevier.)

DEFINITION

A Colles' fracture is a common, extra-articular, dorsally and radially displaced fracture, occurring within 2–3 cm from the distal end of the radius. It is usually caused by a fall on to an outstretched hand (FOOSH) (Fig. 20.2).

INITIAL THOUGHTS

This is a classic presentation of a Colles' fracture. However, other diagnoses should be considered. The patient will require a full assessment following the fall to look for other injuries and any causative factors. It will also be important to look for neurovascular compromise, as this would indicate the need for urgent reduction. Risk factors include increased age, female gender, osteoporosis and high-impact sporting trauma in younger individuals.

DIFFERENTIAL DIAGNOSES

There are many different eponymous fractures of the wrist, as outlined in Table 20.1. In practice it is better to describe the fracture by the displacement seen.

INITIAL INSTRUCTIONS OVER PHONE

Advise the nurse to administer analgesia.

ASSESSMENT AND RESUSCITATION

- End of the bed assessment: the patient is alert and oriented. She is in pain.
- Airway: patent.
- Breathing: RR 19 breaths per minute, SpO_2 98% on room air. On auscultation, there are vesicular breath sounds with good air entry bilaterally.
- Circulation: CRT <2 s, HR 85 bpm, regular. BP 135/84 mmHg, HS I + II + 0, JVP normal.
- Disability: GCS 15/15, PEARL, temperature 36.5°C, CBG 7.20 mmol/L.
- Exposure: abdomen is soft and non-tender. Bowel sounds are normal. The wrist is radially and dorsally

Table 20.1 Common eponymous fractures of the wrist

Colles fracture	Distal radial fracture with dorsal and radial displacement
Smith's fracture	Distal radial fracture with volar displacement (i.e. a 'reverse Colles')
Barton's fracture	Distal radial fracture with involvement of the dorsal rim of the distal radius, in which an oblique intra-articular fracture occurs
Chauffeur fracture	Radial styloid process fracture with intra-articular involvement

deviated (known as a 'dinner-fork' deformity), with bruising, swelling, reduced range of movement and tenderness. On examination of the joint above and below, there is no further tenderness and a good range of movement. There are no open wounds or signs of penetrating trauma. There is no clinical evidence of trauma elsewhere.

INITIAL INVESTIGATIONS

- Haematology: FBC (anaemia or leukocytosis).
- Biochemistry: U&Es (electrolyte imbalance) and CRP (inflammation)
- Radiology: plain wrist X-rays anteroposterior (AP) and lateral fracture (Fig. 20.3) and CT head (if head injury suspected)

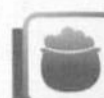

Clinical Tip

Radiological changes to note on X-ray of a Colles' fracture:
- Dorsal angulation
- Dorsal displacement
- Radial deviation of hand
- Proximal impaction

MAKING A DIAGNOSIS

Diagnosis of a Colles' fracture is made based on the history of the causative event, fall onto an outstreched hand (FOOSH) and radiological evidence.
- Symptoms: pain around the wrist
- Signs: tenderness over the radius, dorsal displacement, dorsal angulation and with radial tilt
- Investigations: radiological evidence of fracture – 2.5 cm proximal to radiocarpal joint

MANAGEMENT

Patients with a Colles' fracture are usually haemodynamically stable. The main form of pharmacological intervention they will need is analgesia. It is best to start with simple analgesics, such as paracetamol, and increase according to the recommendations of the World Health Organization (WHO) analgesic ladder if the pain is not controlled.

The orthopaedic team may advise a CT wrist if there is suspicion of intra-articular involvement or an occult fracture.

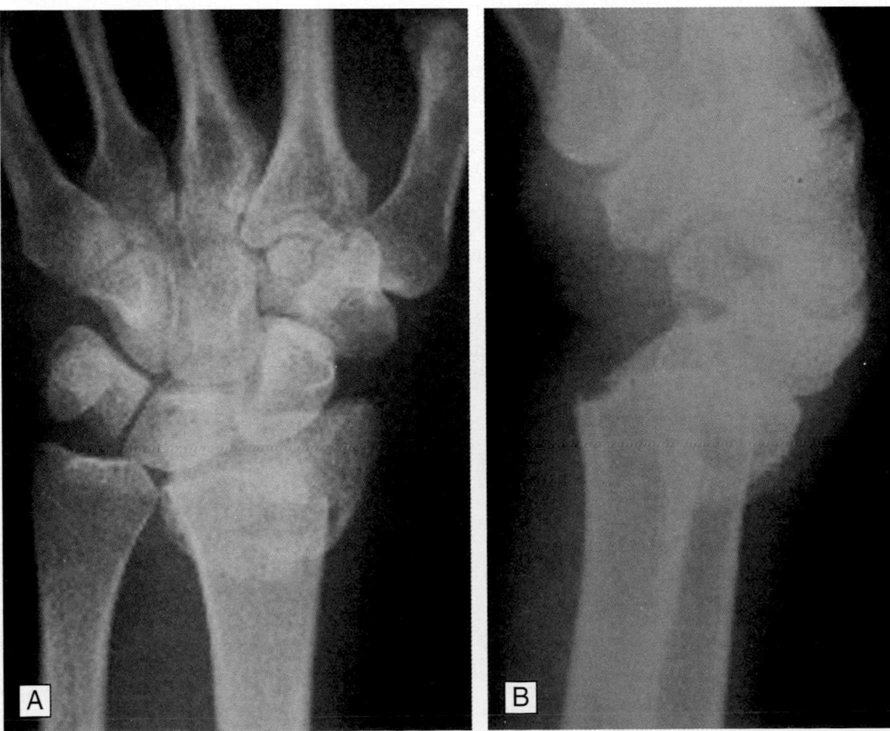

Fig. 20.3 (A) Anteroposterior and (B) lateral radiographs of the wrist revealing a Colles' fracture. (Source: Beredjiklian, P.K., Bozentka, D.J. and Gallant, G. (Eds.) [2021]. *Review of hand surgery*. Elsevier.)

Usually Colles' fractures do not require surgery, and are managed with closed reduction under regional/local anaesthetic and joint immobilisation. Orthopaedics are likely to request a repeat X-ray to confirm satisfactory reduction. Immobilisation is achieved with a Colles' cast or plaster backslab that immobilises the joint with slight flexion and ulnar deviation to counteract the extension and radial deviation of the fracture. The area is then restricted using a cast (from elbow to metacarpophalangeal joint) for 6 weeks. A repeat radiograph after 6 weeks is recommended to assess the level of recovery.

Open reduction is generally only required when closed reduction has not worked, there is intra-articular involvement or when the fracture is unstable (it redisplaces after reduction).

 Clinical Tip

Complications to be aware of include malunion, carpal tunnel syndrome, osteoarthritis and nerve, tendon or vascular injury. For elderly patients, you need to assess the impact of the injury on their activities of daily living. They may require admission for social reasons, awaiting social care to be arranged in the community.

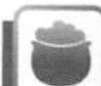 Clinical Tip

If there isn't a known diagnosis of osteoporosis, then this should be investigated in the community by the patient's general practitioner, especially in the elderly population.

ESCALATION

Refer to orthopaedics if open reduction is required. They can give advice on casting the patient in ED, and will follow up the patient in a fracture clinic.

STATION 20.3: ACUTE COMPARTMENT SYNDROME

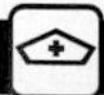 The Bleep Scenario

A 45 year old woman is admitted on the orthopaedic ward postoperatively following nailing of a left tibial fracture. She is complaining of progressive unbearable left calf pain over the last 30 minutes despite analgesia. She has no significant past medical history. Her only medications are paracetamol and prophylactic low-molecular-weight heparin.

Her observations are: HR 95 bpm, BP 130/80 mmHg, RR 20 breaths per minute, SpO_2 98% on room air and temperature of 36.5°C. The ward nurse asks you to review her for further analgesia.

DEFINITION

Acute compartment syndrome is a painful surgical emergency caused by increased interstitial pressure (intracompartmental pressure) within a closed osteofascial compartment resulting in restricted blood flow and tissue hypoxia. It is most common in the legs or forearm but can also affect the hand, foot and buttocks.

INITIAL THOUGHTS

Reviewing analgesia may not always be the top of your jobs list. However, pain out of proportion to the known pathology or injury, especially in the context of long-bone fractures, haemorrhage, compressive circumferential dressings, thermal burns, crush injury or rhabdomyolysis, should raise suspicion of a compartment syndrome – a surgical emergency.

DIFFERENTIAL DIAGNOSES

- Orthopaedics: shin splints (medial tibial stress syndrome), stress fractures, fascial defects or peroneal nerve entrapment
- Vascular: popliteal artery entrapment syndrome or an acute thromboembolic event

INITIAL INSTRUCTIONS OVER PHONE

Advise the nurse to administer analgesia if the patient is reporting significant pain.

 Prescribing Tip

Given the possibility of compartment syndrome, analgesia should only be used if absolutely required as pain is the only reliable symptom. Review the pain requirements over the last few hours and check if the patient had a regional block for surgery which may mask the pain of a compartment syndrome. Carefully document any changes, and if possible speak to a senior colleague before considering strong opiates.

ASSESSMENT AND RESUSCITATION

- End of the bed assessment: the patient is alert and oriented.
- Airway: patent.
- Breathing: RR 20 breaths per minute, SpO_2 98% on room air. On auscultation, there are vesicular breath sounds with good air entry bilaterally.
- Circulation: CRT <2 s peripherally on both upper limbs, HR 95 bpm, regular. BP 130/80 mmHg, HS I + II + 0, JVP normal.

- Disability: GCS 15/15, PEARL, temperature 36.5°C, CBG 6.80 mmol/L.
- Exposure: Abdomen is soft and non-tender. The left lower leg has a tight dressing. There is pain and tightness on palpation of the left calf, which is exacerbated by passive movement. There is also paraesthesia of the affected compartment on examination.

 Clinical Tip

Review the postoperative notes and plan from the operating surgeon as they will help identify any change in examination findings.

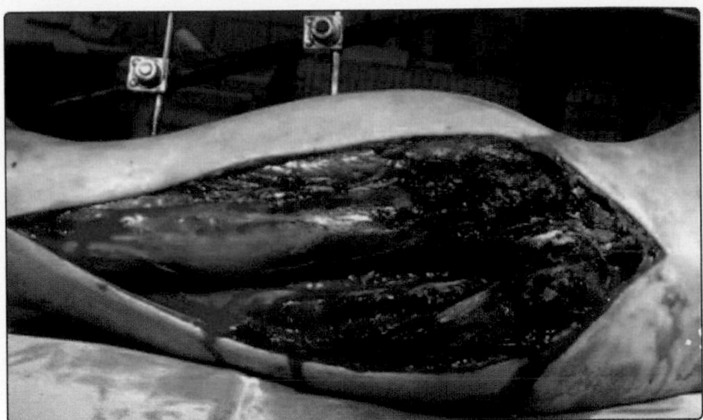

Fig. 20.4 Fasciotomy for acute compartment syndrome of the limb. (Source: Köstler, W., Strohm, P.C., and Südkamp, N.P. [2004]. Acute compartment syndrome of the limb. *Injury*, 35(12), 1221-1227.)

INITIAL INVESTIGATIONS

- Bedside: 12-lead electrocardiogram (ECG: to detect signs of hyperkalaemia in cases of rhabdomyolysis)
- Haematology: FBC (anaemia)
- Biochemistry: U&Es, VBG (raised lactate and potassium – seen in rhabdomyolysis, common in crush injuries) and serial creatinine kinase measurements (to check for evidence of muscle breakdown)

MAKING A DIAGNOSIS

- Symptoms: pain out of proportion to the injury, exacerbated by passive stretching of the muscle groups contained in the involved compartment, is one of the earliest and most sensitive clinical features. In the late stages, pain may be absent.
- Signs: the 5 'P's – pain, paraesthesia, pallor, paralysis and high intracompartment pressure. Pain, tightness and paraesthesia are early signs. Paralysis secondary to prolonged nerve compression and pallor secondary to vascular compromise are late signs.

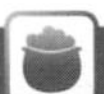 Clinical Tip

An impalpable pulse is not a diagnostic criterion, as peripheral pulses are usually still present despite a high compartment pressure until very late.

MANAGEMENT

The history of a long-bone fracture, compressive dressing, pain out of proportion to the injury and pain on passive movement point towards a diagnosis of an impending compartment syndrome.

This patient should be escalated to the orthopaedic registrar as soon as possible. Keep the patient nil by mouth, as they may deteriorate rapidly and need to go to theatre.

Early management will involve removal of the dressings, maintaining blood pressure and elevation of the limb to the plane of the heart using pillows. Avoid frames as they can worsen symptoms. Split the cast or backslab to the skin and ease it out to relieve compression; beware of removing it completely as it may displace the fracture and worsen the problem. Patients should be monitored closely and reviewed again in 30 minutes. The patient's low molecular weight heparin may also require review, as haemorrhage is a possible cause of compartment syndrome.

This woman has a convincing history of compartment syndrome, therefore the orthopaedic team will likely progress to immediate open fascial decompression (fasciotomy) (Fig. 20.4) if initial conservative steps do not help. If the history was less clear, or the patient was unable to give a history, for example, if shey was critically unwell, then compartment pressure should be measured by a senior member of the orthopaedic team to aid diagnosis.

Following surgery, the wound is left open. It will require re-exploration within 48 hours or earlier if clinically indicated. Input from plastics may be required for appropriate soft-tissue coverage.

In cases of suspected acute compartment syndrome with duration of symptoms > 8 hours and evidence of muscle necrosis, amputation may need to be considered rather than fasciotomy following discussion with the multidisciplinary team.

 Clinical Tip

Upon the decision for open fascial decompression, you will need to inform the emergency theatre coordinator, the ward nurses, the on call anaesthetist and the operating surgeon. Make sure you are aware of information relevant to the case – the team will want to know when the patient will be fasted, if there are any comorbidities, allergies and what tasks are outstanding (i.e. consent, informing next of kin).

Clinical Tip

Intracompartmental pressure monitoring is an important adjunct in the diagnosis of acute compartment syndrome. It is not required for diagnosis and the surgeon may decide to operate on the patient on the basis of history and examination alone. The normal pressure of a tissue compartment falls between 0 and 8 mmHg. In acute compartment syndrome the tissue pressure in the affected compartment is higher. Surgical decompression should be considered if there is a delta pressure (diastolic blood pressure – measured compartment pressure) ≤30 mmHg or an absolute compartment pressure > 40 mmHg with clinical symptoms.

ESCALATION

If the initial conservative steps have not helped reduce the pain or if the diagnosis is unclear, then the patient will require immediate orthopaedic surgical review to restore perfusion.

STATION 20.4: NECK OF FEMUR FRACTURE

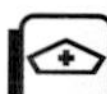

The Bleep Scenario

An 81 year old man has fallen on the ward and is now complaining of right hip and elbow pain. During his admission, he was treated for community-acquired pneumonia, and is now waiting for his package of care to restart. A brief history reveals the patient tripped and fell on his right side. No head injury or loss of consciousness was reported.

His observations are: HR 80 bpm, BP 134/83 mmHg, RR 15 breaths per minute, SpO_2 96% on room air and temperature 36.5°C. You are asked to review him by the ward nurse.

DEFINITION

A neck of femur fracture is a hip fracture across the neck of the femur (NOF).

INITIAL THOUGHTS

A falls assessment and Datix should be completed for this patient. The falls assessment will identify any injuries and risk factors that can be modified to reduce the risk of future falls.

Risk factors for a NOF fracture include older age, female gender, recurrent history of falls, osteoporosis, delirium, dementia, smoking and excess alcohol intake.

DIFFERENTIAL DIAGNOSES

- Orthopaedics: alternative fractures of the pelvis (e.g. pubic ramus fracture), acetabulum, femoral head and femoral diaphysis should all be considered. Pathological fractures should be considered if there is no significant history of trauma
- Rheumatology: osteoarthritis, rheumatoid arthritis, avascular necrosis, trochanteric pain syndrome

INITIAL INSTRUCTIONS OVER PHONE

Ask the nurse to do a full set of observations on the patient, including neurological observations. If possible, carefully transfer the patient back to bed or to a safe area of the ward. He should not mobilise further until imaging has been obtained.

ASSESSMENT AND RESUSCITATION

- End of the bed assessment: the patient is stable, alert and well oriented.
- Airway: patent.
- Breathing: RR 15 breaths per minute, SpO_2 96% on room air. On auscultation there is slightly reduced air entry at the right base.
- Circulation: CRT <2 s, HR 80 bpm, regular. BP 134/83 mmHg with no postural drop. JVP normal, HS I + II + 0.
  - 12-lead ECG: no signs of ischaemia or arrhythmia.
- Disability: GCS 15/15, PEARL, temperature 36.5°C, CBG 4.9 mmol/L, AMTS 10/10.
- Exposure: his abdomen is soft and non-tender. On examination from head to toe, the only signs of trauma are to the right hip and the right elbow, both of which are bruised. Neuological examination and visual acuity testing are normal. The right elbow is bruised over the extensor surface, but with a good range of movement and little pain. The right hip is extensively bruised, but does not feel hot or swollen. The right leg appears shorter than the left, and is held externally rotated. The patient is unable to move the leg at the hip.

Prescribing Tip

Review the patient's drug chart; look for any drugs that may put him at risk of falls, such as sedatives or drugs that can cause postural hypotension, e.g. antihypertensives. Also note if the patient takes any anticoagulants, as it may delay surgery and put him at risk of intracranial bleeds following a head injury.

INITIAL INVESTIGATIONS

- Haematology: FBC (leukocytosis or anaemia)
- Biochemistry: U&Es (electrolyte imbalance), liver function tests (LFTs), bone profile, clotting screen (baseline measurements) and creatinine kinase (if long lie has occurred to assess for rhabdomyolysis)
- Microbiology: urine dip and MC&S (infection)
- Radiology: chest X-ray (to rule out worsening infection), hip X-rays AP and lateral views of affected hip (hip fracture), AP pelvis X-ray (to assess the contralateral normal hip for preoperative planning and templating), full-length femoral X-ray (if there

is suspicion of a pathological fracture) and MRI hip (if there is clinical suspicion of fracture but X-ray is normal).

Clinical Tip

A hip X-ray classically shows a disruption in the continuous Shenton's line that normally bridges the femoral neck and the superior pubic ramus; the femur is flexed and externally rotated (Fig. 20.5).

MAKING A DIAGNOSIS

- Symptoms: recent trauma, pain in the groin, referred pain to the distal femur or upper knee and inability to bear weight on the affected side

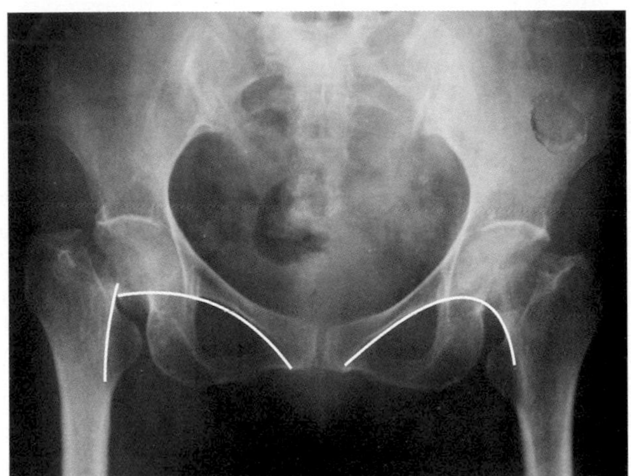

Fig. 20.5 X-ray of fracture of neck of femur with Shenton's line. (Source: Sud, A. and Ranjan, R. [2022]. *Textbook of orthopaedics.* 2nd ed. Elsevier India.)

- Signs: shortened and externally rotated limb on the affected side, inability to perform a straight-leg raise on the affected side
- Investigations: lateral and AP X-ray of the affected hip showing a fracture

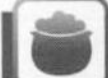

Clinical Tip

Knowledge of hip anatomy is essential to classify NOF fractures. NOF fractures can occur anywhere from the subcapital region of the femoral head to 5 cm distal to the lesser trochanter. There are two distinctive types:

- Intracapsular: from the subcapital region of the femoral head to the intertrochanteric line
- Extracapsular: outside the capsule, subdivided into: (a) intertrochanteric (between the greater and lesser trochanter) and (b) subtrochanteric from the lesser trochanter to 5 cm distal from this point

GARDEN CLASSIFICATION FOR INTRACAPSULAR FRACTURES (FIG. 20.6)

This classification is used to grade intracapsular hip fractures and particularly to identify patients at risk of avascular necrosis.

- Displacement: undisplaced = normal bone alignment; displaced = bone moved from normal alignment
- Completeness: incomplete fracture = the bone is cracked due to the fracture but does not completely break into pieces or separate; complete fracture = the bone breaks or separates into two or more pieces

MANAGEMENT

Primarily ensure the patient is haemodynamically stable. Ensure adequate analgesia is prescribed as NOF fractures are very painful. Prescribe according to the

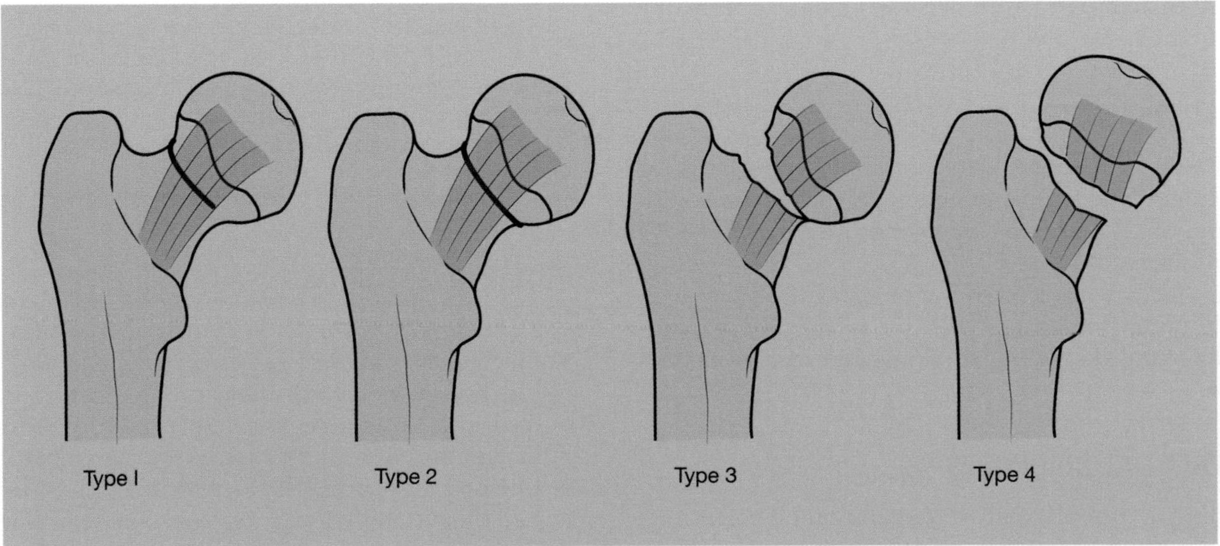

Fig. 20.6 Garden classification for intracapsular neck of femur fractures. Type 1: incomplete fracture without displacement; type 2: complete fracture without displacement; type 3: complete fracture with partial displacement; type 4: complete fracture with full displacement. (Source: Jones, M.S. and Waterson, B. [2020]. Principles of management of long bone fractures and fracture healing. *Surgery*, *38*(2), p. 96.)

recommendations of the WHO analgesic ladder if the pain is not controlled.

Most hospitals will have a hip fracture bundle or care plan to guide management. Definitive management is surgical and will require discussion with orthopaedics once the imaging has been completed. Without prompt definitive management, there is a risk of serious complications, including avascular necrosis of the femoral head.

The specific surgical procedure is dependent on the type of fracture sustained. Generally, intracapsular non-displaced fractures will require internal fixation with cannulated screws. Elderly patients and/or those with intracapsular displaced fractures (unstable fractures) may require hemiarthroplasty or total hip replacement. Extracapsular fractures will need to be reduced and internally fixed with dynamic hip screws. If the fracture extends down further into the femoral shaft then it may require an intramedullary device.

The patient will also require review by the orthogeriatrician, ideally within 72 hours.

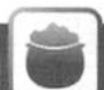 **Clinical Tip**

Upon decision for surgery, you should inform the emergency theatre coordinator, the ward nurses, the on call anaesthetist and the operating surgeon. The team will want to know when the patient will be fasted, if there are any comorbidities and allergies and what tasks are outstanding (i.e. consent, informing next of kin).

ESCALATION

Some patients may require high dependency unit or intensive care unit support following surgical intervention, or even prior to this depending on the degree of trauma they have encountered.

STATION 20.5: OPEN FRACTURES

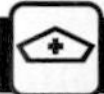 **The Bleep Scenario**

A 32 year old woman has arrived at the ED via an ambulance after being involved in a road traffic accident (RTA). She was hit by a car, which was moving at 15 mph, while crossing the road. It hit the right side of her body, throwing her on to the bonnet of the car. She has a large wound on her right leg with bone protruding through the wound. The patient has no significant past medical history.

Her observations are: HR 93 bpm, BP 122/86 mmHg, RR 18 breaths per minute, SpO_2 98% on room air, temperature 37.3°C and GCS 15/15. You are asked to review her.

DEFINITION

An open or compound fracture is a fracture in which the bone is exposed to the external environment (Fig. 20.7).

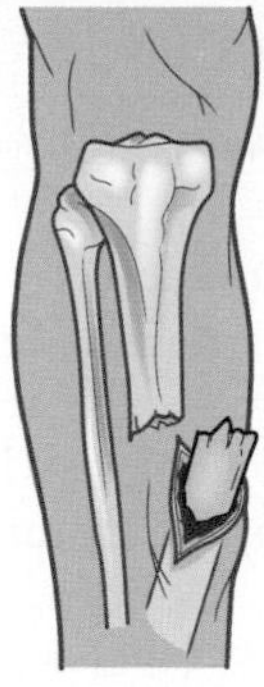
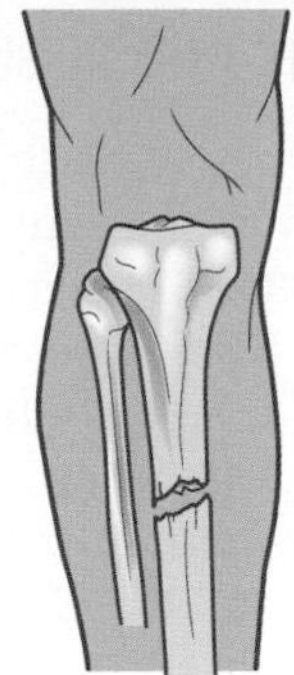

Open fracture Closed fracture

Fig. 20.7 Fracture classification. (Source: Tyerman, J. et al. [2022]. *Lewis's medical-surgical nursing in Canada: assessment and management of clinical problems*. Elsevier.)

INITIAL THOUGHTS

From this brief history, the patient appears to have an open fracture of the leg. These fractures are associated with high-force injury, and in most cases, there will be polytrauma. RTAs and open fractures are usually managed by a dedicated trauma team. The goals are to identify and treat threats to life, then limb and vision, prevent worsening or any additional injuries and return the patient to a level of function as close to their baseline as possible.

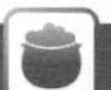 **Clinical Tip: Causes of Open Fractures**

- Trauma: RTAs, firearms, fall from a height, gunshot wounds
- Pathological: minor trauma to already diseased bone, e.g. pre-existing metastatic lesions, bone cysts, advanced osteoporosis

DIFFERENTIAL DIAGNOSES

- Orthopaedics: compartment syndrome, crush syndrome, degloving injury, myositis ossificans or open-joint injury
- Neurology: peripheral nerve injury
- Vascular: vascular injury
- Other: contusion, laceration or rhabdomyolysis

INITIAL INSTRUCTIONS OVER PHONE

Ensure a trauma call has been placed. This should have already been done by ED after the paramedics had alerted them to the incoming trauma case.

 **Clinical Tip**

The Advanced Trauma Life Support (ATLS) algorithm must be adhered to in the management of acute trauma cases. It follows a similar ABCDE approach to the Advanced Life Support (ALS) algorithm but also includes cervical-spine protection in the primary survey.

ASSESSMENT AND RESUSCITATION

- End of the bed assessment: the patient is stable. She is alert and well oriented.
- Airway: patent, cervical spine stable.
- Breathing: RR 18 breaths per minute, SpO_2 98% on room air. On auscultation, there are vesicular breath sounds with good air entry bilaterally. There are no signs of pneumothorax or thoracic trauma.
- Circulation: CRT <2 s, HR 93 bpm, regular. BP 122/86mmHg, JVP normal, HS I + II + 0.
- Disability: GCS 15/15, PEARL, temperature 37.3°C, CBG 6.2 mmol/L, AMTS 10/10.
- Exposure: abdomen is soft and non-tender. The right elbow has significant bruising, but full range of movement and no joint displacement. The right leg is bloody, bruised, tender, deviated medially, with a large open wound laterally beneath the knee with bone protruding out. There is no pallor to the limb and good capillary refill at the toes. Dorsalis pedis and posterior tibial pulses are palpable. She is able to move all toes and has normal sensation.

INITIAL INVESTIGATIONS

- Haematology: FBC (anaemia), clotting screen, group and save (in case of blood loss requiring transfusion)
- Biochemistry: U&Es (electrolyte imbalance), creatinine kinase (rhabdomyolysis or muscle breakdown) and VBG (lactate – in cases of shock)
- Microbiology: wound swab (infection), blood cultures (if there are systemic signs of infection)
- Radiology: plain-film radiograph of affected areas, CT for very comminuted or complex fracture or if head injury is suspected

MAKING A DIAGNOSIS

The Gustilo–Anderson classification can be used to classify open fractures. It grades the fracture according to the energy of injury, extent of soft-tissue damage, level of contamination and comminution of fractures. The higher the grade, the worse the outcome of the fracture.

GUSTILO–ANDERSON OPEN FRACTURE CLASSIFICATION

- Type 1: <1-cm wound, clean
- Type 2: 1–10-cm wound, clean
- Type 3A: >10-cm wound and high energy, but with adequate soft-tissue coverage
- Type 3B: >10-cm wound and high energy, but with extensive soft-tissue loss, usually associated with massive contamination. These will often need further soft-tissue coverage procedures.
- Type 3C: all injuries with vascular injury requiring repair, irrespective of degree of soft-tissue injury

MANAGEMENT

Initial management will require ATLS evaluation to rule out any life-threatening injuries. The patient will require careful fluid resuscitation and a fluid balance chart. If a catheter is to be placed, assessment for urethral injury should be completed first, alongside a rectal and genital exam. Following resuscitation, urgent realignment and splinting to immobilise are required. Remember to reassess and document the neurovascular status after any form of realignment or reduction.

Analgesia should be given for pain management according to the WHO analgesic ladder. A washout is not indicated outside of theatre; instead, a sterile dressing should be placed over the wound to prevent further contamination.

Open fractures carry a high risk of infection and therefore antibiotics should be started promptly in line with local guidance. Broad-spectrum cephalosporins are recommended for initial treatment, as they target gram-positive and negative species. Antibiotics can be reviewed once contaminants are known and microbiology advice has been sought. A tetanus vaccination should be given if the patient is not up to date with vaccinations or there is no evidence of a recent booster.

Alongside these immediate management steps, the patient should be kept nil by mouth so they are ready for theatre. You should prescribe maintenance fluids.

ESCALATION

These cases will be managed by a trauma team, which include an anaesthetist, orthopaedic surgeon, general surgeon and an ED doctor. This may vary depending on your trust.

Following initial management, escalate to the orthopaedic team for definitive surgical treatment. Debridement of the wound and fracture site, removing all necrotic and non-viable tissue, will be required. If there is any vascular compromise, prompt review and surgical intervention by a vascular surgeon would be indicated. Timely management is crucial to ensure optimal outcomes.

STATION 20.6: SEPTIC JOINT

The Bleep Scenario

A 73 year old man has presented to the ED complaining of a painful, hot, swollen right knee that has been getting progressively worse over the last 3 days, and he is now struggling to walk. He reports no history of trauma. He has a background of diet-controlled type 2 diabetes mellitus and osteoarthritis of the knees and hips.

His observations are: HR 98 bpm, BP 99/73 mmHg, RR 18 breaths per minute, SpO_2 96% on room air and temperature of 38.6°C. You are asked to review him.

DEFINITION

A septic joint is an acute monoarthritic inflammation caused by infection, usually bacterial.

Infection routes include: (1) local trauma; (2) haematogenous spread; (3) local spread from nearby affected joint; and (4) sepsis from another source.

INITIAL THOUGHTS

Patients with an acutely swollen, hot, tender joint should be considered to have septic arthritis until proven otherwise, even in the absence of fever if clinical suspicion is high. The history of osteoarthritis, particularly in the joint that is now septic, and diabetes are risk factors for septic arthritis. Other risk factors include immunosuppression, skin ulceration, prosthetic joints, IV drug abuse, trauma and surgery.

DIFFERENTIAL DIAGNOSES

- Orthopaedics: septic arthritis, pre- and infrapatellar bursitis
- Rheumatology: gout, pseudogout, reactive arthritis or psoriatic arthritis

INITIAL INSTRUCTIONS OVER PHONE

Ask the nurse to start supplementary oxygen, aiming for oxygen saturations >94%, obtain IV access and commence fluid resuscitation as per the sepsis protocol.

ASSESSMENT AND RESUSCITATION

- End of the bed assessment: The patient is alert and oriented, showing signs of discomfort and pain.
- Airway: patent.
- Breathing: RR 18 breaths per minute, SpO_2 96% on room air. On auscultation, there are vesicular breath sounds with good air entry bilaterally.
- Circulation: CRT <2 s, HR 110 bpm, regular. BP 99/73 mmHg, JVP normal, HS I + II + 0.
  - Administer 500 mL of crystalloid fluids stat to resuscitate the patient.
- Disability: GCS 15/15, PEARL, temperature 38.6°C, CBG 6.30 mmol/L.
- Exposure: his abdomen is soft and non-tender. Calves are unremarkable. His right knee is erythematous, swollen around the joint with a palpable effusion, and warm to touch. The left knee and other joints appear grossly normal. He is not able to move his right leg at the knee, stating it is too painful. Peripherally he is neurovascularly intact.

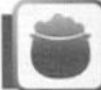

Clinical Tip

Use a marker pen to delineate the area of erythema to help map progress. It is also important to establish early the presence of any metal work in the suspected infected joint, as it will affect management.

INITIAL INVESTIGATIONS

- Haematology: FBC (leukocytosis)
- Biochemistry: CRP (inflammation), U&Es and LFTs (electrolyte imbalance, guide antibiotic choice), VBG (lactate), urate (gout) and rheumatoid factor (only if there is a strong suspicion of systemic rheumatic disease)
- Microbiology: blood cultures and urinalysis (infection), urgent joint aspiration with microscopic analysis and culture of synovial fluid (joint sepsis and crystal-induced arthritis) and polarising light microscopy (crystal arthropathies – gout and pseudogout)
- Radiology: plain-film joint X-ray (baseline), MRI joint (osteomyelitis) (Fig. 20.8), ultrasound hip (assists in the aspiration of a suspected septic hip) and CT (for difficult aspirations or where cartilage or bone may need to be visualised)

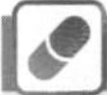

Prescribing Tip

Note that warfarin is not contraindicated for needle aspiration.

MAKING A DIAGNOSIS

- Symptoms: acute history of pain (localised to a joint), made worse by gentle passive motion, joint warm to touch, systemic symptoms of fever, lethargy and malaise
- Signs: fever, swelling and erythema of the joint
- Investigations: raised CRP, raised white cell count, positive gram stain and culture on synovial fluid analysis

MANAGEMENT

The joint should be rested and immobilised. Some ED doctors are trained to aspirate joints. If this is not the case

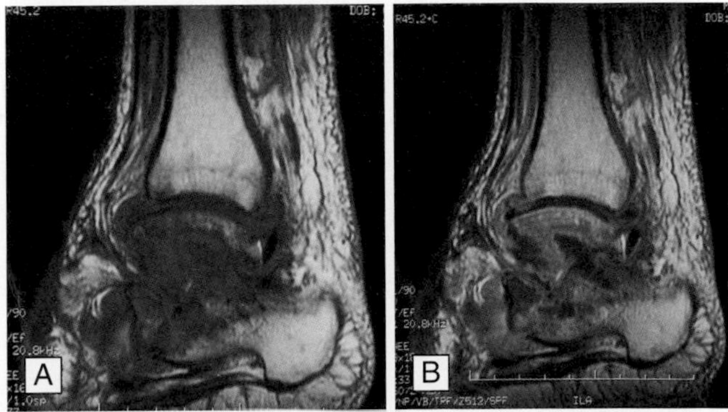

Fig. 20.8 Septic arthritis of an ankle complicated with osteomyelitis. (A) Sagittal view on T1-weighted magnetic resonance imaging (MRI) scan shows severe destruction of the subtalar joint with bone involvement. (B) Contrast-enhanced T1-weighted MRI scan shows a generalised enhancement of both synovial and bone tissues and abscess formation into talus and calcaneus. (Source: Hochberg, M.C. et al. [2011]. *Rheumatology*. 5th ed. St Louis, MO: Elsevier.)

in your trust, the patient will need an urgent review by orthopaedics or rheumatology for joint aspiration and synovial fluid analysis. Antibiotics should be withheld till after the joint has been aspirated. Antibiotic choice is guided by local guidelines and sensitivities.

The most common causative organisms are *Staphylococcus aureus* and *Streptococcus* spp. Flucloxacillin is a common first-line choice as it has good efficacy against both organisms. However, it is important to know whether the joint involved has a prosthesis, whether the patient is at risk of gram-negative sepsis (e.g. elderly, history of recent abdominal surgery or recurrent urinary tract infections), at risk of methicillin-resistant *Staphylococcus aureus* (MRSA: e.g. recent admission or a nursing home resident), an IV drug user or an intensive therapy unit patient. These risk factors predispose to different causative microorganisms, which will in turn influence antibiotic choice and may require discussion with microbiology.

Even if the synovial aspiration is culture-negative, it does not exclude a diagnosis of septic arthritis. Microscopy can also help identify urate crystals (gout), pyrophosphate crystals (pseudogout), blood (trauma or haemarthrosis) and normal fluid (rheumatoid arthritis). If no fluid can be aspirated, then alternative infections such as cellulitis or bursitis should be considered.

ESCALATION

Urgent referral is necessary for joint aspiration if trained staff are not available in the ED. Suspected infection of a prosthesis, hip joint or acute injury with evidence of haemarthrosis should always be escalated to orthopaedics.

FURTHER READING

BMJ Best Practice. *Compartment syndrome of extremities*. Available at: https://bestpractice.bmj.com/topics/en-gb/502/management-approach. [accessed 26 June 2019].

BMJ Best Practice. *Osteomyelitis*. Available at: https://bestpractice.bmj.com/topics/en-gb/354. [accessed 17 April 2021].

Boody, A. R., & Wongworawat, M. D. (2005). Accuracy in the measurement of compartment pressures: A comparison of three commonly used devices. *Journal of Bone and Joint Surgery, 87*, 2415–2422.

British Orthopaedic Association Standards for Trauma (BOAST). (2014). *BOAST 10: Diagnosis and management of compartment syndrome of the limbs*. Available at: www.boa.ac.uk/resources/boast-10-pdf.html. [Accessed 4 January 2022].

Coakley, G., et al. (2006). BSR & BPHR, BOA, RCGP and BSAC guidelines for management of the hot swollen joint in adults. *Rheumatology, 45*(8), 1039–1041.

Hatzenbuehler, J., & Pulling, T. J. (2011). Diagnosis and management of osteomyelitis. *American Family Physician, 84*(9), 1027–1033.

Hindle, P., Davidson, E., & Biant, L. C. (2012). Septic arthritis of the knee: The use and effect of antibiotics prior to diagnostic aspiration. *Annals of the Royal College of Surgeons of England, 94*, 351–355.

LeBlanc, K. E., et al. (2014). Hip fracture: Diagnosis, treatment, and secondary prevention. *American Family Physician, 89*(12), 945–951.

Mathews, C. J., et al. (2007). Management of septic arthritis: A systematic review. *Annals of Rheumatic Disease, 66*(4), 440–445.

McQueen, M. M., & Court-Brown, C. M. (1996). Compartment monitoring in tibial fractures. The pressure threshold for decompression. *Journal of Bone and Joint Surg of Britain, 78*(1), 99.

Mears, S. C. (2014). Classification and surgical approaches to hip fractures for nonsurgeons. *Clinics in Geriatric Medicine, 30*(2), 229–241.

Meena, S., et al. (2014). Fractures of distal radius: An overview. *Journal of Family Medicine and Primary Care, 3*(4), 325–332.

NICE. (2017). *Hip fracture: Management*. CG124. Available at: www.nice.org.uk/guidance/cg124. [Accessed 5 May 2020].

Ovre, S., et al. (1998). Compartment pressure in nailed tibial fractures. A threshold of 30 mmHg for decompression gives 29% fasciotomies. *Archives of Orthopaedic Trauma Surgery, 118*(1–2), 29.

Royal College of Physicians. (2019). *National hip fracture database annual report*. London: Royal College of Physicians.

Schultz, E., et al. (1999). Incomplete intertrochanteric fractures: Imaging features and clinical management. *Radiology, 211*(1), 237–240.

Summers, K., & Fowles, S. M. (2022). *Colles' fracture*. Available at: www.ncbi.nlm.nih.gov/books/NBK553071/. [Accessed 3 January 2022].

Wall, C. J., et al. (2010). Clinical practice guidelines for the management of acute limb compartment syndrome following trauma. *ANZ Journal of Surgery, 80*, 151–156.

White, T. O., et al. (2003). Elevated intramuscular compartment pressures do not influence outcome after tibial fracture. *Journal of Trauma, 55*(6), 1133.

Zalavras, C. G., et al. (2007). Management of open fractures and subsequent complications. *Journal of Bone and Joint Surgery of America, 89*(4), 884–895.

Ear, Nose and Throat

21

Content Outline

STATION 21.1: DYSPHAGIA

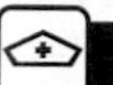

The Bleep Scenario

A 63 year old man has presented to the emergency department (ED) with difficulty in swallowing. It has gradually worsened over the last few months. He is now struggling with both solids and liquids.

His observations are: heart rate (HR) 115 bpm, blood pressure (BP) 126/83 mmHg, respiratory rate (RR) 20 breaths per minute, SpO_2 98% on room air and temperature 37°C. You are asked to review this man.

DEFINITION

Dysphagia is difficulty in swallowing solids and liquids. It can be described as partial or total dysphagia and painful or painless dysphagia.

INITIAL THOUGHTS

The swallowing process can be divided into three phases – oral, pharyngeal and oesophageal. The oral phase refers to the movement of food from the mouth to the oropharynx. The pharyngeal phase is the passage of food from the oropharynx to the oesophagus, and the oesophageal phase is the transfer of food from the oesophagus to the stomach. There are many possible causes of dysphagia, some of which are minor and easily treatable; others can be serious, even life-threatening. A neuromuscular cause is likely in this patient, given the history of progressive difficulty in swallowing solids and liquids.

DIFFERENTIAL DIAGNOSIS

ORAL

- Tonsillar enlargement, oral cavity tumours, or poor dentition

PHARYNGEAL

- Obstructive: goitre, pharyngitis, pharyngeal or laryngeal tumours, pharyngeal pouch, epiglottitis, retropharyngeal abscess, stenosis secondary to prior radiation, surgery or chemical ingestion
- Neurological: stroke, Parkinson's disease or multiple sclerosis
- Muscular: myotonic dystrophy or myasthenia gravis
- Upper oesophageal sphincter: abnormal relaxation

OESOPHAGEAL (FIG. 21.1)

- Obstructive intramural lesions: webs and rings, strictures/fibrosis (secondary to acid reflux, caustic agents, radiotherapy or certain drugs), gastro-oesophageal reflux disease, oesophageal candidiasis, foreign body, malignancy or diverticulum
- Obstructive extramural lesions: mediastinal mass, tortuous aorta or thyroid tumours
- Neurological: Parkinson's disease, stroke or multiple sclerosis
- Muscular: achalasia, scleroderma or diffuse oesophageal spasm
- Congenital: congenital atresia or congenital tracheo-oesophageal fistula

INITIAL INSTRUCTIONS OVER PHONE

Ask the nurse to obtain intravenous (IV) access, take bloods and start IV fluids for resuscitation as required.

Clinical Tip

Your clinical assessment should exclude red flag causes of dysphagia, such as stroke, epiglottitis, retropharyngeal abscess and oropharyngeal carcinoma.

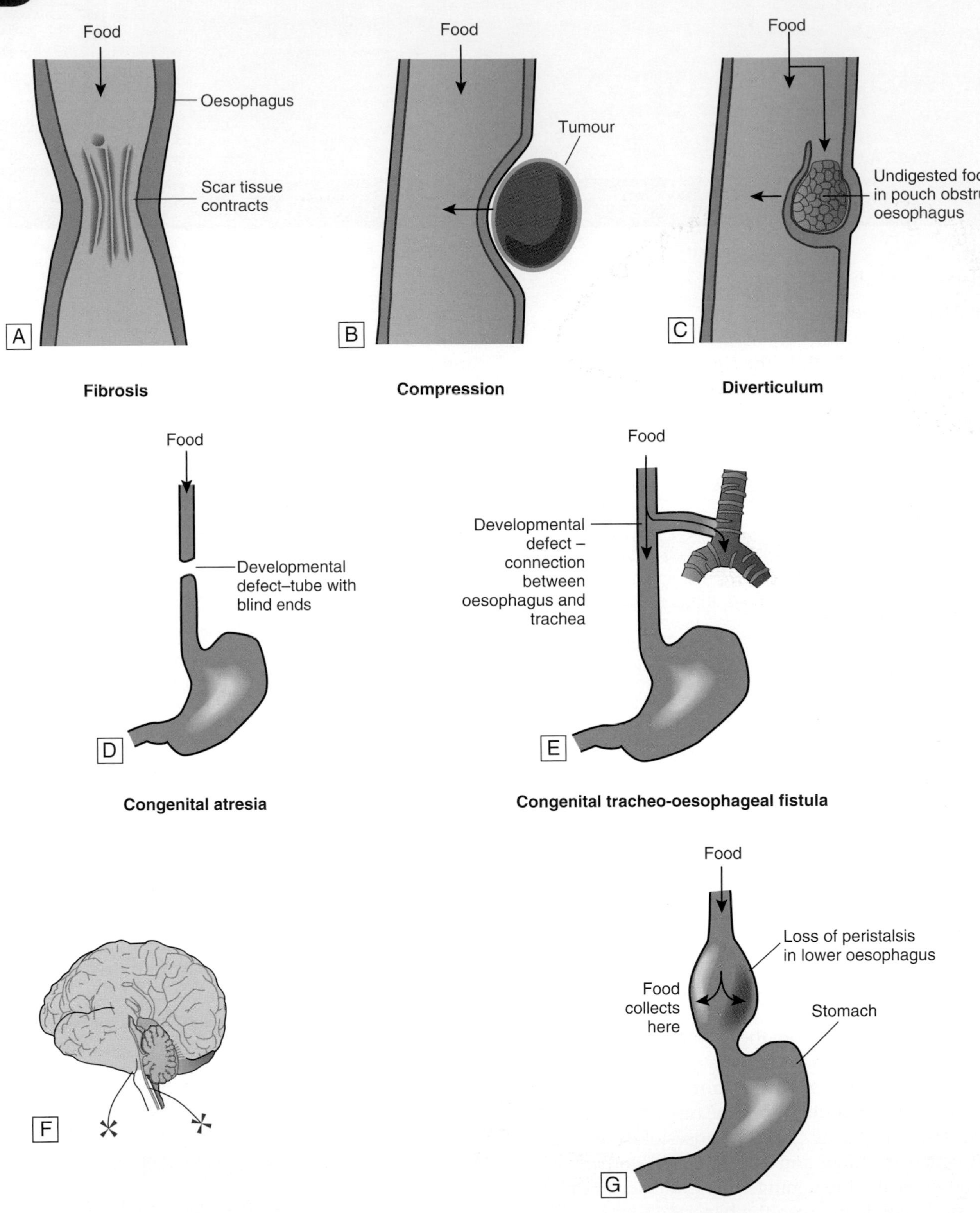

Fig. 21.1 Oesophageal causes of dysphagia. (Source: VanMeter, K.C. and Hubert, R.J. [2022]. Gould's *pathophysiology for the health professions*. Elsevier.)

ASSESSMENT AND RESUSCITATION

- End of the bed assessment: the patient is alert and orientated.
- Airway: patent.
- Breathing: RR 20 breaths per minute, SpO_2 97% on room air. On auscultation, there are vesicular breath sounds with good air entry bilaterally.
- Circulation: capillary refill time (CRT) 3 s, HR 110 bpm, regular. BP 126/83 mmHg. Jugular venous pressure (JVP) normal, heart sounds (HS) I + II + 0. Mucous membranes are dry, skin turgor reduced.
- Disability: Glasgow Coma Scale (GCS) 15/15, pupils equal and reactive to light (PEARL), temperature 37°C, capillary blood glucose (CBG) 7.4 mmol/L.
- Exposure: neurological examination is normal. No other significant findings.

INITIAL INVESTIGATIONS

- Haematology: full blood count (FBC: anaemia or infection)
- Biochemistry: urea and electrolytes (U&Es: electrolyte imbalance), liver function tests (LFTs) and clotting screen
- Microbiology: blood culture, swab or sample microscopy, culture and sensitivity (MC&S).

MAKING A DIAGNOSIS

A thorough history should be taken to identify the aetiology and severity of the dysphagia. The symptom of dysphagia needs to be differentiated from odynophagia (painful swallowing) and globus pharyngeus (sensation of a lump or something stuck in the throat). The following will aid the diagnosis of the underlying pathology and subsequent management:

- Age
- Presence of associated symptoms: coughing or choking when eating or drinking, reflux, heartburn, persistent drooling and recurrent chest infections
- Duration and progression of symptoms
- Nature of the swallowing problem

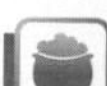

Clinical Tip

Oral dysphagia patients usually report problems initiating the swallow. Pharyngeal dysphagia patients report drooling, postnasal regurgitation, shortness of breath, dysphonia, hoarseness, coughing or choking. Finally, oesophageal dysphagia patients may report food sticking in their lower neck or chest region. However, note that dysphagia is often multifactorial.

MANAGEMENT

The patient is likely to be dehydrated and will need fluid resuscitation. Any electrolyte abnormalities should be corrected. The patient should have a fluid balance chart.

A full swallowing assessment by the speech and language therapists (SALTs) should be requested if dysphagia is suspected to establish safe swallow. The patient needs to be kept nil by mouth (NBM) if there is a risk of aspiration. Following the SALT assessment, further investigations such as a barium swallow may be arranged. In the meantime, the patient should have a nutritional assessment, including weight, body mass index (BMI) and blood tests such as vitamin B_{12}, folate and U&Es. Further investigations to determine the aetiology may also be requested – thyroid function tests (thyromegaly), botulinum toxin assay (botulism), liver enzymes, caeruloplasmin levels (Wilson's disease), creatine phosphokinase (inflammatory myopathies), acetylcholine receptor antibodies (myasthenia gravis) as well as anti-DNA and anti-ANA antibodies (scleroderma).

ESCALATION

Identification of the aetiology will guide further referral. If an anatomical obstruction is suspected, refer to ear, nose and throat (ENT). If neurological dysfunction seems likely, you should refer for neurological and gastroenterological opinions.

STATION 21.2: EPISTAXIS

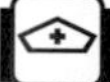

The Bleep Scenario

A 47 year old man has presented to the ED with a nosebleed. The nose has been bleeding for the last 90 minutes. He has a background of hypertension.

His observations are: HR 110 bpm, BP 110/80 mmHg, SpO_2 97% on room air, RR 12 breaths per minute and temperature 37.5°C. You are asked to review the patient.

DEFINITION

Epistaxis is bleeding from the nose, most commonly caused by damage to the Kiesselbach's plexus of vessels in Little's areas on the anterior nasal septum (Fig. 21.2).

INITIAL THOUGHTS

In the majority of cases, epistaxis is self-limiting and does not require medical intervention. However, it can be serious and potentially life threatening. Identifying the cause of the epistaxis is not essential at this time, but in adults you should consider recent nasal surgery and in children consider non-accidental injury.

DIFFERENTIAL DIAGNOSIS

- Idiopathic
- Local: trauma (e.g. nose picking, nasal fractures, foreign body), inflammation (e.g. chronic sinusitis), topical drugs, vascular causes (e.g. granulomatosis with polyangiitis), postoperative bleeding, tumours or nasal oxygen therapy. Cocaine or recreational drug abuse as a cause of epistaxis is on the increase.

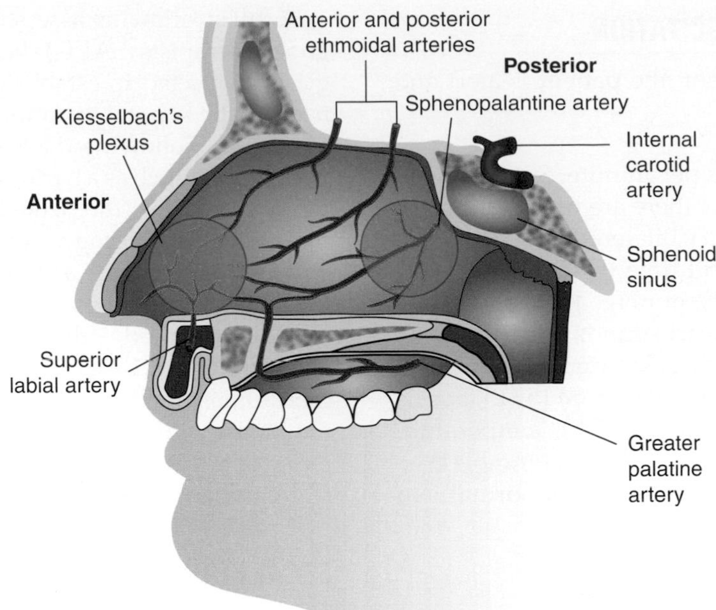

Fig. 21.2 Kiesselbach's plexus. (Source: Lakshmanaswamy, A. [2021]. *Textbook of pediatrics*. Elsevier India.)

- General: atherosclerosis, increased venous pressure from mitral stenosis, haematological conditions (e.g. thrombocytopenia, von Willebrand disease), environmental factors (temperature, exposure to irritants), systemic drugs like aspirin, warfarin or heparin and excessive alcohol consumption

INITIAL INSTRUCTIONS OVER PHONE

Advise the nurse to control the bleeding by positioning the patient with their upper body tilted forward and mouth open, whilst requesting the patient to pinch the lower cartilaginous part of the nose firmly for 15 minutes without releasing the pressure. You should also ask them to obtain IV access with large-bore cannulae, take bloods and start IV fluids for resuscitation as required. Ice packs applied over the bridge of the nose may be helpful.

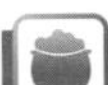 **Clinical Tip**

Complications are more likely if bleeding is severe and/or the patient is elderly and frail. Initial assessment should look for and treat any haemodynamic compromise.

ASSESSMENT AND RESUSCITATION

- End of the bed assessment: the patient is alert and orientated.
- Airway: patent.
- Breathing: RR 24 breaths per minute, SpO_2 94% on room air. On auscultation, there are vesicular breath sounds with good air entry bilaterally.
- Circulation: CRT 3 s. HR 110 bpm, regular. BP 110/60 mmHg. JVP normal, HS I + II + 0.
  - Administer 500 mL of crystalloid fluid stat to resuscitate the patient.
- Disability: GCS 15/15. PEARL. Temperature 37°C. CBG 7.4 mmol/L.
- Exposure: abdomen soft and non-tender.
  - Examine both nasal passages with a nasal speculum and look for a bleeding point.
  - Ensure nasal pressure is applied.

 **Clinical Tip**

Suspect a posterior bleed in cases where bleeding is significant from both nostrils, the bleeding site cannot be identified on speculum exam and/or if bleeding first started down the throat. However, note that if the patient is supine, the blood is likely to drain to the throat regardless of the bleeding point.

 **Prescribing Tip**

Ensure that you review the patient's drug chart to look for any drugs that may cause or exacerbate the epistaxis, e.g. topical cocaine, decongestants, corticosteroids, anticoagulants or antiplatelets.

INITIAL INVESTIGATIONS

- Haematology: FBC (anaemia) and group and save, cross-match (if transfusion is necessary)
- Biochemistry: U&Es (biochemical baseline) and LFTs (unexplained clotting abnormalities)

MAKING A DIAGNOSIS

Managing haemodynamic instability should take precedence. If the patient is haemodynamically stable, take a focused history to establish the diagnosis and further management:

- Duration of symptoms
- If individual or both nostrils are affected

- The volume of blood loss: if significant, ask the patient to estimate it as cups of blood loss (each equates to approximately 250 mL)
- Previous history of epistaxis, nasal trauma, nasal surgery or bleeding disorders
- Any packing trialed at home to stop bleeding
- Any associated symptoms: nasal obstruction, rhinorrhoea, facial pain, hearing loss or cranial nerve palsy.

MANAGEMENT

The priority is to resuscitate the patient and ensure they are haemodynamically stable. Identify and address any causative factors. If the bleeding does not stop after 10–15 minutes of nasal pressure, the next step is nasal cautery if the bleeding point can be seen, and the patient tolerates it.

Before cauterisation, prepare the site with a local anaesthetic spray, preferably with a vasoconstrictor. Wait 3 minutes for the full effect, then identify the bleeding site. Apply the silver nitrate stick to the bleeding point for 3–10 seconds until a grey-white colour develops and only cauterise one side of the septum to minimise the risk of septal perforation. Apply a topical antiseptic cream such as Naseptin to the site (unless the patient is allergic to neomycin, peanuts or soya). This should be continued four times a day for 10 days.

If the epistaxis stops, the patient should be monitored in ED for at least an hour to ensure it doesn't start again and advised to avoid strenuous activity, blowing or picking the nose, lying flat, heavy lifting and drinking alcoholic or hot drinks for 24 hours. If nasal cautery fails to stop the bleeding, the next step is nasal packing.

The two most common nasal packs are Merocel (nasal tampon) and Rapid Rhino (inflatable nasal pack) (Fig. 21.3). Anaesthetise the nostril with topical local anaesthetic spray, again waiting for 3 minutes for the full effect. With Merocel, the blood should wet the sponge, and it will expand. If using Rapid Rhino, once the pack is inserted, a syringe full of air should be attached and used to inflate the pack until the pilot cuff becomes rounded and feels firm when squeezed. Secure the package and ensure there is no pressure on the cartilage or bleeding into the oropharynx. If there is bleeding into the oropharynx, you may have to pack the other nostril to tamponade the postnasal space.

If these two techniques fail, the next pack to try is bismuth iodoform paraffin paste, which will require escalation to the ENT team.

ESCALATION

If the above measures have failed, there is severe uncontrolled bleeding or a history of recurrent episodes of bleeding, involve the ENT registrar early as the patient may need to go to theatre to control the bleeding surgically. Contact the paediatric registrar if epistaxis is seen in a child.

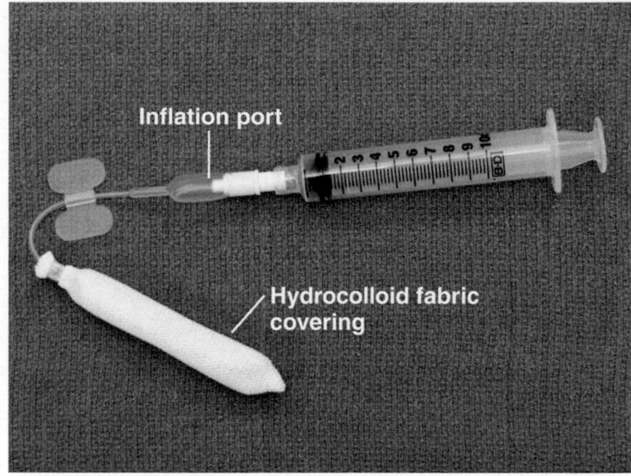

Fig. 21.3 The Rapid Rhino epistaxis device shown here has an air-inflatable balloon covered by a hydrocolloid fabric covering that allows easy insertion and removal. Various lengths and configurations are available. (Source: Roberts, J.R. [2019]. *Roberts and Hedges' clinical procedures in emergency medicine and acute care*. Elsevier.)

STATION 21.3: FOREIGN BODY IN THE NOSE

The Bleep Scenario

A 15 year old girl with learning disabilities has been brought into the ED by her mum with 5 hours history of right nasal discharge, pain and irritation. Her mum reports she has lodged objects into her nostrils in the past and she is concerned that this may be the case again.

Her observations are: HR 102 bpm, BP 125/78 mmHg, RR 15 breaths per minute, SpO_2 97% on room air and temperature 36.8°C. You are asked to review the patient.

DEFINITION

A foreign body in the nose is an external object that has entered the nose; this is most often seen in children.

INITIAL THOUGHTS

The history is suggestive of a nasal foreign body. Common foreign bodies in children include beads, buttons, seeds, peas and parts of toys. Button batteries, magnets and living foreign bodies are especially harmful. Metallic button battery foreign bodies are treated as surgical emergencies and require prompt removal. If left even for a few hours, they can leak and cause widespread damage to the lining of the nose.

DIFFERENTIAL DIAGNOSIS

- ENT: sinusitis, nasal polyps, malignancy or unilateral choanal atresia
- Respiratory: upper respiratory tract infection

INITIAL INSTRUCTIONS OVER PHONE

Ask the nurse to administer analgesia if indicated.

ASSESSMENT AND RESUSCITATION

- End of the bed assessment: the patient is alert and orientated.
- Airway: patent.
- Breathing: RR 16 breaths per minute, SpO_2 99% on room air. On auscultation, there are vesicular breath sounds with good air entry bilaterally.
- Circulation: CRT 2 s, HR 90 bpm, regular. BP 120/80 mmHg. HS I + II + 0.
- Disability: GCS 15/15, PEARL, temperature 37°C, CBG 7.5 mmol/L.
- Exposure: abdomen soft and non-tender. There is no evidence of discharge from the nose. Examination of the nasal cavity shows a bead lodged below the inferior turbinate.

 **Clinical Tip**

Examination may be tricky in a young child. Children should be examined in a sitting position to allow optimal visualisation. It may be better to use your thumb rather than a speculum to push the nose upward, to reduce patient anxiety.

 **Clinical Tip**

The most common location of a nasal foreign body is anterior to the middle turbinate or below the inferior turbinate in the right nostril, as most people are right-handed.

INITIAL INVESTIGATIONS

- Radiology: plain radiography to detect a metallic foreign body, if the type of nasal foreign body is unknown and cannot be visualised (Fig. 21.4).

MAKING A DIAGNOSIS

History is key to making a diagnosis; often, the patient will report a foreign body being lodged in the nostril. It is important to establish the type of foreign body and whether there is unilateral or bilateral involvement.

- Symptoms: nasal discharge, epistaxis, recurrent sneezing or pain
- Signs: visualisation of the foreign body on physical examination

MANAGEMENT

Trial positive pressure for large occlusive foreign bodies first. This involves forced exhalation through the nostril, with the unaffected nostril occluded.

Only attempt foreign body removal if the foreign body can be visualised on examination and there is a reasonable probability of extraction. Start by using a nasal anaesthetic spray in the affected nostril. The best equipment to use depends on the type of foreign body. If the object is smooth and round, it is best to insert a hook behind it and flick it out, rather than using forceps which may push it further in. Foreign bodies such as paper and sponge are best removed with suction or crocodile forceps. Always warn the patient that there may be bleeding from the nose.

After successful removal of the foreign body, examine the affected side for sinusitis, which is commonly seen if the foreign body has been present for a long time.

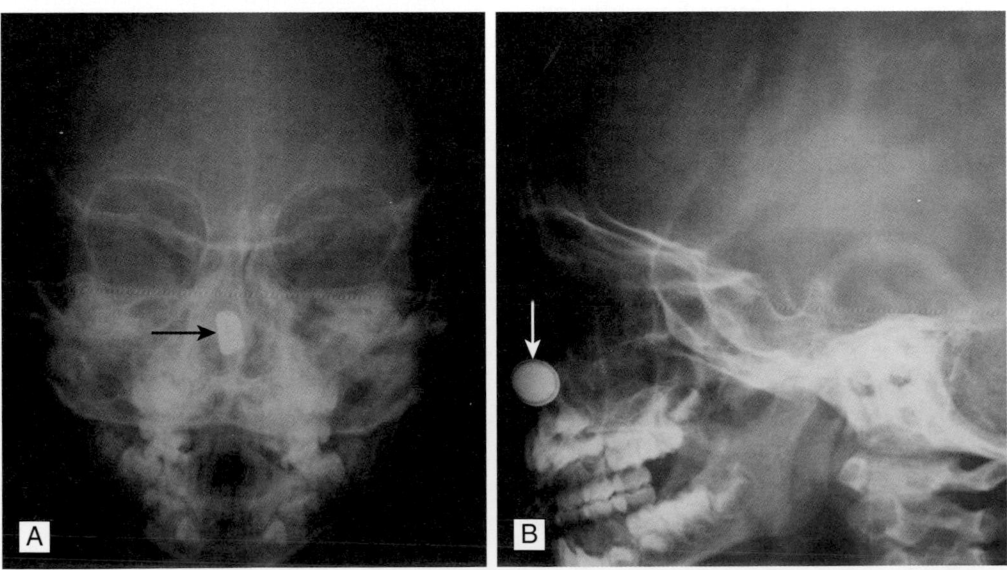

Fig. 21.4 (A) Frontal and (B) lateral radiographs of the nasal airway show a metallic foreign body in the right nasal cavity (arrows). (Source: Coley, B.D. [2019]. *Caffey's pediatric diagnostic imaging*. Elsevier.)

ESCALATION

If the foreign body cannot be visualised, is located in a posterior position or cannot be removed under local anaesthetic, escalate immediately to the ENT or surgical registrar as there is a risk of aspiration.

STATION 21.4: POST-TONSILLECTOMY BLEED

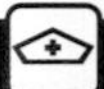

The Bleep Scenario

A 15 year old girl has presented to the ED, with her mother, after expectorating blood over the last 4 hours. The patient had a tonsillectomy a week ago.

Her observations are: HR 115 bpm, BP 105/80 mmHg, RR 13 breaths per minute, SpO_2 98% on room air and temperature 37°C. You are asked to review her.

DEFINITION

Post-tonsillectomy bleed is fresh bleeding from the throat that occurs after a tonsillectomy.

INITIAL THOUGHTS

Primary post-tonsillectomy bleeds occur within 24 hours of the operation. Secondary post-tonsillectomy bleeds usually occur 5–10 days postoperatively. Post-tonsillectomy bleeds are normally secondary to infection of the tonsillar fossae. They often start as mild bleeds but can rapidly deteriorate. Therefore, even if the patient has stopped bleeding after spitting out a small amount of blood, you should be aware that this could progress quickly into a life threatening condition.

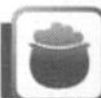

Clinical Tip

It is important to note that younger children may only present with increased swallowing and tachycardia.

DIFFERENTIAL DIAGNOSIS

- ENT: Post-tonsillectomy bleed
- Gastroenterology: oesophagitis, gastritis or peptic ulcer disease
- Haematology: bleeding disorders

INITIAL INSTRUCTIONS OVER PHONE

Ask the nurse to obtain IV access with two large bore cannulae, take bloods and start IV fluids for resuscitation as required. The patient should be kept nil by mouth.

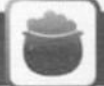

Clinical Tip

It is important to assess the quantity of blood loss using the patient's vital signs, capillary refill time and skin pallor. You should also ask the patient if possible.

ASSESSMENT AND RESUSCITATION

- End of the bed assessment: the patient is alert and orientated.
- Airway: patent.
- Breathing: RR 24 breaths per minute, SpO_2 99% on room air. On auscultation, there are vesicular breath sounds with good air entry bilaterally.
- Circulation: CRT 3 s, HR 120 bpm, regular. BP 110/82 mmHg. HS I + II + 0.
  - Administer 500 mL of crystalloid fluids stat to resuscitate the patient.
- Disability: GCS 15/15, PEARL, temperature 37°C, CBG 7.0 mmol/L.
- Exposure: abdomen soft and non-tender. Examination of the tonsillar fossae shows a clot over the tonsillar bed and signs of active bleeding. No other sites of blood loss.

INITIAL INVESTIGATIONS

- Haematology: FBC (anaemia, infection), group and save and cross-match (if transfusion may be necessary)
- Biochemistry: U&Es (biochemical baseline) and coagulation profile (clotting abnormalities)

MAKING A DIAGNOSIS

The history should establish when the patient had the tonsillectomy, if there were any complications before, during or after surgery, the quantity of blood loss and what the patient has eaten.

- Symptoms: expectoration of blood from the mouth
- Signs: evidence of active bleeding or clot formation over the tonsillar beds. It is often normal to identify white slough over the tonsils

MANAGEMENT

The priority is to resuscitate and ensure the patient is haemodynamically stable. This patient should be escalated to the ENT registrar as soon as possible. The patient should be kept nil by mouth, as she may deteriorate rapidly and need to go into theatre. Following resuscitation, the patient will require maintenance IV fluids. Start a fluid balance chart.

If there is no active bleeding or clot formation, the patient should be admitted for IV antibiotics. IV benzylpenicillin is a typical choice but you should be guided by your trust's antimicrobial guidelines. Symptomatic relief would include analgesia (avoid non-steroidal anti-inflammatory drugs) and mouthwash (hydrogen peroxide gargle if available) every 4 hours.

If a clot is seen in the tonsillar fossa but there is no active bleeding, do not dislodge the clot as it may cause severe bleeding.

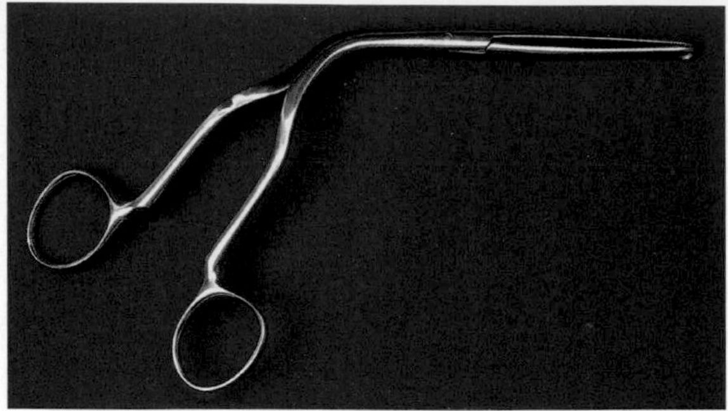

Fig. 21.5 Magill's forceps. (Source: Davey, A. and Diba, A. [2012]. *Ward's anaesthetic equipment*. Elsevier.)

If a clot is seen and there is active bleeding, you should try and remove the clot. This can be done with a Magill's forceps (Fig. 21.5) or a Yankauer sucker. Another approach is to cauterise the area with silver nitrate.

If there is no bleeding after the clot has been removed, admit the patient for IV fluids, IV antibiotics and hydrogen peroxide gargle every 4 hours.

In some cases, the patient starts bleeding quickly after removal of the clot. Be prepared for this and make sure the ENT registrar has been contacted. Soak some gauze with 1:1000 adrenaline, then with the Magill's forceps push the gauze into the fossa and hold it there for as long as the patient can tolerate. Lean the patient forward so she can spit out any blood or saliva.

ESCALATION

Patients with post-tonsillectomyy bleeding should be escalated to the ENT registrar as soon as possible. The patient may need surgical intervention. In the event of active bleeding, most commonly following removal of a clot, it is imperative to contact the ENT registrar and the anaesthetist urgently as well as to notify theatres.

STATION 21.5: QUINSY

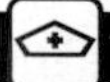 **The Bleep Scenario**

A 17 year old boy has presented to the ED with fever, difficulty opening his mouth and right sided throat pain. He also reports ear pain for the last few days on the right side, and his mum has noticed that his voice has changed. He is known to have a history of recurrent tonsillitis.

His observations are: HR 124 bpm, BP 120/80 mmHg, RR 13 breaths per minute, SpO_2 98% on room air and temperature 38.3°C. You are asked to review him.

DEFINITION

Quinsy is an abscess (collection of pus) that forms between one of the tonsils and the lateral pharyngeal wall. It is also known as a peritonsillar abscess.

INITIAL THOUGHTS

There are two important differentials to consider given the presentation: epiglottitis and tonsillitis. The preceding ear pain combined with the unilateral mouth pain makes tonsillitis more likely. Tonsillitis exists as a spectrum of forms – isolated tonsillitis, tonsillitis with peritonsillar cellulitis and tonsillitis with peritonsillar abscess.

DIFFERENTIAL DIAGNOSIS

- ENT: tonsillitis (and associated forms), epiglottitis or glandular fever

INITIAL INSTRUCTIONS OVER PHONE

Ask the nurse to obtain IV access, take bloods and commence fluid resuscitation as required. Advise analgesia.

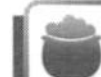 **Clinical Tip**

Prompt diagnosis is key. Untreated quinsy can result in airway compromise, parapharyngeal or retropharyngeal abscess, aspiration pneumonia or sepsis.

ASSESSMENT AND RESUSCITATION

- End of the bed assessment: the patient is alert and orientated.
- Airway: patent; he has a characteristic 'hot-potato voice'.
- Breathing: RR 20 breaths per minute, SpO_2 98%. On auscultation, there are vesicular breath sounds with good air entry bilaterally.
- Circulation: CRT 4 s, HR 110 bpm, BP 115/80 mmHg. HS I + II + 0.
  - Administer 500 mL of crystalloid fluids stat to resuscitate the patient.
- Disability: GCS 15/15, PEARL, temperature 38.6°C, CBG 7.6 mmol/L.
- Exposure: the abdomen is soft and non-tender. Examination of the tonsillar fossae shows an inflamed tonsil on the right side, deviation of the uvula to the left and an erythematous palate and mucosa. There are also swollen and painful lymph nodes in the neck.

INITIAL INVESTIGATIONS

- Haematology: FBC (infection)
- Biochemistry: U&Es (biochemical baseline) and C-reactive protein (inflammation)
- Microbiology: Gram staining and culture of aspirate (infection), glandular fever screen (Epstein–Barr virus) and blood cultures (infection)

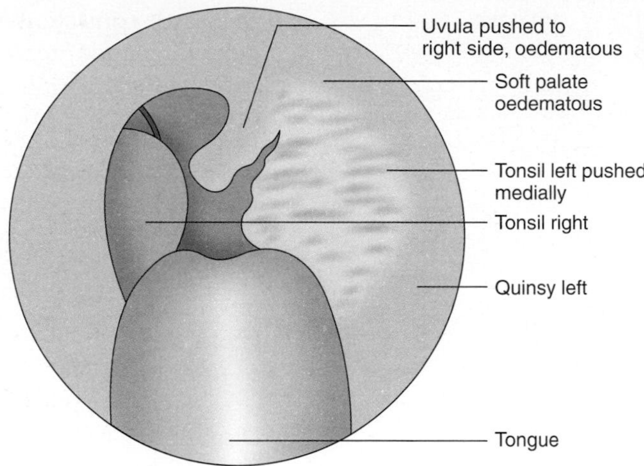

Fig. 21.6 Quinsy. The left tonsil is asymmetrically inflamed and swollen; there is displacement of the uvula to the opposite side. (Source: George, S. [2016]. *Smart study series – ENT and head & neck surgery*. Elsevier.)

MAKING A DIAGNOSIS

- Symptoms: severe throat pain, fever, drooling of saliva, fetor, painful swallowing, trismus, earache on the affected side, neck stiffness, headache and general malaise
- Signs: pus collection lateral to the tonsil, deviation of the uvula away from the affected side and an erythematous palate and mucosa on the affected side. There will be associated cervical lymphadenopathy involving the upper deep cervical lymph nodes. If there is quinsy, there will be associated trismus. The patient also has a characteristic 'hot-potato voice'. An isolated swollen tonsil is suggestive of tonsillitis

MANAGEMENT

Examination of the mouth can be difficult if there is significant trismus. In this case, it is reasonable to admit the patient, commence antibiotics, provide symptomatic relief and then re-examine. IV benzylpenicillin is a typical choice but follow the local antimicrobial guidelines at your hospital trust. Symptomatic relief should include regular analgesia, which may incorporate a topical analgesic spray. If the patient is unable to swallow, you may have to consider an alternative route of administration of analgesia. Following resuscitation, the patient will require maintenance IV fluids and a fluid balance chart.

Peritonsillar swellings require aspiration. You should only perform this procedure if you have performed it under supervision and feel confident; otherwise escalate it to your senior. Ensure there is good lighting and have the patient sitting up. Spray the throat with a local anaesthetic and then inject the surface mucosa overlying the swelling with lignocaine. Wait for 3 minutes for the local anaesthetic to take effect. Then use a 5-mL syringe and a large-bore needle or IV cannula to perform a three-point aspiration. Send the aspirate to microbiology. Incision and drainage may be used in recurrent cases or if the abscess fails to resolve within 24 hours (Fig. 21.6).

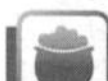

Clinical Tip

Caution is required when aspirating a peritonsillar swelling due to its close proximity to the carotid artery. The normal position of the carotid artery is lateral and posterior to the tonsil. Therefore, it is essential that an incision is not made too deeply or laterally. Some patients have anatomical variants where the carotid artery is located more towards the midline and are in danger of iatrogenic injury during aspiration.

ESCALATION

Escalate immediately to the ENT registrar if there are any signs of airway compromise.

STATION 21.6: STRIDOR

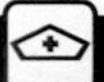

The Bleep Scenario

A 60 year old man has been brought to ED by his daughter with difficulty in breathing, with a harsh high pitched sound on inspiration. He is very drowsy. He is known to be a heavy smoker and reports a history of gastro-oesophageal reflux disease.

His observations are: HR 104 bpm, BP 120/80 mmHg, RR 24 breaths per minute, SpO_2 92% on room air and temperature 37.0°C. You are asked to review him.

DEFINITION

Stridor is the term given to the harsh high pitched sound through a partially obstructed airway at the level of the supraglottis, glottis, subglottis or upper trachea. It is more common in children.

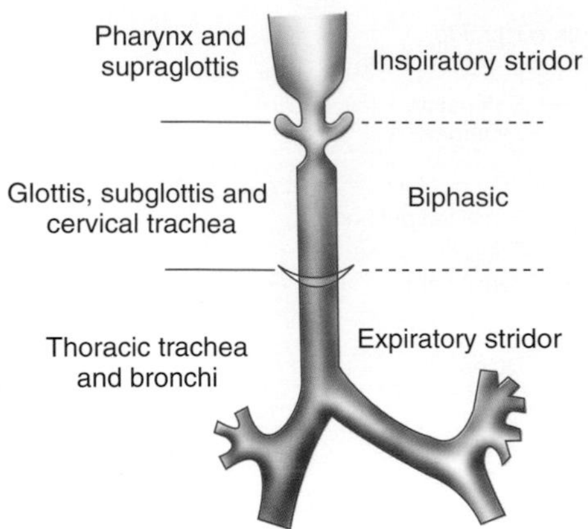

Fig. 21.7 Types of stridor. (Source: Dhingra, P.L. and Dhingra, S. [2022]. *Diseases of ear, nose and throat*. Elsevier India.)

INITIAL THOUGHTS

The priority is to determine how acute the airway obstruction is and whether the patient will need to go to theatre to secure the airway. Confirm whether the patient has stridor or wheeze as they are easy to confuse. Identifying the cause of stridor is not essential at this time. It is more important to treat the upper-airway obstruction as soon as possible and then once the airway is secure, a cause can be identified and managed.

 Clinical Tip

Stridor is a sign of upper-airway obstruction at or above the vocal cords (supraglottic/epiglottic and glottis areas) and is usually an inspiratory noise. Biphasic stridor (both inspiratory and expiratory) is usually heard at the glottis or subglottic areas. Expiratory stridor is characteristic of a high tracheal lesion (Fig. 21.7).

DIFFERENTIAL DIAGNOSIS

- Congenital: laryngomalacia, vocal cord web, bilateral vocal cord palsy, subglottic stenosis, subglottic haemangioma or bronchomalacia
- Acquired: trauma, foreign body, epiglottitis or supraglottitis, croup, carcinoma or airway compression

INITIAL INSTRUCTIONS OVER PHONE

Ask the nurse to start supplementary oxygen, aiming for oxygen saturations >94%, obtain IV access, take bloods and start IV fluids for resuscitation as required.

ASSESSMENT AND RESUSCITATION

- End of the bed assessment: the patient is alert and orientated. A faint inspiratory high pitched thrill can be heard, consistent with stridor. Supraclavicular indrawing and intercostal recession are present.
- Airway: patent.
- Breathing: RR 24 breaths per minute, SpO_2 94% on 15 L oxygen via non-rebreather mask. Increased respiratory effort: mild supraclavicular indrawing, some subcostal and intercostal recession present. On auscultation, there are vesicular breath sounds with good air entry bilaterally.
- Circulation: CRT 3 s, HR 110 bpm, BP 100/60 mmHg. HS I + II + 0.
    - Administer 500 mL of crystalloid fluids stat to resuscitate the patient.
- Disability: GCS 15/15, PEARL, temperature 37°C, CBG 7.8 mmol/L.
- Exposure: Throat examination is unremarkable.

INITIAL INVESTIGATIONS

- Haematology: FBC (infection)
- Biochemistry: U&Es (to check for acute kidney injury secondary to dehydration, electrolyte imbalance), C-reactive protein (inflammation)
- Microbiology: Gram stain and culture of swabs (if infection suspected)
- Radiology: chest X-ray (if foreign body suspected)

MAKING A DIAGNOSIS

A thorough history should be taken to identify the aetiology of the stridor. You should ascertain the following information:

- Age of onset, duration, severity and progression of stridor
- Precipitating factors
- Positioning
- Quality and nature of crying in children
- Associated symptoms: aphonia, cough, history of foreign body aspiration, difficulty feeding, drooling and fever

It is important to assess the severity of the stridor as it will guide management:

Mild stridor may present with minimal recession and cough. The patient will be able to eat and drink normally, and the oxygen saturation will be normal.

Moderate stridor may present with some subcostal and intercostal recession but only mild supraclavicular indrawing. The stridor noise is often loud, with a barking cough. Oxygen saturation is often normal.

Severe stridor presents with marked supraclavicular indrawing, subcostal and intercostal recession and reduced air entry. Be aware, the stridor itself may not be loud if the airway is compromised. Oxygen saturation < 92% is a sign of extremely severe disease.

MANAGEMENT

Patients with moderate to severe stridor should be kept nil by mouth and escalated immediately to your senior, as well as the anaesthetic and ENT teams. In the meantime, allow the patient to stay in whatever position is most comfortable.

If the patient is distressed, you should defer examination until seniors are present for emergency airway management. In a child with stridor, any distress (e.g. any intervention) may precipitate acute laryngospasm and further airway compromise. Therefore, interventions are best done in theatre in a controlled environment with the appropriate staff. In all cases, regularly monitor oxygen saturations and titrate oxygen accordingly. Nebulised salbutamol can be considered if oxygen saturations remain low.

After securing the airway and resuscitating the patient, treatment should address the underlying cause. For example, children presenting with stridor secondary to epiglottitis will need oxygen and IV antibiotics and some may require steroids.

ESCALATION

If there are signs of moderate or severe stridor, immediately escalate to the ENT registrar and the anaesthetist. Further management of the underlying cause once the patient is stabilised will require input from ENT, and if the patient is a child, the paediatric team.

STATION 21.7: TRACHEOSTOMY ASSESSMENT

The Bleep Scenario

A 57 year old man is currently on the respiratory ward and has a tracheostomy in situ. The tracheostomy has been present for the last 48 hours, since he came off invasive mechanical ventilation.

His observations are: HR 124 bpm, BP 129/87 mmHg, RR 20 breaths per minute, SpO_2 98% on room air and temperature 36.3°C. You are asked to assess his artificial airway.

DEFINITION

A tracheostomy is a surgically created opening through the neck into the trachea to allow direct access to the airway. A tube is usually placed through this opening to provide an airway and remove secretions from the lungs (Fig. 21.8).

INITIAL THOUGHTS

It is important to ascertain the indication for the tracheostomy. There are many possible indications for a tracheostomy: upper airway obstruction, prolonged ventilation, protection against pulmonary aspiration, tracheobronchial toilet, major head and neck surgery or to aid early weaning from a ventilator.

Patients with a tracheostomy are usually managed in critical care, respiratory or ENT wards, to ensure they receive the specialised nursing care they require. All patients with a tracheostomy should have a tracheostomy emergency box by their bedside.

INITIAL INSTRUCTIONS OVER PHONE

Ensure that the tracheostomy emergency box is with the patient.

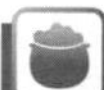

Clinical Tip

Review the sign at the head of the bed (Fig. 21.9); it will have the details of the type of artificial airway in situ and whom to call in case of emergency.

ASSESSMENT AND RESUSCITATION

- End of the bed assessment:the patient is alert and orientated. A green tracheostomy sign is noted.
- Airway: patent. Assess the mouth and the tracheostomy: no air leaks, snoring, stridor or grunting are noted.

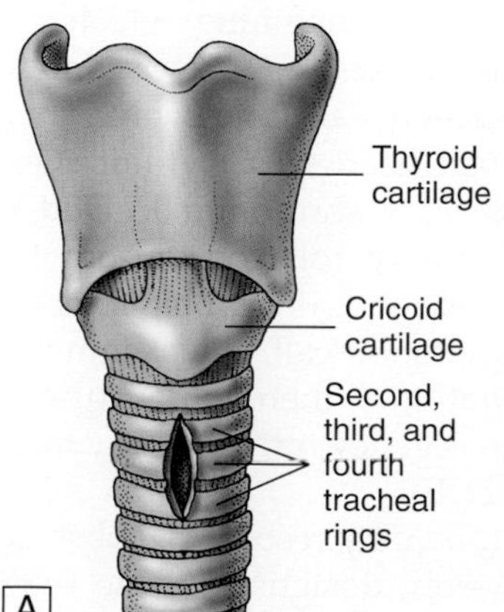

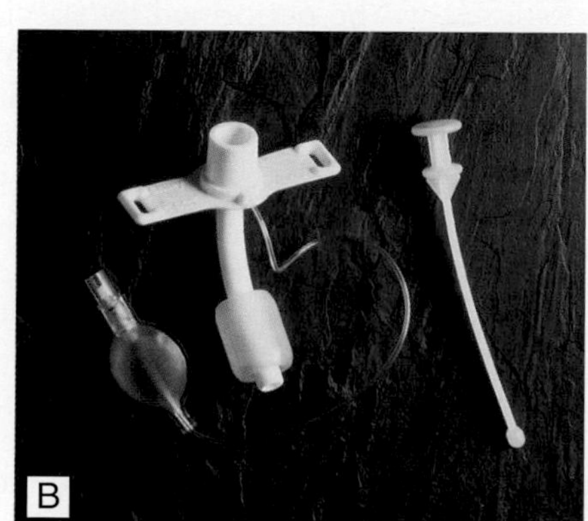

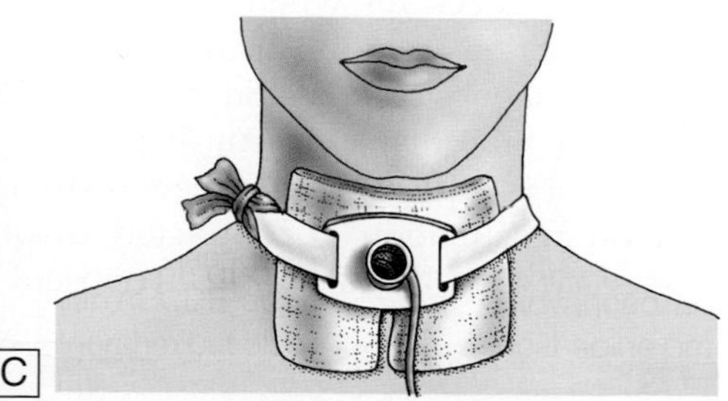

Fig. 21.8 (A) Vertical tracheal incision for a tracheostomy. (B) Tracheostomy tube. (C) Placement of gauze and tie around a tracheostomy tube. (Source: Zenith [2017]. *Medical assisting module D textbook: Cardiopulmonary systems, vital signs, electrocardiography and CPR*. Elsevier.)

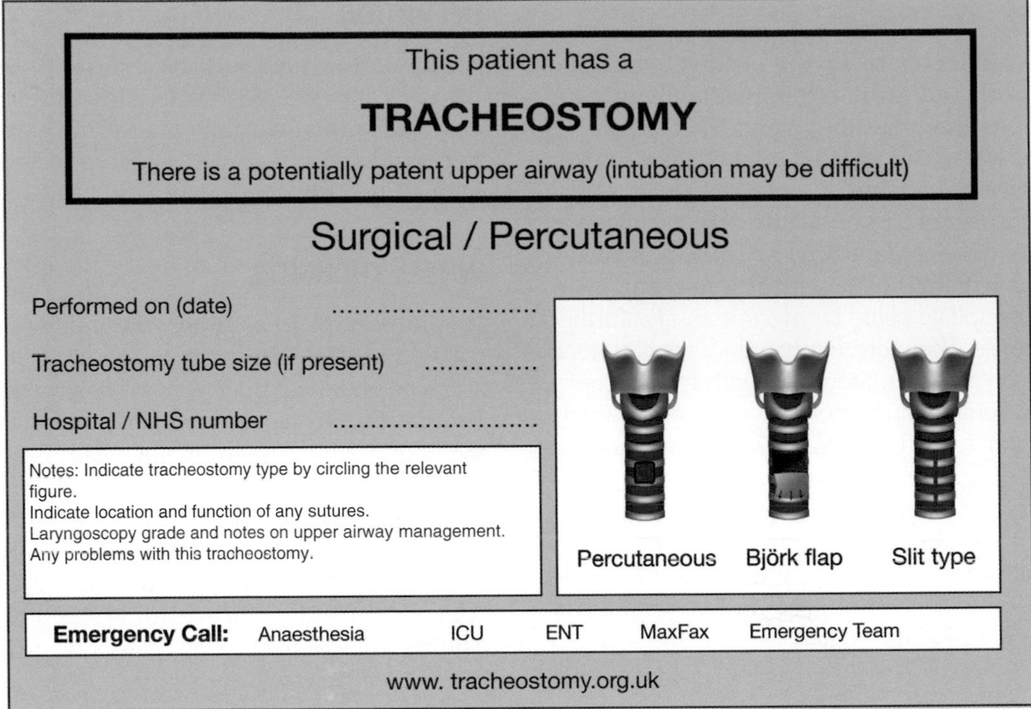

This patient has a

TRACHEOSTOMY

There is a potentially patent upper airway (intubation may be difficult)

Surgical / Percutaneous

Performed on (date) ....

Tracheostomy tube size (if present) ....

Hospital / NHS number ....

Notes: Indicate tracheostomy type by circling the relevant figure.
Indicate location and function of any sutures.
Laryngoscopy grade and notes on upper airway management.
Any problems with this tracheostomy.

Percutaneous Björk flap Slit type

Emergency Call: Anaesthesia ICU ENT MaxFax Emergency Team

www. tracheostomy.org.uk

Fig. 21.9 National Tracheostomy Safety Project (NTSP) tracheostomy bed head sign. (Source: McGrath, B. A., Bates, L., Atkinson, D., & Moore, J. A. (2012). Multidisciplinary guidelines for the management of tracheostomy and laryngectomy airway emergencies. *Anaesthesia*, 67(9), 1025–1041.)

- Breathing: RR 21 breaths per minute, SpO_2 98% on room air. Normal respiratory effort. On auscultation, there are vesicular breath sounds with good air entry bilaterally. No whistling noises or noisy breathing audible.
- Circulation: CRT < 2 s. HR 120 bpm, regular. BP 134/82 mmHg. HS I + II + 0.
- Disability: GCS 15/15, PEARL, temperature 36.3°C. CBG 7.7 mmol/L.
- Exposure: abdomen soft and non-tender. No other findings.

 Clinical Tip

Red flags to look out for include a visibly displaced tracheostomy tube, blood or blood stained secretions around the tube, increased discomfort/pain or requiring a lot of air to keep the cuff inflated, which may be secondary to a damaged cuff, air leak or tube displacement.

MAKING A DIAGNOSIS

There are two major tracheostomy complications that you should check for when you review the patient: tube obstruction and tube dislodgement.

- Signs of tube obstruction: stridor and difficulty breathing
- Signs of tube displacement: if partially displaced, the chest is expanding and there is still good air entry on auscultation. If completely displaced, chest expansion and breath sounds are absent

 Clinical Tip

Waveform capnography is a useful tool to assess tracheostomy patency and should be used where available. Exhaled carbon dioxide indicates a patent or partially patent airway.

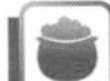 Clinical Tip

Complications of Tracheostomy

- Immediate (<24 hours): haemorrhage, injury to trachea, larynx and neighbouring structures, air embolism or displacement of tube and loss of airway
- Early (1–14 days): subcutaneous emphysema, pneumothorax, pneumomediastinum, tube displacement and blockage, wound infection, tracheal necrosis, tracheomalacia and secondary haemorrhage
- Late (> 2 weeks): haemorrhage, tracheo-oesophageal fistula, laryngeal or tracheal stenosis

MANAGEMENT

Regular assessment is essential for patients who have a tracheostomy. This involves tracheostomy tube care, humidification, stoma care and suctioning, which will be performed by specialist nurses. If airway compromise is suspected, immediately call for airway expert help as detailed on the bed head sign. If the patient is breathing, high flow oxygen should be applied to both the face and tracheostomy, following which the tracheostomy patency is assessed. If the patient is not breathing, put out a resuscitation call, and commence cardiopulmonary resuscitation if there is no pulse or signs of life. Follow the emergency tracheostomy management algorithm (Fig. 21.10).

Removal of the inner tube may resolve the obstruction in some cases. However, designs of these tubes vary, with some requiring replacement of the tube after cleaning to allow connection to breathing circuits. A soft suction catheter should be used to minimise the risk of creating a false passage if the trachea tube tip

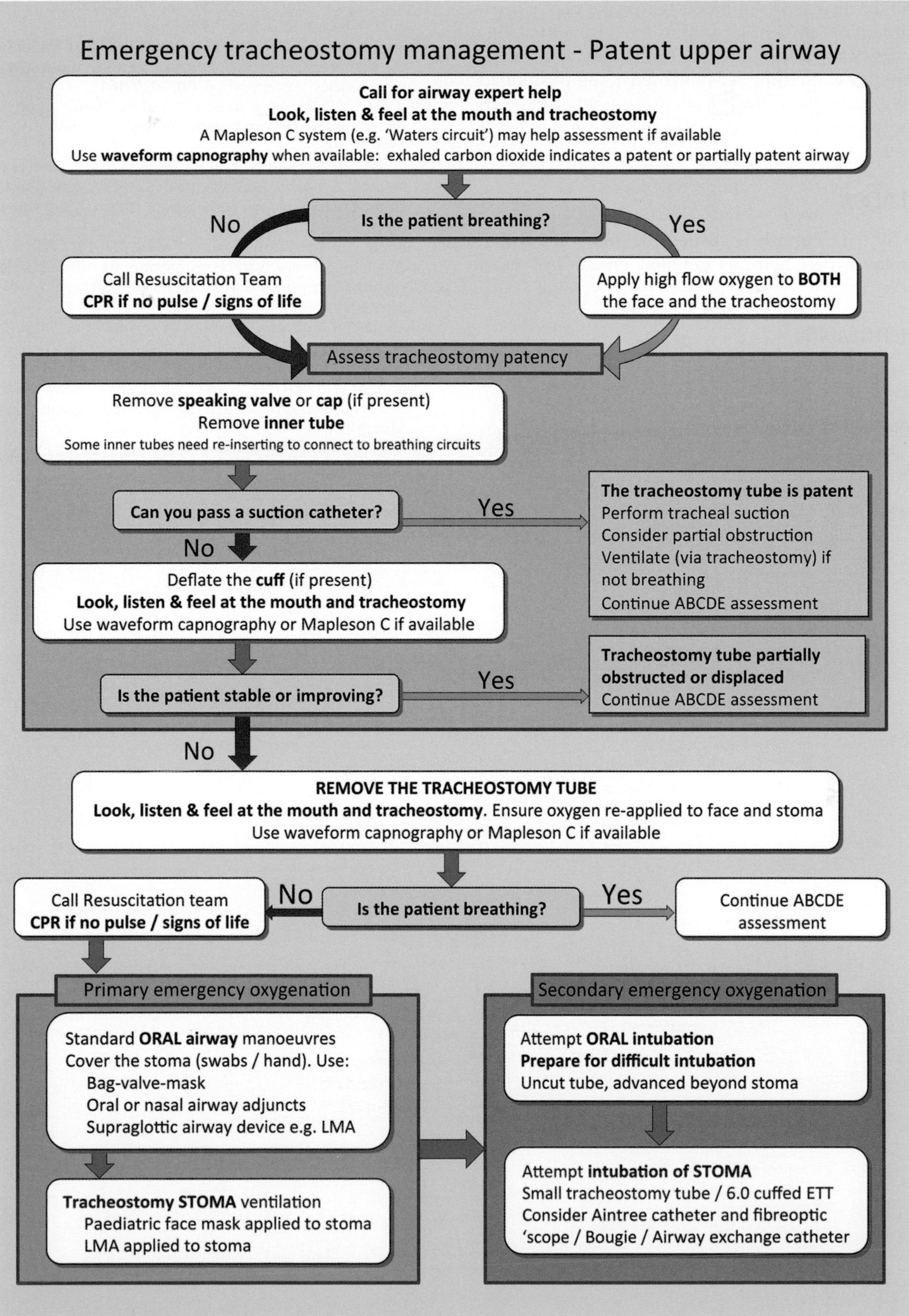

Fig. 21.10 Emergency tracheostomy management algorithm. CPR, cardiopulmonary resuscitation; ETT, endotracheal tube; LMA, laryngeal mask airway. (Source: McGrath, B. A., Bates, L., Atkinson, D., & Moore, J. A. (2012). Multidisciplinary guidelines for the management of tracheostomy and laryngectomy airway emergencies. *Anaesthesia*, 67(9), 1025–1041.)

is partially displaced. Do not attempt the above measures if you are unfamiliar with the equipment as this may cause more harm. Do not ventilate via the tracheostomy unless the tube is confirmed to be positioned correctly and patent using a suction catheter. In addition, only gentle hand ventilation is recommended if required.

ESCALATION

If airway compromise is suspected, immediately call for airway expert help, as detailed on the bed head sign.

FURTHER READING

BMJ Best Practice. *Assessment of dysphagia*. Available at: https://bestpractice.bmj.com/topics/en-gb/226/diagnosis-approach (accessed 15 October 2021).

Corbridge, R., & Steventon, N. (2019). *Oxford handbook of ENT and head and neck surgery* (3rd ed.). New York: Oxford University Press.

Crouch, R., et al. (2016). *Oxford handbook of emergency nursing* (2nd ed.). New York: Oxford University Press.

Lyons, M., & Singh, A. (2005). *Your first ENT job: a survivor's guide*. Oxford: Radcliffe Publishing.

McGrath, B. A., et al. (2012). Multidisciplinary guidelines for the management of tracheostomy and laryngectomy airway emergencies. *Anaesthesia, 67*(9), 1025–1041.

Medscape. (2021). *Nasal foreign bodies*. Available at: http://emedicine.medscape.com/article/763767-overview. (Accessed 2 May 2020).

National Tracheostomy Safety Project (n.d.) *Emergency care (adults)*. Available at: www.tracheostomy.org.uk/healthcare-staff/emergency-care/emergency-algorithm-tracheostomy (accessed 7 May 2020).

National Tracheostomy Safety Project. (2013). *NTSP manual*. Available at: www.tracheostomy.org.uk/storage/files/Emergency%20tracheostomy%20management.pdf. (Accessed 7 May 2020).

NICE. (2019). *Epistaxis (nosebleeds)*. Available at: https://cks.nice.org.uk/epistaxis-nosebleeds#!scenario. (Accessed 1 May 2020).

Omran, M. L. (2001). *Dysphagia*. Available at: www.thedoctorwillseeyounow.com/content/aging/art2074.html. (Accessed 1 May 2020).

Parker, R., Thomas, C., & Bennett, L. (Eds.). (2007). *Emergencies in respiratory medicine*. Oxford: Oxford University Press.

Warner, G., et al. (2009). *Otolaryngology and head and neck surgery*. New York: Oxford University Press.

Ophthalmology

22

Content Outline

STATION 22.1: ACUTE ANGLE CLOSURE GLAUCOMA

The Bleep Scenario

A 60 year old man presents to the emergency department (ED) reporting a red, painful left eye, associated with reduced vision, headache and nausea. He is known to be hypermetropic and reports no past medical history.

His observations are: heart rate (HR) 100 bpm, blood pressure (BP) 126/87 mmHg, respiratory rate (RR) 17 breaths per minutes, SpO_2 98% on room air and temperature 37.6°C. You are asked to review him.

DEFINITION

Acute angle closure glaucoma (AACG) is a rise in intraocular pressure secondary to obstruction of aqueous humour flow from the ciliary body to the trabecular meshwork.

INITIAL THOUGHTS

Acute angle closure is the key diagnosis to consider in a patient over the age of 50 presenting with a painful, red eye with reduced vision. This patient demonstrates symptoms of systemic upset – headache, nausea and vomiting – which will further support this diagnosis. Failure to recognise and treat this condition promptly can result in irreversible sight loss secondary to optic nerve damage. Risk factors of AACG include increased age, female gender, family history of glaucoma, presence of cataract and hypermetropia.

DIFFERENTIAL DIAGNOSIS

- Infection: endophthalmitis, conjunctivitis, infectious uveitis or corneal ulcer
- Inflammation: uveitis, marginal keratitis, scleritis, episcleritis or blepharitis
- Trauma: foreign body, blunt or penetrating trauma
- Raised intraocular pressure (IOP): AACG

INITIAL INSTRUCTIONS OVER THE PHONE

Ask the nurse to lay the patient supine, as this may help the passage of aqueous humour into the trabecular meshwork. Administer analgesia and antiemetics. Request that the patient's vision is checked using a Snellen chart.

ASSESSMENT AND RESUSCITATION

- End of the bed assessment: the patient is distressed and has a sick bowl in front of him.
- Airway: patent.
- Breathing: RR 16, SpO_2 96% on room air. On auscultation, there are vesicular breath sounds with good air entry bilaterally.
- Circulation: capillary refill time (CRT) < 2 s, HR 90 bpm, regular. BP 137/89 mmHg, heart sounds (HS) I + II + 0.
- Disability: Glasgow Coma Scale (GCS) 15/15. Right pupil equal and reactive to light (PEARL). The left pupil is poorly reactive and mid-dilated. Temperature 37.5°C, capillary blood glucose (CBG) 7.7 mmol/L.
- Exposure: best-corrected visual acuity right eye 6/6 and left eye 6/48. Ideally, a slit-lamp examination should be conducted at this point. A cloudy cornea, ciliary injection and high intraocular pressure are noted on examination of the left eye.

Clinical Tip

Factors that cause pupillary dilatation can precipitate AACG; for example, a dark room, pharmacological mydriatics, adoption of a semiprone position, acute emotional stress and occasionally certain systemic medications, e.g. parasympathetic antagonists, sympathetic agonists, motion sickness patches and cold/flu remedies.

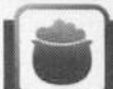

Clinical Tip

History is crucial in an ophthalmic assessment. The main ophthalmic symptoms to enquire about are redness, blurred vision, discharge, pain, photophobia, photopsia, floaters and systemic upset. It is also important to enquire about his past ocular history (especially history of glaucoma or refractive error), past medical history, drug history (including over-the-counter medications) and family history.

INITIAL INVESTIGATIONS

- Biochemistry: urea and electrolytes (U&Es: to check renal function before commencing a carbonic anhydrase inhibitor (acetazolamide) to lower IOP).

Clinical Tip

In AACG, the peripheral iris may restrict the drainage of aqueous humour by coming into contact with the trabecular meshwork – plateau iris mechanism. Alternatively, there may be blockage of flow from the posterior chamber into the anterior chamber at the pupillary margin, most likely secondary to a cataract - pupil block mechanism (Fig. 22.1). As aqueous humour continues to be produced, the pressure within the eye increases, resulting in optic nerve damage and subsequent vision loss.

MAKING A DIAGNOSIS

- Symptoms: acute red, painful eye, reduction in vision, systemic upset (e.g. headache, nausea, vomiting)
- Signs: conjunctival hyperaemia, hazy cornea, mid-dilated pupil, raised intraocular pressure ± optic disc swelling/atrophy

MANAGEMENT

If AACG is suspected, the patient should be seen by ophthalmology on an urgent basis. In the meantime, position the patient so that he is lying supine without any pillow support, as this may relieve the pressure on the iridocorneal angles. Symptomatic relief is also advised, such as analgesia and antiemetics.

The ophthalmologists will treat the patient with pilocarpine, steroid and intraocular pressure-lowering drops, alongside either oral or intravenous acetazolamide to reduce aqueous humour production. In addition, check for history of renal disease and sulphonamide allergy before commencing acetazolamide. With prompt treatment, the outlook is good.

ESCALATION

AACG is an ophthalmic emergency and requires an urgent referral to ophthalmology to reduce intraocular pressure and prevent irreversible sight loss.

STATION 22.2: AMAUROSIS FUGAX

The Bleep Scenario

A 60 year old man presents to the ED with a 45 minute history of transient visual loss in his right eye. He is known to have a background of hypertension and atrial fibrillation.

His observations are: HR 80 bpm, BP 166/91 mmHg, RR 18 breaths per minutes, SpO_2 98% on room air and temperature 37°C. You are asked to review him.

DEFINITION

Amaurosis fugax is a transient ischaemic attack (TIA) of the ophthalmic circulation. It is characterised by transient monocular visual loss, usually of embolic origin.

INITIAL THOUGHTS

The patient's presentation is suggestive of amaurosis fugax: a history of transient monocular visual loss with a background of cardiovascular risk factors. Patients often describe it as a curtain coming down over their vision, with a gradual recovery in the same pattern as loss. Risk factors include a history of hypertension, diabetes, carotid artery stenosis, atrial fibrillation,

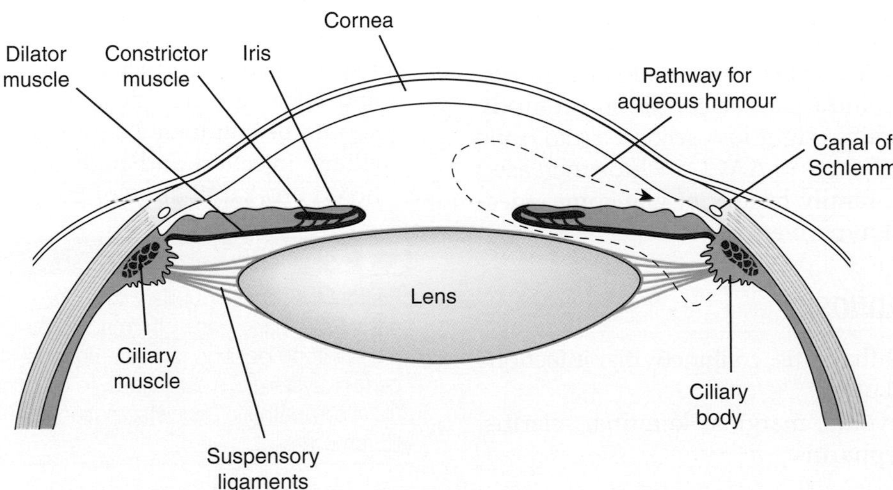

Fig. 22.1 The drainage pathway of aqueous humour in the anterior segment of the eye. (Source: Rang, H.P. et al. [2020]. *Rang & Dale's pharmacology*. Elsevier.)

smoking, hypercoagulable state, advanced age and a family history of stroke.

DIFFERENTIAL DIAGNOSIS

- Systemic: migraine and hypoglycaemia
- Ophthalmic: amaurosis fugax, central retinal artery occlusion, central retinal vein occlusion, retinal detachment, vitreous haemorrhage, arteritic ischaemic optic neuropathy and non-arteritic ischaemic optic neuropathy

 Clinical Tip

The following information will aid diagnosis: the duration of symptoms, whether the visual loss is complete/partial, any association with pain, photopsia or floaters, presence of systemic symptoms (e.g. jaw claudication, headache, neurological symptoms) or cardiovascular risk factors.

INITIAL INSTRUCTIONS OVER THE PHONE

Advise the nurse to check the patient's vision using a Snellen chart and take initial bloods.

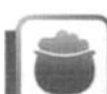 Clinical Tip

The attack may sometimes be accompanied by an ipsilateral cerebral TIA, with contralateral neurological features. Therefore, assessment should always include a complete neurological exam.

ASSESSMENT AND RESUSCITATION

- End of the bed assessment: the patient looks comfortable.
- Airway: patent.
- Breathing: RR 18, SpO_2 98% on room air. On auscultation, there are vesicular breath sounds with good air entry bilaterally.
- Circulation: CRT < 2 s, HR 85 bpm, irregular, BP 164/93 mmHg, HS I + II + 0. On auscultation of the carotid arteries, a bruit is noted on the right side.
  - 12-lead electrocardiogram: sinus rhythm.
- Disability: GCS 15/15, PEARL, temperature 37.1°C, CBG 7.0 mmol/L.
- Exposure: no neurological deficit was noted on neurological and cranial nerve examination. Best-corrected visual acuity 6/9 right and left. Undilated direct ophthalmoscopy shows a normal red reflex and healthy optic discs bilaterally.

INITIAL INVESTIGATIONS

- Haematology: full blood count (FBC) (hypercoagulable state or anaemia)
- Biochemistry: random glucose, HbA_{1c} and lipid profile (cardiovascular risk factors). Erythrocyte sedimentation rate (ESR) and C-reactive protein (CRP) (giant-cell arteritis [GCA])

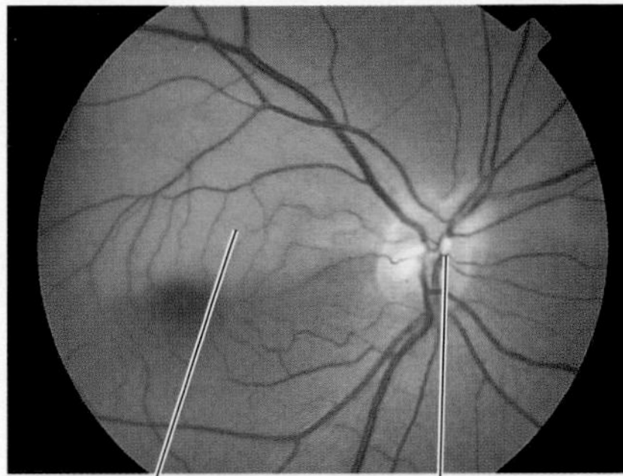

Fig. 22.2 Fundoscopy image of the right eye showing a Hollenhorst plaque. In this image, the superior half of the fundus appears pale and oedematous which indicates ischaemia. Persistant ischaemia in this distribution is suggestive of a branch retinal artery occlusion. (Source: Friedman, N.J., Kaiser, P.K. and Pineda II, R. [2021]. *The Massachusetts Eye and Ear Infirmary illustrated manual of ophthalmology.* Elsevier.)

MAKING A DIAGNOSIS

- Symptoms: transient visual loss, which completely resolves within 24 hours of onset and cannot be explained by another condition, e.g. hypoglycaemia
- Signs: normally ocular examination is unremarkable; however, sometimes a Hollenhorst plaque is noted on fundus examination (Fig. 22.2). Carotid bruit may be audible on auscultation of carotid arteries

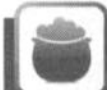 Clinical Tip

It is crucial to rule out arteritic ischaemic optic neuropathy associated with GCA in these patients, as it can result in rapid, irreversible sight loss without intervention. It should be suspected in any patient over the age of 50 presenting with transient or persistent visual loss. A history of temporal tenderness, headache or jaw claudication and bloods showing raised CRP or ESR will also support this diagnosis.

MANAGEMENT

The management of amaurosis fugax is similar to a TIA. The patient should be given an antiplatelet drug such as 300 mg aspirin if not already taking antiplatelets or warfarin. If the patient already takes low-dose aspirin regularly, continue the current dose of aspirin until a specialist reviews him. Any immediate cardiovascular risk factors should also be managed in the interim. Patients should also be commenced on a statin as long as there are no contraindications. The patient should be advised not to drive. The duration will vary depending on the type of driving license they hold.

 Prescribing Tip

Discuss with a senior before prescribing high-dose aspirin, in the context of previous peptic ulcer disease, uncontrolled hypertension or bleeding disorders.

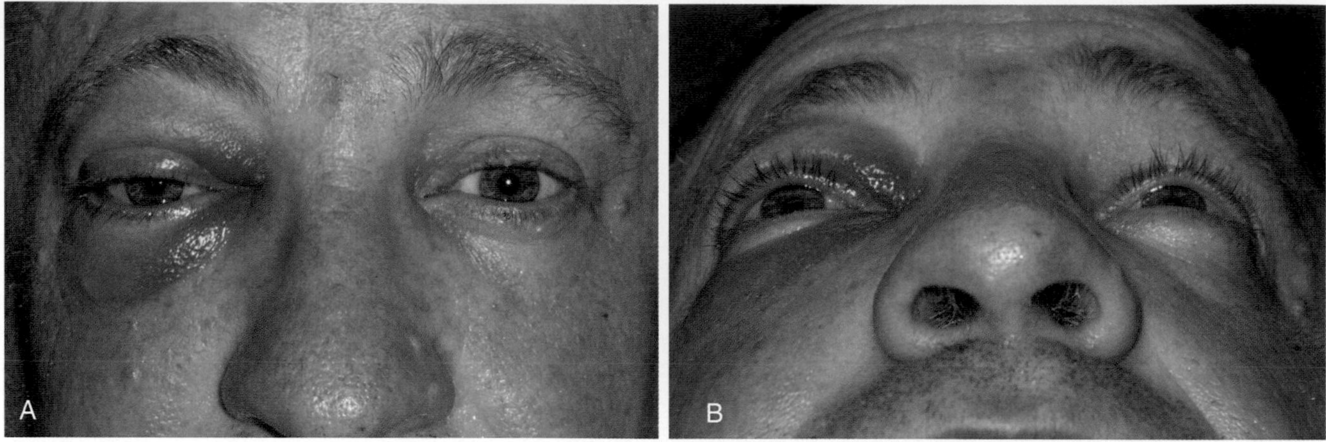

Fig. 22.3 (A) Right orbital cellulitis with swollen and erythematous eyelids. (B) Right orbital cellulitis with proptosis. (Source: Nerad, J.A. [2021]. *Techniques in ophthalmic plastic surgery: A personal tutorial.* Elsevier.)

ESCALATION

The patient should be referred to the stroke team for specialist assessment and they should be seen within 24 hours of symptom onset. The patient should also be discussed with ophthalmology; they will complete a dilated fundus exam to look for emboli and rule out other causes of visual loss.

STATION 22.3: ORBITAL CELLULITIS

The Bleep Scenario

A 37 year old male has presented to the ED with worsening pain, redness and swelling around the right eye. He has recently been treated for sinusitis by his general practitioner.

His observations are: HR 115 bpm, BP 120/80 mmHg, RR 15 breaths per minutes, SpO_2 96% on room air and a temperature of 38.6°C. You are asked to review him.

DEFINITION

Orbital cellulitis is an infection of the soft tissues posterior to the orbital septum within the orbit.

INITIAL THOUGHTS

Preseptal and orbital cellulitis are the main differentials to consider given the history of recent sinusitis and worsening pain, erythema and swelling around the eye. This patient may be septic; follow your local sepsis protocol when assessing him. Possible sources of infection include the paranasal sinuses (especially the ethmoidal sinus), preseptal cellulitis, dacryocystitis (inflammation of the lacrimal sac), midfacial skin/dental infection, haematogenous spread, trauma or surgery.

DIFFERENTIAL DIAGNOSIS

- Systemic: trauma, mucormycosis (fungal infection), sarcoidosis or malignancy
- Ophthalmic: preseptal or orbital cellulitis, retrobulbar haemorrhage, dysthyroid exophthalmos, viral/allergic conjunctivitis or insect bite/sting
- Neurology: cavernous sinus thrombosis

INITIAL INSTRUCTIONS OVER THE PHONE

Ask the nurse to consider supplementary oxygen, aiming for oxygen saturations > 94%. Obtain intravenous access, take initial bloods, give analgesia and start intravenous fluids for resuscitation as required. Request that the patient's vision be checked using a Snellen chart.

ASSESSMENT AND RESUSCITATION

- End of the bed assessment: the patient looks sweaty and clammy. The right eye is closed, and the eyelids are swollen and erythematous (Fig. 22.3).
- Airway: patent.
- Breathing: RR 20 breaths per minutes, SpO_2 96% on room air. On auscultation, there are vesicular breath sounds with good air entry bilaterally.
- Circulation: CRT < 3 s. HR 125 bpm, regular. BP 100/70 mmHg. HS I + II + 0.
  - Administer 500 mL of crystalloid fluids stat to resuscitate the patient.
- Disability: GCS 15/15, PEARL. Right eye relative afferent pupillary defect (RAPD). Temperature 38.5°C, CBG 7.5 mmol/L.
- Exposure: best-corrected visual acuity right eye 6/36 and left eye is 6/6 on the Snellen chart. External eye examination shows swollen, erythematous right upper and lower eyelids and proptosis. On assessing extraocular movements, restriction of ocular motility, with pain and diplopia reported. The conjunctiva is hyperaemic and chemotic. Visual fields are full on confrontation. Assess colour vision if Ishihara plates are available.

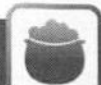

Clinical Tip

Mark the area of cellulitis, as it will help to detect any further progression.

INITIAL INVESTIGATIONS

- Haematology: FBC (anaemia or leukocytosis)
- Biochemistry: U&Es (acute kidney injury, electrolyte imbalance), CRP (inflammation), venous or arterial lactate (sepsis screen)
- Microbiology: blood cultures, urinalysis, conjunctival and nasal swabs (infection)
- Radiology: contrast-enhanced computed tomography (CT) orbit, sinus and brain (confirm the diagnosis of orbital cellulitis, aetiology and exclude a subperiosteal or intracranial abscess)

MAKING A DIAGNOSIS

- Symptoms: acute onset of unilateral swelling and erythema of conjunctiva and lids, pain and restriction of extraocular movement, reduction in vision, diplopia or fever
- Signs: reduced visual acuity, proptosis, chemosis, lid swelling and erythema, restricted eye movements, reduced colour vision, RAPD, optic disc swelling, pyrexia, systemic upset
- Investigations: contrast-enhanced CT orbit, sinus and brain confirming orbital cellulitis

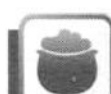

Clinical Tip

Indications for Imaging

- Suspected central nervous system involvement
- Signs of orbital cellulitis: proptosis, restriction of/pain on eye movement, chemosis, RAPD, reduced visual acuity/colour vision/visual fields, optic nerve swelling
- Failure to improve or continued pyrexia after 36–48 hours of intravenous antibiotics

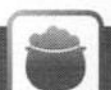

Clinical Tip

It is crucial to exclude a diagnosis of retrobulbar haemorrhage in these patients; this is another sight-threatening emergency. This condition typically presents with pain and reduction in vision, associated with proptosis, restricted eye movements, RAPD and high intraocular pressures, in the context of trauma. Immediate lateral canthotomy and cantholysis to decompress the orbit is required, as there is a risk of sight loss secondary to optic nerve compression.

MANAGEMENT

The patient has symptoms and signs suggestive of orbital cellulitis. Management of orbital cellulitis will require a multidisciplinary team approach, with urgent review by the ophthalmologists, ear, nose and throat (ENT) team and, if the patient is a child, the paediatricians. Intravenous antibiotics should be given immediately, initially broad-spectrum with anaerobic cover. Ensure you check your trust's antimicrobial guidelines. The most common causative organisms are *Streptococcus pneumoniae, Staphylococcus aureus, Streptococcus pyogenes* and *Haemophilus influenzae*. After blood culture results are known, antibiotics can be tailored to sensitivities. Further discussion with microbiology may be necessary if the patient is immunocompromised or does not respond to initial antimicrobial therapy. The patient will also need nasal decongestants, such as Otrivine nasal drops twice daily, if the infection is secondary to sinusitis. If the orbital cellulitis is secondary to trauma, it is important to ascertain the patient's tetanus immunisation status. If an orbital collection is identified on imaging, drainage may be considered by the ENT or maxillofacial surgeons depending on the location of the collection.

ESCALATION

Any intracranial complications should be discussed with neurosurgery and microbiology.

FURTHER READING

BMJ Best Practice (n.d.) *Peri-orbital and orbital cellulitis*. Available at: https://bestpractice.bmj.com/topics/en-gb/734/management-approach. (accessed 11 May 2020).

Bowling, B. (2016). *Kanski's clinical ophthalmology*. China: Elsevier.

ENT UK (n.d.) Orbital cellulitis management guideline for adults & paeds. Available at: www.entuk.org/sites/default/files/files/ENT%20UK%20Revised%20Orbital%20Cellulitis%20Flow%20Chart%202017.pdf. (accessed 11 May 2020).

NICE. (2019a). *Glaucoma*. Available at: https://cks.nice.org.uk/glaucoma. (Accessed 10 May 2020).

NICE. (2019b). *Stroke and transient ischaemic attack in over 16s: Diagnosis and initial management*. NG128. Available at: www.nice.org.uk/guidance/ng128. (Accessed 10 May 2020).

The College of Optometrists (n.d.) *Cellulitis, preseptal and orbital clinical management guidelines*. Available at: www.college-optometrists.org/guidance/clinical-management-guidelines/cellulitis-preseptal-and-orbital.html. (accessed 11 May 2020).

Index

Note: Page numbers followed by 'f ' indicate figures those followed by 't' indicate tables and 'b' indicate boxes.